SCHISTOSOMIASIS – the St Lucia project

The research and Control Department situated on Morne Fortune, St Lucia. Cul de Sac valley and banana plantations can be seen in the background. (Photograph by M. A. Prentice & G. Barnish.)

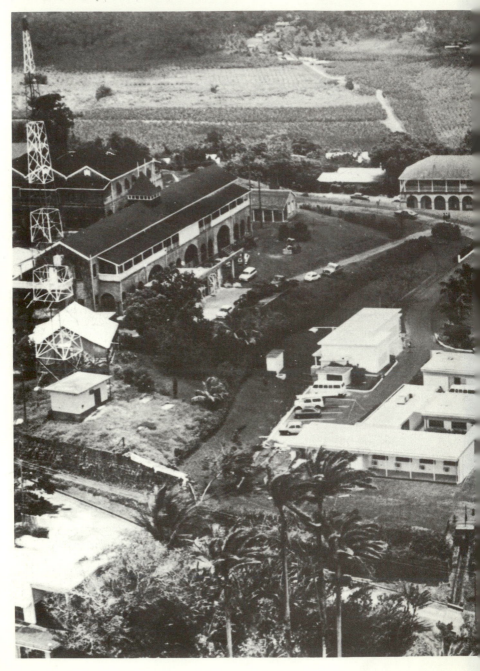

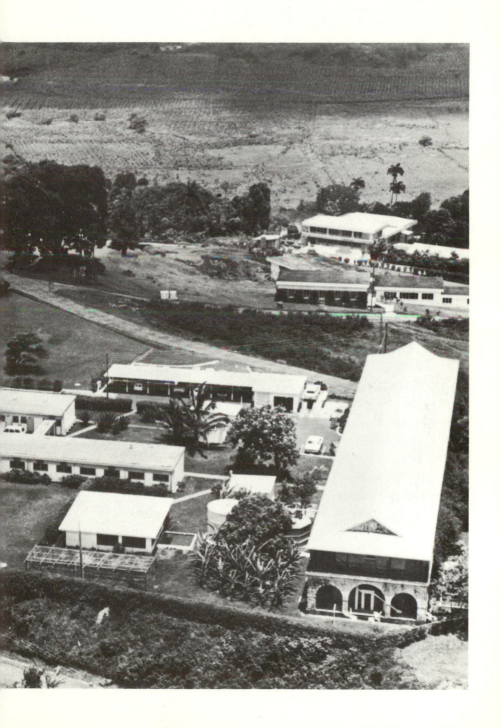

SCHISTOSOMIASIS

The St Lucia Project

PETER JORDAN, CMG

*Formerly Director of the Research and Control Department
Ministry of Health, St Lucia; Member of Expert
Advisory Panel on Parasitic Diseases,
World Health Organisation*

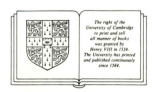

The right of the
University of Cambridge
to print and sell
all manner of books
was granted by
Henry VIII in 1534.
The University has printed
and published continuously
since 1584.

CAMBRIDGE UNIVERSITY PRESS

Cambridge

London New York New Rochelle

Melbourne Sydney

Published by the Press Syndicate of the University of Cambridge
The Pitt Building, Trumpington Street, Cambridge CB2 1RP
32 East 57th Street, New York, NY 10022, USA
10 Stamford Road, Oakleigh, Melbourne 3166, Australia

First published 1985

Printed in Great Britain by the University Press, Cambridge

Library of Congress catalogue card number: 85–406

British Library cataloguing in publication data

Jordan, Peter, 1924–
Schistosomiasis – the St Lucia Project.

1. Schistosomiasis – Saint Lucia
I. Title
614.5′53   RC182.S24

ISBN 0 521 30312 5

CONTENTS

PREFACE

This is an account of work carried out by staff and visiting workers at the Research and Control Department of the Ministry of Health in St Lucia between 1966 and 1981.

Although most of it has been described in nearly 150 published papers, this volume attempts to bring them together and to emphasise the continuity of the longitudinal studies. It is hoped that workers in developing countries, many of whom do not have access to international journals, will find various aspects of the work described of use and that it may stimulate new lines of enquiry.

In compiling this account published work has been referred to, but extensive use has been made of unpublished work from the Annual Reports prepared for the Rockefeller Foundation and the Medical Research Council.

The volume is in two sections – the first deals with the different approaches to control of schistosomiasis that formed the main part of the work of the department; the second section describes other related investigations that invariably had a bearing on the control activities.

I am grateful to the Rockefeller Foundation and the Medical Research Council for their support during the project, for providing the opportunity to write this book, for continued support and encouragement, particularly from Dr K. S. Warren, and for the financial assistance from the Foundation for its publication.

I am indebted to Dr D. Colley for reviewing the work of his and other teams of visiting immunologists, to Dr J. Christie for his contribution on TBTO, and to past staff of the New York office and the Research and Control Department for reading various chapters – Dr J. M. Weir, Dr V. C. Scott, Dr J. A. Cook, Dr R. F. Sturrock, Mr M. A. Prentice, Mr G. Barnish, Mr G. O. Unrau and, particularly, Mr R. F. Bartholomew who, being near at hand, reviewed more than his fair share; thanks also to Dr Angela Taylor and

Dr K. E. Mott for assisting with manuscript reading. I am grateful to Mr Unrau for preparing numerous maps and to my son, Mr A. J. Jordan, for assisting, and to Mr J. W. Block, illustrator at the National Institute for Medical Research, for preparing graphs and histograms. The editors of the *Transactions of the Royal Society of Tropical Medicine and Hygiene*, the *Annals of Tropical Medicine and Parasitology*, the *American Journal of Tropical Medicine and Hygiene*, the *Bulletin of the World Health Organisation*, the *Journal of Immunology*, the *International Journal of Parasitology* and Heinemann Medical Books gave permission to use previously published tables and figures; their co-operation is gratefully acknowledged.

I wish to thank also Prof M. Healy of the London School of Hygiene and Tropical Medicine for putting the epidemiological data on to computer tape, Ms Allison Douglas for carrying out analysis and Dr M. Goddard for similar work with water contact study data.

The St Lucia project could not have been carried out without the co-operation of the Ministry of Health and the loyal support, for which I am most grateful, of the St Lucian staff and the scientists from overseas. A special word of thanks must go to Mr O. F. Morris, my Administrator, and his staff who, amongst their numerous other 'behind the scene' activities, kept the vehicles moving for the field work.

Lastly I wish to thank my sister, Mrs M. Robb, for her patience in typing and re-typing the manuscript, and to Dr F. Bendall and Dr Rachel Meller of Cambridge University Press for their help and guidance.

FOREWORD

DR J. M. WEIR
Former Director, Medical and Natural Sciences Programme, The Rockefeller Foundation

As staff members of the Rockefeller Foundation and members of the Department of Parasitology of the Peking Union Medical College (established by the Rockefeller Foundation in 1921), Ernest Carroll Faust and Henry Meleney studied and described the cycle of *Schistosoma japonicum* in its molluscan host *Oncomelania hupensis hupensis* and in the Chinese population of the Yangtze flood areas. However, the Foundation's first active interest in the disease of schistosomiasis occurred when Dr Claude Barlow and a sanitary engineer, Mr Joseph C. Carter, were assigned to a programme to combat hookworm disease in Egypt in 1929. The major emphasis of the programme was the sanitation of Egyptian villages using bored hole latrines, but Barlow continued an interest in schistosomiasis, developed when he was in China, and studied the use of copper sulphate for the control of snails in the canals. The Foundation closed its programme in hookworm control in 1940, but Barlow stayed on as a consultant to the Egyptian Government until the 1950s. From 1947 through 1952, I was a member of the International Health Division of the Rockefeller Foundation and with Egyptian colleagues studied the prevalence of schistosomiasis in a rural population in five villages of Qualyub Province as part of a controlled study of sanitation. Again schistosomiasis was not the main concern and no co-ordinated studies were made to investigate the biology of the snail or its control.

Though officers of the Foundation had followed the various attempts by the World Health Organisation (WHO) and others to study the natural history and the increasing prevalence and importance of schistosomiasis associated with the development of large lakes and irrigation schemes, particularly in Africa, a programme to make broad based research studies of the problem was not considered until 1958–59. At that time, the Director of the Agricultural Sciences of the Rockefeller Foundation, Dr J.

George Harrar, and I were asked by the National Academy of Sciences to participate in a study of development problems and needs of many of the newly independent nations of Africa. We were deeply impressed with the gravity of schistosomal disease as a threat to an orderly development of the economy and improved agriculture, and health in Africa. A portion of the report made to the National Academy of Sciences of the United States and to the British Government expressed the need for an integrated study of ways and means of controlling schistosomiasis by snail control, sanitation and treatment of infected humans.

Officers of the Rockefeller Foundation agreed that some attempt should be made to find an area in which careful field research on the biology and natural history of the snail vector could be combined with studies of the disease and evaluation of various treatment regimes in humans. From 1960 through 1964 visits were made to Africa, Brazil and Puerto Rico to look at possible sites for such a study. For a variety of reasons none of the programmes under way at that time appeared to provide the essential basis for the study of the type of programme envisaged. Conferences were held at the London School of Hygiene and Tropical Medicine and the Liverpool School of Tropical Medicine, at Harvard with the group studying schistosomiasis under Dr T. Weller, and with groups at the University of Michigan and the National Institute of Health. Professors George Macdonald and Brian Magraith (London and Liverpool Schools of Tropical Medicine), Dr Raymond Lewthwaite (Colonial Office, London), and Sir Harold Himsworth of the Medical Research Council in London met with Foundation staff and, in general, agreed on the desirability of such a programme and stressed the importance of finding an area with both *S. mansoni* and *S. haematobium*. While this was ideal, in the end it did not prove feasible to carry out the studies in an area that had both parasites and also met other criteria.

Fortunately the Minister of Health of St Lucia in the West Indies came to the Rockefeller Foundation office in New York in 1964 to see Dr Robert B. Watson, seeking assistance in meeting some of the health problems of that island. Watson told the Minister of our interest in a careful study of schistosomal disease in a natural laboratory setting, and the Minister invited Dr Watson to visit the area and see the opportunities offered by the island of St Lucia for such a study.

After discussion with the New York officers and visits again to programmes in Puerto Rico and Brazil, Watson was asked to go to St Lucia with Dr Edward Michelson of Weller's Department at the Harvard School of Public Health. They visited the island in October 1964 to see what the prospects were for a successful study of all facets of schistosomiasis. Both were impressed with the topography of the island: the central thrust of the mountains dividing the island into more or less discrete valleys with individual water sheds that would allow trials of various techniques for abating transmission. Data available at that time, although limited, indicated a high prevalence of infection and it seemed likely that one or two of the valleys would be amenable for installing some type of piped water supply as one phase of the study. The Government seemed genuinely interested in a co-operative programme of the type we had in mind (and on the whole, in retrospect, this seems to have been true).

I was perhaps the one person in the Rockefeller Foundation at that time who had had any significant experience with the disease and its treatment and control and who had also visited most of the studies being undertaken at that time. As far as I was concerned, no other area offered the natural topography for controlled studies, an administrative government structure that was apparently eager to implement such a programme, a high generalised prevalence of infection, and was situated where it would be agreeable to live for relatively long periods of time without undue stress or physical hardships.

The schistosomiasis problem was not associated with canals or rice paddies but there were banana drains and swamps and slow and fast running streams harbouring populations of *Biomphalaria glabrata*. They were used by the human population, with a low level of sanitation, for drinking, bathing, laundering and swimming – all the essential elements for establishing and maintaining transmission of schistosomiasis in any endemic area. No single area is a prototype for all forms, but the principles of snail control and the problems associated with changing people's habits are similar in all endemic areas, though details of strategy may vary. Certainly chemotherapy trials are alike wherever they are tried for *S. mansoni* and the general methodology would be the same for *S. haematobium* or *S. japonicum* even though response might vary. The point in favour of the use of St Lucia for the type of studies done there was the ability to do controlled studies, evaluate them properly and do adequate cost studies of a variety of approaches.

It was on this basis that the officers and the Board of Trustees of the Rockefeller Foundation decided to undertake the programme in St Lucia.

INTRODUCTION

Historical background

Schistosome worms were discovered in 1852 by the German pathologist, Theodore Bilharz; he was performing an autopsy in Cairo and found them in the portal vein. Originally named *Distomum haematobium*, it was later found that only one of the suckers had an oral cavity and Weinland renamed it *Schistosoma*, referring to the cleft (*schistos*), and body (*soma*), of the male worm. Cobbold suggested the name *Bilharzia* for the worm but rules of nomenclature gave *Schistosoma* priority; however, the infection is now commonly known as schistosomiasis, bilharziasis or bilharzia.

Bilharz reported both terminal and lateral spined eggs in the oviduct of the female worm, but Harley (1864), in the Cape of Good Hope, could find only terminal spined eggs in the urine of his patients and thought he had a different species which he called *Schistosoma capense*. Manson (1902) found only lateral spined eggs in a patient who had lived on the Caribbean islands of St Kitts and Antigua. He wrote: 'Possibly there are two species of *Bilharzia*, one with a lateral spined ova depositing its eggs in the rectum only, the other haunting the rectum and bladder indifferently'. This view was supported by other workers, and in 1907 Sambon named the lateral spined species after Sir Patrick Manson.

It was realised that trematode worms usually have snail intermediate hosts, but they were not identified until 1915 when Leiper worked out the life cycles of *S. haematobium* and *S. mansoni* in Egypt. His report (Leiper, 1915) remains a classic to this day and the preventive measures he suggested, based on the new-found knowledge of the life cycle, are not unlike those currently recommended. (It is of historical interest to note that in his annual report on Egypt in 1913, Lord Kitchener expressed the view that 'it is high time that serious steps should be taken to prevent the continuity of infection [schistosomiasis] that has been going on for so long in this country' (quoted by Leiper, 1915).

After Manson's discovery of schistosomiasis in the West Indies the infection was reported from many Caribbean islands in the first decade of the century, but although a St Lucian working on the Panama Canal was found to be infected (Monroe, 1916), it was not until 1924 that an autochthonous case was reported in the island.

In the Rockefeller Foundation hookworm campaign on St Lucia (1914–22) nearly 50 000 stools were examined and although helminth ova, still widespread, were reported, no mention was made of *S. mansoni*. R. B. Watson, however (personal communication), has pointed out that when the same technique of stool examination was used in the Brazilian hookworm campaigns, no *S. mansoni* ova were found in Maranhão or Minas Gerais where the infection is now known to be common. In Bahia, where prevalence of *S. mansoni* is now very high, it was found in only 317 of 10 411 persons examined. Since the stool examination techniques used in these campaigns are now recognised as inefficient methods for detecting *S. mansoni* ova, the non-reporting of the parasite in St Lucia cannot preclude the possibility of the infection having been present. One report by the Director of the St Lucia project, Dr Rolla B. Hill, is of interest – in a survey of the police force he reported 15% with unidentified eggs; but the question remains, could these have been *S. mansoni*?

Reports of the Medical Department of St Lucia between 1924 and 1931 make no mention of schistosomiasis, but a 10% prevalence of infection was found by Dr Gresham, District Medical Officer, amongst 1509 school children at Soufriere, and *Biomphalaria glabrata* (the snail intermediate host) were infected with the parasite. As a result of these findings the Colonial Office arranged for Dr J. J. C. Buckley of the London School of Hygiene and Tropical Medicine to visit St Lucia. Later, when there was concern about the situation, Professor Leiper noted, in a letter to the Colonial Office, that

> the control of bilharzia disease can be obtained in one of two ways, either by treatment of all carriers or by the eradication of the water snails which act as intermediaries. Neither method is simple or effective unless sustained over a long period, for the treated persons are afterwards liable to re-infection and measures for eradication which have been suggested as a result of laboratory experiments have not yet been properly tested in the field.

Understandably nothing was done.

Over the next 30 years schistosomiasis spread, and an island-wide stool and skin test survey showed the infection to be common in most parts of the island (Panikkar, 1961); additionally, tourists were infected (Most & Levine, 1963).

WHO consultants (Dr Louis Oliver, Dr E. Malek and Mr Z. J. Buzo) visited the island in 1962 and 1963 and confirmed that *B. glabrata* was widespread. They considered that 'the prevalence of bilharzia is sufficiently high to justify consideration of a comprehensive control programme'.

A start in this direction was made in 1964 when Dr R. E. M. Lees, the Medical Officer of Health, obtained a grant from the Standing Advisory Committee for Medical Research in the British Caribbean to investigate the infection but, in 1965, after rapidly concluded negotiations between the Government and the Rockefeller Foundation, the Research and Control Department of the Ministry of Health was formed. The object was to provide for co-operation between the St Lucia Government and the Rockefeller Foundation for the study of 'matters affecting the health of the people, and, more specifically, schistosomiasis'. As a result of this agreement all patients with schistosomiasis were referred from hospitals, health centres and private practitioners to physicians of the Department for treatment.

Rockefeller Foundation provided funds for the building of houses and the laboratory on land provided by the St Lucia Government. The Government supported some local staff with grants from the Commonwealth Development and Welfare (CD & W) funds, and later from the Medical Research Council through the Overseas Development Administration, but apart from this the Rockefeller Foundation was responsible for all recurrent expenditure. Construction of buildings started at the end of 1965 and the laboratories were formally opened by Mrs Gerald Bryan, wife of the Administrator of St Lucia, in November 1966.

The Memorandum of Understanding between the Rockefeller Foundation and the Government was extended twice, the agreement finally terminating on 31st December 1981 when the keys of the laboratory were handed to the St Lucia Minister of Health.

Schistosomiasis control in 1965

When the St Lucia project started, successful schistosomiasis control schemes were in operation only in Venezuela and Japan. In Venezuela public health control had been started in 1942 with mollusc-iciding, chemotherapy (with miracid D), washing units, sanitation and education. Over the years these combined measures reduced prevalence of

S. mansoni (Jove & Marszewski, 1961; Faria, 1972). In Japan a national schistosomiasis control programme, launched in 1950, drastically reduced prevalence over the next 15 years. Control was mainly through habitat modification with emphasis on cement lining of canals, reclamation of swampy areas by drainage and filling, the use of molluscicides, and general improvement in living conditions (Yokagawa, 1972). In both these public health schemes measures were directed against as many points in the life cycle of the parasite as was practicable at the time. Although they were not research schemes, and the role of each component in achieving success was unknown, they are still probably the best long term programmes to have been reported.

Efforts elsewhere concentrated on field trials with different molluscicides. Copper sulphate was evaluated in the WHO-assisted Egypt-10 project but was considered too costly for wide application (Van der Schalie, 1958), although it was later used extensively in Rhodesia and the Sudan. Sodium pentachlorophenate was evaluated in different parts of the world and results of short term pilot control schemes in Egypt (Wright, Dobrovlny & Berry, 1958) and Rhodesia (Clarke, Shiff & Blair, 1961) suggested that prevalence of infection was reduced. In the Patillas areas of Puerto Rico this chemical was used in combination with limited chemotherapy, biological control with *Marisa* and *Thiara* and habitat modification. The prevalence of *S. mansoni* was reduced, but the same was true in uncontrolled comparison areas (Palmer, Colon, Ferguson & Jobin, 1969).

WHO-assisted projects were established in Syria and Egypt in 1952, in Iraq in 1956 and Iran in 1959, but apart from official reports to WHO there are few published results. The schemes had varied objectives, but seem to have had common problems with staff, budget, transport and, in some cases, difficulties in collaborating with governments.

In a review of the status of molluscicides in the control of schistosomiasis, Paulini (1958) considered that the effect of snail control on the incidence and severity of bilharziasis in man was inconclusive. The following year niclosamide (Bayluscide) was introduced (Gönnert & Schraufstatter, 1959) and field trials in many parts of the world indicated the supremacy of this chemical over other molluscicides. Two years later, in 1961, WHO initiated Egypt–49 as a major effort to evaluate the role of a molluscicide (niclosamide) in control of the parasite, and five years later there was evidence that transmission had been interrupted (Farooq, Hairston & Samaan, 1966a). Except for limited trials with triphenmorph (Frescon®) in the 1960s, niclosamide has remained the main molluscicide in use.

Meanwhile, the WHO scheme on Leyte in the Philippines (1953–61), probably the first in-depth study on a scientific basis of a schistosomiasis control scheme, showed that over a two-year period environmental efforts against the snail intermediate host of *S. japonicum* were successful in reducing transmission in an area unsuited to the use of molluscicide (Pesigan & Hairston, 1961).

In the 1950s and 1960s, emphasis was on snail control. The drugs then available were antimonial preparations (in use after Christopherson showed the curative value of antimony sodium tartrate in 1918), and lucanthone hydrochloride. These were generally considered too toxic for widespread use as control tools although antimony was used in a compulsory treatment project in Egypt between 1953 and 1959 (Abdallah, 1973), and, combined with molluscicide (sodium pentachlorophenate), on Vieques Island, Puerto Rico, from 1954 (Ferguson, Palmer & Jobin, 1968).

Various attempts were made to reduce toxicity. Alves (1946) proposed a one-day course of antimony to produce a 'public health cure' (i.e. to reduce egg output but not necessarily obtain a parasitological cure), but it was never used on a large scale. Friedheim & De Jongh (1959) introduced the concept of suppressive management using 'Astiban' (potassium antimony dimercaptosuccinate, TWSb) in monthly injections for 5 or 6 months. The egg output of patients was reduced significantly (Davis, 1961; Jordan & Randall, 1962) but the method fell far short of what was considered necessary for successful transmission control by chemotherapy, and only one large scale project was carried out in Egypt in 1964–65 (Sherif, El Sawy, Madary & Barahat, 1970).

Lucanthone hydrochloride alone (Davis, 1963; Lees, 1968) and combined with Astiban® (Jordan, 1966) and niridazole (McMahon, 1966) were evaluated as suppressive regimes of treatment: although egg output remained low for some months after treatment, such regimes were impracticable for adults or children not attending school and were never used in control.

Improved sanitation and water supplies were integral parts of the successful public health scheme in Venezuela, but as control tools in their own right these measures had received scant attention, although latrine campaigns in Egypt (Scott & Barlow, 1938; Weir *et al.*, 1952) are frequently quoted as showing they have no effect on transmission of *S. mansoni*. However, critical review of these papers suggests that insufficient data were provided on which to form a valid opinion, while Pitchford (1970) noted that 'any number of them [latrines] will not prevent human beings urinating when they get into water nor will they stop indiscriminate defaecation'.

Until recently, community rural water supplies were installed more for political and utilitarian purposes than for their health benefits. However, such benefits are sometimes appreciated and the piped water supply may be chlorinated for controlling bacterial diseases (typhoid and gastro-enteritis). This does not reduce schistosome infections acquired from washing and bathing in infested streams and ponds, but in the epidemiological studies in the Egypt-49 scheme it was noted that the prevalence of infection was lower in villages with water supplies (Farooq *et al.*, 1966*b*).

In 1959 work started to provide water and simple swimming facilities and to prevent access to infected water in a village in South Africa. (Pitchford, 1966). The use of environmental methods for controlling schistosomiasis was prompted by the poor and costly results obtained with molluscicide several years earlier. In Brazil a similar environmental programme with community water supplies, laundry and shower units, and household latrines started in 1964 (Barbosa, Pinto & Souza, 1971). Results of these schemes, published several years later, suggested a lowering of transmission.

Over the years WHO was responsible for stimulating and encouraging research through their Expert Committee reports and the activities of the Bilharziasis Advisory Board under the leadership of Dr D. McMullen, but in 1965 the only really successful control schemes were those in Japan and Venezuela. Since a variety of measures had been used, it was impossible to estimate what the different measures had contributed to the results, but as most countries afflicted by the infection are economically poor it was important that an attempt be made to evaluate the relative costs, advantages and disadvantages of their different components, so that countries with limited resources would be better able to select the method or methods most likely to succeed in their particular conditions.

This the St Lucia project aimed to do.

Part I: Experiments in Control

I

The island of St Lucia

Topography and climate

St Lucia is a rugged island of volcanic origin covering approximately 616 km². It lies between Martinique to the north and St Vincent to the south in latitude 14° N and longitude 60° W (Fig. 2.1)

The southern and central regions are of more recent origin than the northern end and are characterised by numerous peaks covered by dense rain forest and rising to over 600 m; the highest, Mount Gimie, reaches 950 m. From these highland areas rivers radiate to enter the Caribbean Sea and Atlantic Ocean on the west and east side of the island respectively. In the south-west, valleys are deep with steeply sloping walls (Fig 1.1), and while those running south and east start in steep rugged mountain country, nearer the coast the land is less hilly and stream flow much reduced.

The older northern end of the island has been eroded leaving a hilly terrain, with a central mountain ridge – the Barre de L'Isle – joining the highland area in the south. Rivers flow west or east through wide alluvial flat-bottomed valleys, usually having well-defined valley walls separating one valley from the next. In general there is only limited contact by footpath between adjacent valleys which have been intensively cultivated since the earliest days of colonisation; changes in them have been a major influence in all spheres of the island's development.

The pattern of rainfall is related to the physical features of the island with the highland areas averaging over 3000 mm a year and less than 1500 mm being recorded in the low-lying northern and southern parts of the island. Since the prevailing winds are the north-east trade, the leeward side (the west) has generally more rain than the windward side, but there is considerable variation within the valleys, the least rain being recorded near the coast (Fig 1.2).

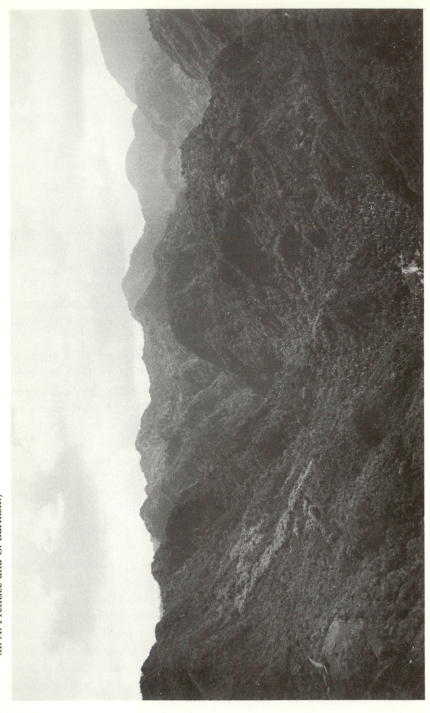

Fig.1.1. Rugged, uninhabited mountainous country in the southwest of St Lucia. (Photograph by. M. A. Prentice and G. Barnish.)

Fig.1.2. Distribution of rainfall in St Lucia.

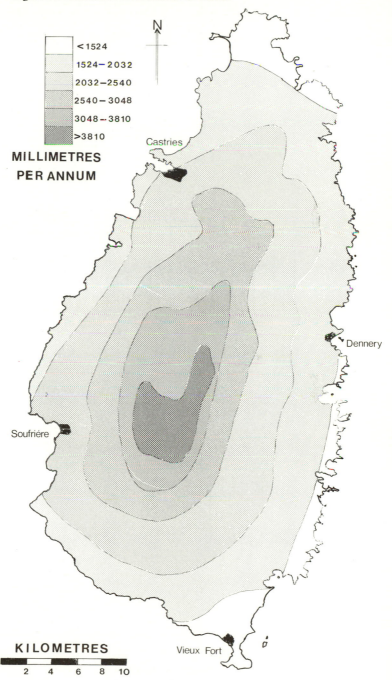

Fig.1.3. Mean monthly rainfall in Cul de Sac valley. (Data from Geest Industries (WI) Ltd for period 1952–1981.)

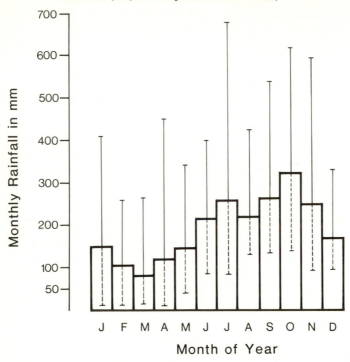

Fig.1.4. Annual rainfall, 1952–1981, with mean and 3-point moving average.

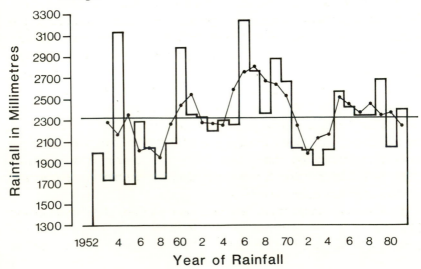

January to June are the drier months, but extreme variations in rainfall occur by the month and year: between 1952 and 1981 annual rainfall in Cul de Sac valley ranged from 1700–3250 mm (Figs. 1.3 and 4). Variation from year to year is similar in the different valleys and is an important factor in the population dynamics of *B. glabrata* and the transmission of *S. mansoni*. Data from Cul de Sac valley for 1952–81 show that the 1950s were abnormally dry years, in the early 1960s rainfall was average, the late 1960s were abnormally wet, the early 1970s again dry, and the late 1970s average to wet (Fig 1.4).

Apart from occasions when the island may be hit by a hurricane or suffer a 'near miss', tropical storms cause flooding of river systems with destruction of their snail colonies; however flooding of banana fields can occur and lead to dispersal of *B. glabrata* and the development of colonies over a wide area (Fig 1.5 and 1.6).

Maximum shade temperatures from May to October are generally between 29 and 35 °C: in the cooler months the day temperature rarely falls lower than 24 °C. Relative humidity ranges from 60 to 95% depending on the season and time of day.

The people

At some time in the past, Arawaks from South America came to the Caribbean islands, spreading northwards through the Lesser Antilles and eventually occupying Puerto Rico, Jamaica, Haiti, Cuba and the Bahamas. They were followed by the Caribs, who conquered many of the more southerly islands.

Although the date of discovery of St Lucia by Europeans is not known, the island appears to have been mapped as early as 1512–1513 and is referred to in a document dated 23rd December 1511 in which His Most Catholic Majesty the King of Spain gave permission for war to be waged against the Caribs in St Lucia. In 1593 or 1594 a privateer expedition led by George, 3rd Earl of Cumberland, visited the island to 'water and refresh themselves' and in 1603 a ship bound for Virginia arrived at St Lucia in mistake for Bermuda. Those on board were well received by the natives, but two years later, when a ship bound for the Guianas was blown off course and put into the island, only 19 out of 67 passengers who elected to stay in St Lucia survived treacherous attacks by the Indians and escaped to South America in an open boat.

The first real attempt at English colonisation was in 1638 when nearly 400 men arrived from Bermuda and St Kitts – the supposed cradle of England's West Indian colonies. For 18 months they survived without

Fig.1.5. Cul de Sac river before tropical storm. (Photograph by G.Barnish.)

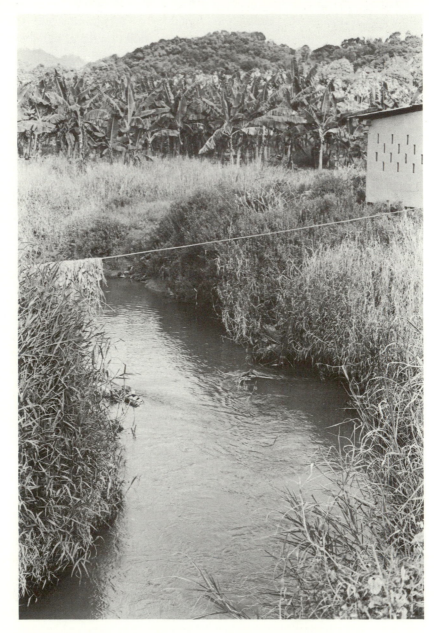

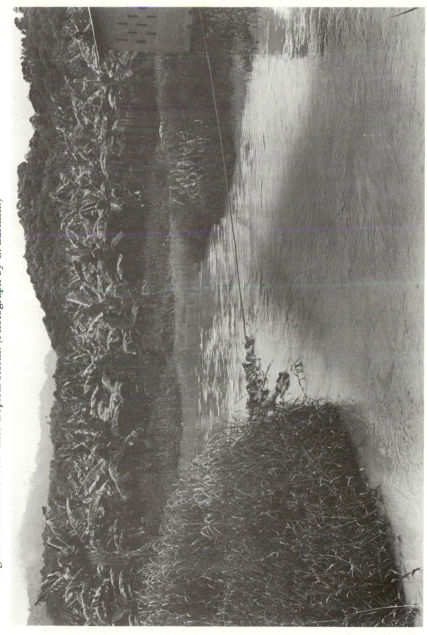

Fig.1.6. Cul de Sac river after tropical storm. (Photograph by G. Barnish.)

interference from the Caribs, but in August 1640 the colony was practically exterminated by the Caribs of the island and their neighbours.

In 1651 an expedition of about 40 Frenchmen, the first of many, arrived from Martinique. The leader had married a Carib woman and the colony did well until 1654, but in the following few years three French Governors died through Carib treachery. There can be little doubt that many Caribs were killed in the early days of French and British settlement, but the principal factor which led to their extermination was the spread amongst them of newly introduced diseases, smallpox, measles and influenza, to which they had no resistance (Guerra, 1966). By the end of the decade the colony was prospering, and repulsed an English attempt to land in 1659.

Morne Fortune, overlooking Castries harbour, became a key point in the struggles between the two European powers, and between 1663 and 1803 control of the island passed between the French and the British fourteen times. During this period it was settled by families of both nationalities. Parishes were established and their boundaries remain virtually unchanged to this day. Similarly the names of the original plantations are still used. This was the time of the slave trade and slaves came to St Lucia via Barbados or the French islands of Martinique and Guadeloupe. The tribal origins of the Negro population are therefore very mixed. A slave register from one plantation in the island listed their origins as Ibo and Aruba (probably Yoruba) from Nigeria, Mandino (probably Mandingo) from Sierre Leone and Guinea, and Corymantyn (Fanti and Ashanti) from Ivory Coast and Ghana, who were embarked at Koromantin on the Ghana coast. Moco and Copoloan are also listed; no tribes exist with these names and it is likely they refer to slaves embarked at the ports of Mocamedes (Angola) and Coppolani (Mauritania). A further tribal origin is given as Congo. This single slave register indicates the vast area of West Africa from which only a fraction of St Lucians originate. It is almost certain therefore that many tribes are represented in the population. By 1789 nearly 17 000 slaves were in the island with 1200 whites and nearly 2000 coloureds (Breen, 1844).

In 1803 the British stormed the island for the last time and the island was finally ceded to Britain in 1814.

Emancipation in 1838 created a need for additional labour and East Indians (mainly from the Bombay area) were brought to the island as indentured labourers; descendants of many remain in St Lucia to this day. French remained the official language until 1842 and a French patois is still spoken in rural districts.

The island remained a British colony until 1967 when it became an

Associated State, with Britain responsible only for defence and foreign affairs. In 1979 the island became fully independent within the British Commonwealth.

The Government is elected every five years, with all persons aged 18 or more having a vote. A Prime Minister heads the ruling party in the 17-seat

Fig.1.7. Increase in island population since records began.

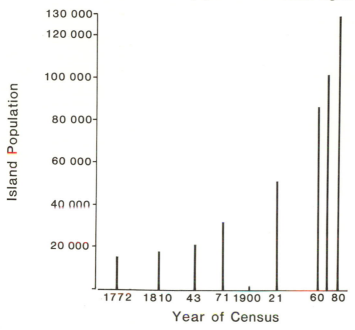

Fig.1.8. Population structure in rural areas based on census data from surveys in control valleys.

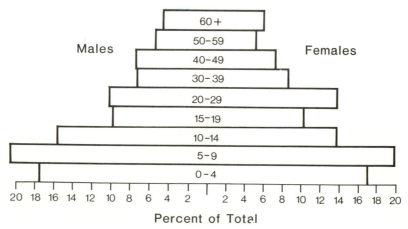

House of Assembly. An upper house, the Senate, consists of 11 nominated members. On the recommendation of the Prime Minister, a Governor-General is appointed by the Queen as her representative in the island.

In spite of an outbreak of cholera in 1854, as well as frequent epidemics of yellow fever and malaria, hurricanes, earthquakes and fires, the population gradually increased. Malaria was eradicated in the late 1950s (Wells, 1961), and by 1960 the population was 86 000; 20 years later it was nearly 130 000 (Fig. 1.7). About half the population are under 15 years of age (Fig. 1.8); about half live in the main urban centres of Castries, Soufriere, Vieux Fort and Dennery. Although the population is predominantly of Negro origin, descendants of the East Indians comprise 8–9%, with Caucasians forming a small fraction, of the total population.

Social conditions

The location of early settlements in St Lucia was dependent on the topography of the island and consequent agricultural expansion. The mountainous terrain made settlement in the interior of the island difficult except in the valleys, so that urban development from the outset was around the coast in sheltered bays in which sailing ships were loaded with sugar from the canefields. Smaller settlements appeared in the valleys and, in some cases, on ridges between them.

Houses were invariably built of wood and such homes predominate to

Fig.1.9. A better class wooden house, typical of rural St Lucia.

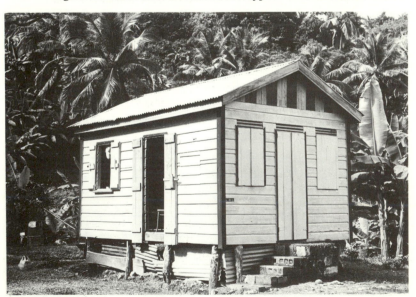

this day, but after disastrous fires in Castries (1948) and Soufriere (1955) many houses were rebuilt in brick. Rural wooden houses are usually small two-roomed constructions, raised about 300 mm from the ground, and housing an average of between 5 and 6 persons. There is usually an outside shelter where food is prepared on a small charcoal-burning 'coalpot' (Fig. 1.9).

Villages vary considerably in size, some having about twenty houses, others several hundred. They are usually located close to a river or stream which provides water for all domestic and other requirements, being carried to the home in buckets or other suitable receptacles.

When piped water is available it is used primarily for drinking purposes. While in most cases the source of water is safe, intakes have been seen in cercariae-infected water. An alternative source is often roof water collected and stored in an oil drum. Clothes are usually washed in the nearby river or stream at a popular 'washing site' where women congregate with their friends for a gossip. Young children invariably accompany their mother to the river, in which they play and may be exposed to prolonged water contact.

Sanitation campaigns in recent years have been based on the use of pit latrines, but many are serviceable for a short time only. They are used mainly by adults as children are frequently accused of soiling them and young children are afraid of falling in. In the absence of pit latrines (with a riser on top of a concrete slab), a simple hole in the ground may be used for faecal disposal. These flood in the rains, spreading faecal matter over the adjacent ground. Septic tanks are built for the better standard brick-built houses that are now appearing.

About 90% of the population is Catholic and there is usually a Catholic church in each valley and adjacent to it a Government school. Schooling to the age of 12 years is, in theory, compulsory, but in practice there are insufficient places for the rapidly growing numbers of children. Secondary education is now available at all the main centres of population in the island.

Agriculture and the economy

The early settlers grew ginger, cotton and tobacco, but from 1765 sugar became of increasing importance and by 1830 80 sugar factories were operating and no less than 50 177 tons were exported. At that time, there were 13 000 slaves in the island, but after emancipation in 1838 sugar production appears to have declined, due possibly to a lower price and to the freed slaves finding their own employment or emigrating. Although 2000 East Indians were brought in as indentured labourers, many of the large plantations had to be split up and exports fell. In the 1900s production never approached that of the previous century and was generally less than 10 000 tons annually.

After a prolonged and costly strike in 1957 the last three sugar factories were forced to close – Dennery (in Richefond valley) in 1958, Cul de Sac in 1959 and the Roseau factory in 1962, thus ending the sugar era in St Lucia. The banana industry, which had begun to compete with sugar, took over as the mainstay of the economy and the largest source of employment (F. J. Carasco, personal communication).

The growing of bananas began seriously at the beginning of the 20th century, but Panama disease in the 1930s led to declining exports, which ceased during the Second World War. A start was made after the war with a strain resistant to the disease, and exports gradually increased, reaching a peak of 85 000 tons for the British market in 1969. Low rainfall in subsequent years led to a drastic decline in production and in 1982 only 42 000 tons were exported.

Approximately two-thirds of the bananas produced are grown on small holdings of up to 5 acres, the majority being less than an acre in extent. The remaining third come from larger plantations of up to 750 acres and include the old sugar fields in Cul de Sac, Roseau and Richefond valleys. Since banana trees need abundant water at all times, and rainfall has been low for the last 10 years, overhead irrigation is used on some estates, and small dams (so far not infected with *B. glabrata*) have been built to provide the water. Before 1973 the bananas were exported on stems but banana hands are now washed, treated for fungus and boxed at packing stations around the island.

No sanitary facilities exist in the banana fields and the sporadic finding of infected *B. glabrata* indicates that on occasions either drain cleaners, banana cutters or carriers defaecate in the fields.

Until the early part of the 1970s banana exports formed about 90% of the total exports of the island and were the mainstay of the island's economy. The industry is still important, but is severely affected by variation in rainfall, nematode disease and the need to fertilise the plants. The whole island crop, along with coconuts, was destroyed by Hurricane Allan in 1980.

Other crops of less importance include coconuts, mangoes, cocoa, coffee, nutmeg, citrus and spices. Plantains, breadfruit, cassava, sweet potatoes, pigeon peas, tannias, eddoes and dasheen are grown for local consumption on small holdings or 'gardens' – dasheen is grown in marshy situations frequently containing *B. glabrata*.

While there has tended to be a one-crop economy in the past, since the early 1970s considerable progress has been made to diversify the agriculture and to develop the tourist industry. A number of luxury hotels (with over 2000 beds) have been built, mainly in the south and on the north-west coast of the island, and tourist revenue in 1979 amounted to US $15.5 million.

Notices have been posted in hotels warning tourists of the danger of *S. mansoni* in the pleasant looking mountain streams, but the original focus of transmission, a waterfall at a drive-in volcano near Soufriere where American tourists became infected (Most & Levine, 1963), was eliminated during geothermal drilling through the river bed! It is hoped that cheap electricity will be provided from this source and that the development of light industries in the south of the island will be encouraged. By 1979 these included the manufacture of cardboard cartons, textiles, electrical parts and beer.

A major boost to the economy came in 1977 when the giant American conglomerate Amerada Hess commenced its 201 million gallon oil terminal on 700 acres at the mouth of the Cul de Sac river. A deepwater harbour, built at a cost of US $30 million, accommodates the largest supertankers in operation today. While the project is not expected to provide jobs for many of the island's unemployed, it is expected to contribute significantly to the economy in the future.

Future development plans include the construction of a dam (surface area 40–50 acres) in Roseau valley to supplement the now inadequate water supplies of Castries. The project is a potential hazard as far as schistosomiasis is concerned, and recommendations to reduce the danger have been made to the Government.

The local currency issued by the East Caribbean Currency Board (ECC) is the dollar. Until 1976 this was tied to sterling at £1 to $4.80 ECC (US $1.00 equivalent to $2.00 ECC). From 1976 the currency has been tied to the US dollar at $2.70. The national income per person in the island in 1979 was reported as approximately US $700 (*The Economist*, 1980).

Development of health services

From all accounts St Lucia used not to be a healthy place, the rapid succession of Governors in the 18th and 19th centuries being an indication of the high mortality due to malaria and yellow fever; and, as recently as the 1960s, the infant mortality was over 100 per 1000. The situation is now very different with the disease pattern being more that of a developed country rather than a developing one. Malaria control, and later eradication, probably contributed more than any other single event to the change in the health profile of the island, but other specific and non-specific disease

preventive measures, improved health coverage throughout the island, and
the development of water supplies must all have played a part.

Mosquito control

In the past, malaria was of major importance with *Plasmodium
falciparum*, *P. malariae* and *P. vivax* being encountered in that order of
frequency. *Anopheles aquasalis*, found in marshes round the coast, and
A. argyratarsis, in seepages and streams, were the main vectors.

Table 1.1. *Some milestones in the history of St Lucia (with emphasis on
health)*

1838	Emancipation
1839	Yellow Fever epidemic. Island hit by earthquake
1842	Yellow Fever
1854	Cholera epidemic
1884	Colonial Hospital, Castries burned down
1887	Victoria Hospital opened
1898	Hurricane hit the island
1899	'*Filaria demarquaii* in St Lucia, West Indies' by Dr O. Galgey published in *British Medical Journal*
1903/4	'Sulphur Dermatitis' from Mt Pélee eruption in Martinique
1906	Earthquake
1913	First motor vehicle imported
1915	Rockefeller Foundation Hookworm Campaign to 1922. Sanitary regulations introduced by the Board of Health
1922	Alastrim epidemic
1924	First recorded case of *S. mansoni*
1927	Castries fire
1938	98 persons killed in landslides following heavy rains. Nutritional survey: 10% of school children undernourished
1942	Public Health Engineering Unit (PHEU) formed
1946	First Health Centre established
1948	Castries fire: four-fifths of town destroyed
1951	10% of Soufriere school children found infected with *S. mansoni*
1954	First laundry unit built at Soufriere with CD & W funds
1955	Soufriere fire
1957	Yaws eradication campaign (using penicillin)
1959	Environmental Sanitation Programme launched
1961	Panikkar Survey – *S. mansoni* widespread
1962	Expanded Nutrition Programme
1963	Central Water Authority established. St Lucia officially declared malaria free
1965	Research and Control Department formed
1966	Hurricane Beulah
1967	Associated Statehood
1979	Independence
1980	Hurricane Allan
1981	Research and Control Department closed

In 1942, when the malaria mortality rate was 33 per 10 000, the Public Health Engineering Unit (PHEU) was established and carried out extensive anti-malarial swamp reclamation work. In 1950 annual DDT residual spraying of houses in the valleys started and workers were encouraged to take prophylactic quinine. Later, with assistance from WHO, UNICEF and CD & W funds, all houses in the island were sprayed on a 6-monthly cycle for the control of *Aedes aegypti*. The programme had a marked effect on malaria mortality, which fell from 13.2 per 10 000 in 1952 to 6.1 in 1955 (Wells, 1961). The emphasis then changed from malaria control to eradication. Increased DDT doses were applied, the blood of all febrile patients was examined for parasites, and chloroquine or Daraprim® treatment was given. By 1960 no malaria deaths were reported and St Lucia was declared malaria free in 1963.

The drainage of swampy areas to control *Anopheles* mosquitoes, particularly in the low-lying areas round the larger coastal villages, probably had a marked effect on *S. mansoni* transmission. At Anse la Raye, south of Castries, where land reclamation and drainage were initiated in 1960, Panikkar (1961) reported that 36% of school children were infected with *S. mansoni* on stool examination, but in a survey in 1975 prevalence was only 1%, although a small focus of *B. glabrata* had been known to exist for some years close to the village (Fig. 1.10). (See also Table 8.1.)

A WHO/PAHO *A. aegypti* campaign has been operating for many years, and, while not having eradicated the mosquito, their numbers have presumably been reduced. Dengue is occasionally diagnosed clinically, and a serological survey carried out in 1974 showed that 10% of children in the 1–5 year age group and 25% of those under 25 years of age had antibodies by the complement fixation test (Evans *et al.*, 1979).

Filariasis was of interest at the turn of the century as there was uncertainty as to the species present, but there seems little evidence that elephantiasis and hydrocoele, due to *Wuchereria bancrofti*, were ever serious problems in the island. The microfilariae found in blood slides were probably *Mansonella ozzardi* – described as *Filaria demarquaii* by Dr O Galgey in 1899. The vector, *Culicoides furens*, is still present and a nuisance to the tourist industry. A successful scheme to alleviate the problem in the north of the island involved opening up to the sea the main marsh where flies were breeding, and developing it as a marina for yachts. Microfilariae were seen regularly when microscopists examined blood for malaria parasites but are now infrequently noted.

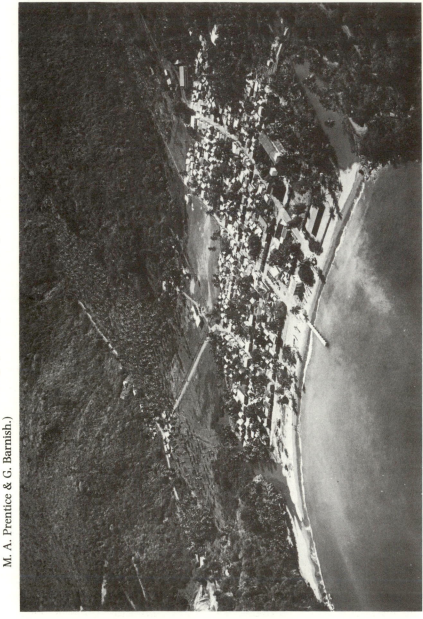

Fig.1.10. Anse la Raye: a coastal village where land reclamation and drainage as anti-mosquito measures on the outskirts of the village probably controlled *B. glabrata* populations. (Photograph by M. A. Prentice & G. Barnish.)

Yaws control

At the end of the last century yaws was common and a yaws hospital was established on Rat Island just north of Castries. Most of the patients were children who were compelled to bathe in the sea every day.

A campaign to eradicate yaws and control venereal disease with penicillin was carried out in 1957 but was considered 'abortive' as only 60% of the population was reached. Although prevalence of yaws fell, there was a rapid return to the pre-control levels, but over the years yaws has been practically eliminated (Lee & De Bruin, 1963; Lees, 1973), whereas venereal disease is still very common.

Intestinal parasites, sanitation and water supplies

From the 1904 report of the Medical Department, and others, it is apparent that *Ascaris* infections were a serious problem: 'Everyone suffers, adults as well as children – sudden deaths amongst the latter are due to extensive infection'.

Hookworm infections were also associated with severe disease, and limited studies have recently incriminated *Necator americanus*. The Rockefeller Foundation hookworm campaign from 1914–22 did much to alleviate the problem, at least temporarily. During the campaign, the whole island was surveyed and nearly 50 000 persons were examined; 64% were found infected, of whom 84% received two or more treatments with oil of chenopodium or carbon tetrachloride.

Regulations were introduced in 1915 by the Board of Health in the island to improve the standard of sanitation, and the Sanitary Department provided fly-proof latrine seats to fit the top of a wooden box placed over a 4 ft deep pit. The pits often overflowed during heavy rains and became breeding places for mosquitos (Branch, 1922).

Intestinal parasites continued to be a major problem and in 1959 a new Environmental Programme was launched with support from WHO, UNICEF and CD & W funds. The aim was to provide an estimated 10 000 latrines of new design to households and schools and to develop communal water supplies in rural areas. The work was carried out by the Sanitary Department and the PHEU (Public Health Engineering Unit). The new latrine consisted of a pre-cast concrete slab, a concrete riser and a hinged wooden seat cover. They were distributed free but superstructures were constructed by householders. In 1963, when the objective of 10 000 units had been achieved, a charge of $4.50 ECC (US $1.88) was made for additional latrines. Over the next few years approximately 250 units were sold annually so that by 1971 there should have been about 12 000 rural latrines, used by a population of approximately 60–65 000. In spite of this intestinal helminths have remained all too common, although there was some evidence from the schistosomiasis project that prevalence has declined slowly over the past 15 years, possibly as a result of improved and more readily available treatment. However, the importance of *Trichuris* infections in young children is thought by some paediatricians to have been underestimated in the past and this is now being investigated (E. Cooper, personal communication).

S. mansoni was not referred to in reports of the Medical Department until 1924; subsequent findings in relation to this parasite are described in Chapter 2.

Entamoeba histolytica is rarely seen in St Lucia.

Although data suggest pit latrines had been provided in a high proportion of rural homes, a survey in Roseau in 1966 (unpublished data) showed that only 15% of them were maintained and used regularly. Campaigns to promote latrines were launched without any health education to explain why and how they should be used and maintained. Whether such a programme would have changed the situation is debatable, but the above survey does indicate the general unacceptability and short life of this type of latrine in St Lucia and the need for an improved system of excreta disposal.

Cost of latrines has steadily increased from the 1963 price of $4.50 ECC ($1.88 US) to $20 ECC ($7.40 US) in 1976 and $40 ECC ($14.80 US) in 1982.

Latrines are provided in schools but often in inadequate numbers and some children must question the sincerity of those teaching health education relative to proper excreta disposal in these circumstances. Public latrines have been provided alongside laundry and shower units in the urban coastal villages in the past but until recently they were rarely provided in rural settlements.

Piped water has been available in the main urban towns for many years and, in an attempt to control exposure to *S. mansoni*, the first public laundry, shower and toilet facility was built in Soufriere in 1954 with a grant from CD & W funds. Sceptics apparently did not expect that the laundry would be used, but it proved popular and is in use to this day. Rural water supplies, however, have been developed only within the last two decades. These entailed the digging or drilling of wells, the collection of surface waters or the protection of springs. By 1962 work had been completed in 30 rural settlements initially selected for such supplies. Other schemes followed, but wells frequently supplied less than 5000 l of water a day and there were problems with maintenance of hand pumps. Although the supply of water from protected springs in a 24-hour period may have been better, its storage was usually inadequate for maximum daytime use. Some larger schemes using petrol and diesel driven pumps with medium sized storage tanks were also completed. One such scheme became operational in the Desruisseau area where water was pumped to a 31 500 l storage tank for gravity distribution to communal standpipes, but washing and bathing continued in the rivers.

In 1963 the Central Water Authority was established with sole jurisdiction in all matters relating to potable water supplies in the island.

In 1966 plans were prepared for the first large rural water supply scheme in Richefond valley at an estimated cost for materials of over $150 858 (ECC) or, at the time, US $62 857. The scheme became operational on the north side of the valley in 1969 and provided 15 communal standpipes for a population of approximately 4000 people. The area included all the settlements used for comparison with the experimental schistosomiasis control schemes of the Research and Control Department when the water supply in the area was shown to do nothing to prevent schistosomiasis (Chapter 4).

A further major scheme was developed in 1974 to improve the system in the Desruisseau area. Surface water was piped four miles by gravity from hills near the centre of the island. The Research and Control Department collaborated with Government in the distribution system (see Chapter 7).

This brief review is not intended to cover the development of water schemes over the whole island, but it shows that although development of water supplies in rural areas has been a major consideration of Government in recent years, owing to financial constraints the supplies have generally been inadequate for *S. mansoni* control and maintenance frequently unsatisfactory. Laundry and shower units were not initially part of the facilities provided, but they are now being constructed in rural areas. By 1981 possibly 90% of the population had access at some time to piped water but the systems rarely provided a *reliable* and *adequate* source of water so that populations had, of necessity to go to the nearest stream, river or pond for domestic supplies when the water supply failed, and, in the normal course of events, for washing purposes.

Nutrition

In 1974 the Caribbean Food and Nutrition Institute made a detailed study of the nutritional state of the population (Anon., 1976). The most important sources of energy foods were cereals, sugar, oils and local crops; wheat (*Triticum aestivum*), wheat products, salted codfish, fresh fish and beef provided protein, and cooking oil provided most of the fat in the diet.

Using the Gomez classification of malnutrition, amongst children under 5 years of age, 33% were in Gomez grade one, (slightly underweight) 9% in grade two (children definitely underweight), and 1.9% in grade three (severely underweight), while 56.1% showed no sign of malnutrition.

Anaemia occurred amongst all age groups. It was generally mild but 33% had a haemoglobin level less than 10 g% and 4% less than 8 g%. Iron deficiency was the major type of anaemia although only 8% of the households sampled had iron intakes of less than 80% of the recommended level. The high prevalence of hookworm suggested this was an important contributory cause of anaemia (Anon., 1976).

In an attempt to overcome these deficiencies the nutritional programme of the Government aims at better education of mothers, co-ordinated with a community agricultural programme to teach what foods to grow and to help with small-animal raising projects. In addition, basic nutrition is taught to primary school children and school gardens are encouraged, with the use of fertilisers being demonstrated.

Health services in the 1980s

The medical department has expanded considerably in recent years. Since 1955 the total health budget has increased from $153 000 US to more than $4½ million in 1981 and *per caput* expenditure from $1.58 to $35.6. As a percentage of the National Budget, health expenditure has varied in the last 20 years between 9% and 14% but does not show any consistent trend. Data on actual expenditure for 5-year periods from 1951–80 are shown in Table 1.2.

Table 1.2. *Total and Health Services expenditure of Government of St Lucia in 5-year periods 1951–1980*

(Eastern Caribbean currency)[a]

Period	Total budget (in $1000)	Health Services (in $1000)	% of total	Mean expenditure per caput/year	
				$ECC	$US
1951–55	17 666	1260	7.1	3.2	1.6
1956–60	26 787	2365	8.8	5.6	2.8
1961–65	35 436	4307	12.2	9.5	4.7
1966–70	57 968	7358	12.7	15.1	7.5
1971–75	126 912	13 827	10.9	25.3	12.6
1976–80	282 320	30 136	10.7	41.3	15.3

[a] Data from 'Government Estimates'

Victoria Hospital, with 260 beds, is located at Castries. St Jude's Hospital, with 100 beds, is run by the Sisters of Sorrowful Mother, with Government assistance, and is near Vieux Fort at the southern end of the island. Small Government hospitals with 40 and 23 beds are located at Soufriere and Dennery respectively. In total there is one bed per 423 population.

Health Centres in the rural areas (and in Castries) are each staffed by a State Registered Nurse/Midwife and are visited once or twice weekly by District Medical Officers. At these centres ante-natal and child welfare clinics are held regularly. The number of these centres has risen from 13 in 1960 to 27 in 1981.

Staff in the medical department has increased and at the end of 1981 there were 33 doctors (1 per 4000 population), 37 district nurses, 73 community aides, 23 environmental officers (Public Health Inspectors) and 65 environmental health aides.

Cadres of Community and Environmental Health Aides have been formed within the last five years. Personnel are selected from the areas that they will serve and are to assist Public Health and District Nursing staff in the delivery of basic primary health care at the community level.

Vital statistics

The infant mortality rate of 31.9 per 1000 in 1979, although higher than the previous few years, has shown a dramatic decline over the last 20 years (107.1 in 1960), due largely to the Expanded Nutrition Programme (Lees, 1966) (Table 1.3). There has been a marked change in the death rate of young children: in 1963, 50% of all deaths occurred in children under 2 years of age, mainly from gastro-intestinal infections and malnutrition, but by 1977 only 15.5% of deaths were in children

Table 1.3. *Vital statistics for the year 1979*[a]

Birth rate	30.3 per 1000
Infant mortality	31.9 per 1000
Toddler mortality rate (1–4 years)	1.9 per 1000
Stillbirths	14.5 per 1000
Neonatal death rate	18.5 per 1000
Crude death rate	6.8 per 1000
Fertility rate (15–44 years)	165 per 1000
Rate of natural increase	23.5 per 1000
Population doubling time	29.8 years

[a] This table and much information in this section was obtained from a dissertation by Mr G. Barnish entitled 'St Lucia, with emphasis on the Health Services' prepared for the degree of Master of Community Health at the Liverpool School of Tropical Medicine.

below the age of 5 years. These changes have no doubt been brought about by significant improvements in the delivery of health care, particularly the rural health services, and by the development of water supplies. While the majority of deaths in children below the age of 2 are still due to gastro-enteritis, it has been demonstrated that the diarrhoea attack rate is less in homes with an individual household water supply than in those served by a community standpipe (Henry, 1981).

Although there has been a decline in the prevalence of communicable diseases, measles, tuberculosis and typhoid are not infrequently reported. A survey for antibodies to poliomyelitis was carried out in 1959 when, in the 5–9 year age group, 91% were positive for Type I, 100% for Type II and 97% for Type III (Wells, 1959). Results of a similar survey in 1981 showed a decline in the percentage with antibodies to Type I (70%) but little change in Types II (99%) and III (86%) (Anon., 1982a).

In the Expanded Programme of Immunisation, between 1979 and 1981, over 10 000 children under one year old were immunised against poliomyelitis, 8500 against diphtheria, pertussis and tetanus, and 7250 with BCG. Measles immunisation started in 1981 and 682 immunisations were performed. It is anticipated that by 1984 80% coverage will be achieved.

With the reduction in infant mortality and the decline in deaths from communicable diseases, the mortality pattern resembles that of a developed country, with diabetes and hypertension occurring in the middle-aged and older age groups as recently confirmed by rural surveys (Tee-Kaw & Rose, 1982).

The most common causes of death are now:

(1) Heart disease – other than ischaemic
(2) Cerebro-vascular disease
(3) Neoplasm
(4) Ischaemic heart disease
(5) Pneumonia
(6) Cirrhosis
(7) Bronchitis, emphysema and asthma
(8) Enteritis and diarrhoeal diseases
(9) Hypertensive diseases.

2

*Snail intermediate hosts and schistosomiasis in the Caribbean**

Within two years of Manson's 1902 report of bilharzia in St Kitts or Antigua (the patient had lived in both islands), the infection was reported from Martinique and Puerto Rico (Letulle, 1904; Gonzales-Martinez, 1904), from Guadeloupe and Venezuela in 1906 (Holcomb, 1907; Faria, 1972), from Brazil in 1908 (Paulini, de Freitas & Aguirre, 1972) and from Surinam in 1911 (Flu, quoted by van der Kuyp, 1961) (Fig. 2.1). Eventually it was found in most of the islands to the north of St Lucia, but in none to the south although it occurs on the South American mainland.

Intermediate hosts

The snail intermediate host of *S. mansoni* in the Caribbean is *B. glabrata*, but although the latter is present in Dominica and Haiti, *S. mansoni* occurs in neither country. In Dominica snails were found in a localised area of Roseau valley in 1970 and are believed to have been introduced to an ornamental pond on lilies from St Lucia. In 1973 they were found in marshes and watercress beds over a wide area in the same valley. Amateur aquarists, it is thought, are potentially liable to spread the snail around the island (Prentice, 1980). Although occasional cases of *S. mansoni* are reported, there are no reports of autochthonous infections, but the Dominican strain of *B. glabrata* was shown to be susceptible to St Lucian *S. mansoni* (Sturrock & Sturrock, 1970b). Until recently the Dominican Republic was thought to be the north-western limit of *B. glabrata* in the Caribbean, but they have now been found in Haiti although *S. mansoni* is not as yet being transmitted (Robart, Mandahl-Barth & Ripert, 1977).

B. glabrata is not found in islands to the south of St Lucia but is the main intermediate host on the South American mainland. *B. straminea* is

* The subject has been recently reviewed by Bundy (1984).

Fig.2.1. The Caribbean region.

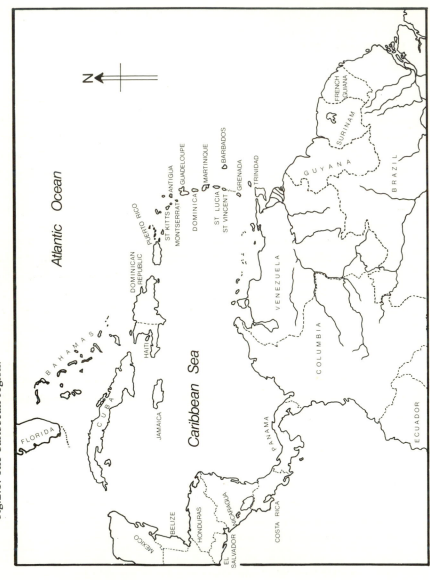

responsible for transmission in north-east Brazil; it is also found in Martinique (W. L. Paraense, personal communication), Trinidad and Grenada (Richards, 1973; Ferguson & Buckmire, 1974), though its taxonomic status in Grenada has been questioned by Malek (1975), who believes it to be *B. havanensis.* In Martinique *B. straminea* is thought to be replacing *B. glabrata* and *S. mansoni* transmission is now at a very low level (Pointier, 1982). *B. straminea* is generally less susceptible to *S. mansoni* infection than *B. glabrata.*

Strains from Trinidad, Grenada and Martinique could not be infected with St Lucian *S. mansoni* but juvenile snails from Grenada were infected with the Puerto Rican strain (Richards, 1973). *B. straminea* from Martinique showed a low level of susceptibility when exposed to *S. mansoni* from Belo Horizonte (W. L. Paraense, personal communication) and little importance is attached to this snail in that island, although some have been found naturally infected (Paraense, 1975).

Neither *B. glabrata* nor *B. straminea* have been found in St Vincent only 20 miles south of St Lucia and 20 miles north of Grenada. The soils of St Vincent are well drained compared with those in St Lucia so that marshy areas (such as those colonised by *B. glabrata* in St Lucia) are less numerous. This may account for the absence of the snail, but extensive investigations provided no reason why it could not colonise some sites if it were introduced. Apart from *Lymnaea cubensis* and *B. glabrata*, all other species of freshwater snail found in St Lucia were present in St Vincent (Harrison & Rankin, 1978). Snails resembling *B. glabrata* were found on one occasion; they were identified by Paraense as an eco-phenotype of *Helisoma duryi.* When cultured in St Lucia, the adult snails added new shell and assumed a *Helisoma*-like shape; offspring of the snails had typical *H. duryi* shells (Prentice, Barnish & Christie, 1977).

B. helophila has been reported from Puerto Rico, Cuba, Barbados, Jamaica and Haiti. Specimens from Puerto Rico were shown in the laboratory to be susceptible to *S. mansoni* (Richards, 1963) (the snail at the time was identified as *Tropicorbis albicans*), but infected snails have not been found in the field. *B. havanensis* (formerly *Tropicorbis riisei*) have also been found in Puerto Rico. Although field infections have not been reported, laboratory infections were obtained (Cram & Files, 1946).

Schistosomiasis in the islands

Manson's original patient had lived in St Kitts but schistosomiasis was not mentioned in reports of the Medical Department until 1918; (Anon., 1918) hepatosplenic cases were however later reported to be common (Jones, 1932). The endemic area was small, and when the affected streams were subsequently used for town and village piped water supplies, the source of infection was adversely affected, so by 1935 only low numbers of schistosomiasis cases were being reported. In 1937 it was noted that the water supplies had resulted in dry water courses where formerly there had been streams, though deforestation may have been a further cause of their drying. Whatever the reason, there seems to have been a gradual natural abatement of the infection in the island (Ferguson, Richards, Sebastian & Buchanan, 1960). St Kitts also provided the first evidence that animals in the wild could be a reservoir of *S. mansoni* infection – green monkeys (*Cercopithecus sabeus*) were found to be infected (Cameron, 1928).

Manson's original patient had lived in Antigua as well as St Kitts, and Antiguans working on the Panama Canal were found infected. The Rockefeller Foundation hookworm survey in the island in 1924 found an 18% *S. mansoni* prevalence rate in the St Thomas Parish. Several cases of schistosomiasis were reported in 1926, and *Planorbis antiguensis* (later identified as *B. glabrata*) (Anon., 1967) were found in Bendel's stream in 1928; however over the next few years cases were seen less frequently. Body Pond's dam was built to provide water for St John's, the capital, and while it, newer reservoirs and ponds throughout the island are infested with *B. glabrata*, human contact with them is limited (Prentice, 1980). A recent survey showed less than 5% of children under 14 years of age were infected, but 30% of those 15–24 years were excreting *S. mansoni* ova (Tikasingh, 1982). While there may be low grade transmission there seems little danger of a resurgence of transmission unless the reservoirs become important recreation sites (Prentice, 1980).

In surveys in Montserrat, *B. glabrata* were found (Prentice, 1980); 4% of children under the age of 14 years and less than 20% of adults were excreting ova (Tikasingh *et al.*, 1982). The findings from Antigua and Montserrat are of interest as they indicate that even when *B. glabrata* are widespread, transmission can be at a low level.

In Puerto Rico, biological control of *B. glabrata*, some mollusciciding, limited chemotherapy and the effect of general development have done much to reduce *S. mansoni* prevalence (Haddock, 1981), but in the Dominican Republic, where the infection was first reported in 1945, *B. glabrata* and *S. mansoni* have been found over a wide area of the country (Etges & Maldonado, 1969). Although limited attempts have been made at chemical and biological control (with *Marisa*), no major schemes have been implemented.

In parts of Guadeloupe the infection is considered an important public health problem (Golvan *et al.*, 1977). *Rattus rattus* and *R. norvegicus* have been found to harbour *S. mansoni* (Mongeot & Golvan, 1977; Théron, Pointier & Combes, 1978) and the possibility of biological control by trematode antagonism using *Ribeiroia marini guadeloupensis* has been investigated (Nassi, 1978; Nassi, Pointier & Golvan, 1979; Pointier, Toffart & Nassi, 1981).

In Martinique, although *S. mansoni* is endemic, transmission is now probably declining (Pointier, 1982).

St Lucia is the most southerly island in the Caribbean chain in which *B. glabrata* and schistosomiasis are found, although, as discussed above, the potential molluscan host, *B. straminea*, is found on some islands to the south.

Schistosomiasis on the mainland

Venezuela is the only country in South or Central America bordering on the Caribbean where *S. mansoni* is found, but the distribution of *B. glabrata* and *S. mansoni* in Surinam warrants comment in that they are restricted to well-defined areas of the coastal belt characterised by calcareous sands and alkaline waters of shell-ridges (van der Kuyp, 1961). In Surinam also, the great anteater and squirrel monkey have been found naturally infected with *S. mansoni* (Rijpstra & Swellengrebel, 1962; Swellengrebel & Rijpstra, 1965). *B. glabrata* are found in French Guyana, but could not be infected with St Lucian strain of *S. mansoni* (Sturrock & Sturrock, 1970a) and van der Kuyp (1961) believes transmission does not occur there.

Neither schistosomiasis nor its molluscan hosts have been recorded from Guyana.

Origin and spread of schistosomiasis in St Lucia

The origin of the infection in St Lucia must be a matter of conjecture. It would seem reasonable to assume it was brought to the island during the slave trade, the presumed source of infection in the rest of the New World, but if this were so it is difficult to understand its limited distribution until recently. Apart from the slave trade there was much contact with Martinique, where the infection was reported in 1906, and which must be considered an additional potential source of infection.

If, as seems likely, *S. mansoni* was not introduced directly from Africa, the question must be asked 'why not?' It was not introduced into Barbados, St Vincent and other islands to the south of St Lucia as there are no efficient snail intermediate hosts. If this were true of St Lucia in the 18th century, and that *B. glabrata* were later introduced to the island, then potential sources of recent infection must be considered.

It was suggested by the late Sir Frederick Clarke (former Chief Medical Officer and later Governor of St Lucia), that the infection may have been introduced by Jamaican army personnel who had been in Egypt and were later stationed in St Lucia in 1888. The troops were, however, garrisoned in the north of the island and are thus unlikely to have introduced the infection to Soufriere in the south unless they had gone to the nearby Sulphur Springs for the health-giving properties of the hot water. St Lucian

Fig.2.2. Towns and areas noted in the spread of *S. mansoni* in St Lucia. (See also Table 2.1.)

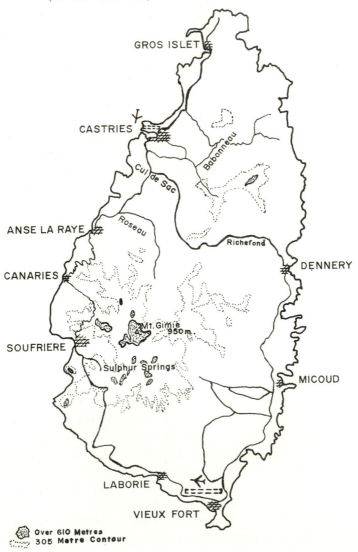

troops were in Egypt in the First World War and could, in theory, have introduced the infection on their return, but this seems unlikely in view of Monroe's case of a St Lucian being found infected in 1916 in the Panama Canal zone.

The possibility of the infection having been brought from Martinique cannot be excluded, but a source further afield should be considered.

At the turn of the century Castries, with a fine natural harbour, was, in terms of tonnage handled, the fourteenth most important port in the world (Morris, 1963): it was the chief coaling station in the West Indies for ships from South America *en route* to Europe. At the time, the fertile area near Soufriere was noted for farming which provided produce for Castries. There was no road link between the two but a regular shipping service operated. It is possible that *S. mansoni* was brought to St Lucia by seamen from South America and that initially it was spread around Castries and later to Soufriere.

Whatever the origin, the presence of *S. mansoni* in St Lucia, before its 'discovery' in 1924, is not doubted. It was probably at a low level of intensity and is not mentioned again in reports of the Medical and Sanitary Department of the Government until the 1930s when reference is made to its being found in a low percentage of stools routinely examined at Victoria Hospital, those from Soufriere being specifically mentioned. The record book for results of examinations made between 1940 and 1961 was

Table 2.1. *Numbers of stools examined (and positive) for* S. mansoni *from different areas of St Lucia (1940–61)*[a]

	1940–44	1945–49	1950–54	1955–59	1960–61
Soufriere	74 (24)	77 (22)	71 (15)	174 (28)	529 (49)
Castries	667 (20)	422 (13)	718 (20)	743 (28)	1159 (148)
Canaries	28 (6)	15	22 (2)	37 (4)	76 (16)
Babonneau	74	58 (1)	132	114 (1)	201 (24)
Vieux Fort	50	15 (1)	38	46 (1)	412 (68)
Roseau	85	49	225 (2)	140 (4)	180 (48)
Dennery	61	20	107	93 (5)	168 (75)
Cul de Sac	139	95	203	110 (4)	375 (136)
Anse La Raye	41	14	52	46	132 (5)
Gros Islet	53	21	88	33	119 (7)
Laborie	20	9	21	27	68 (9)
Micoud	50	43	44	55	135 (18)
Total	1352 (50)	838 (37)	1721 (39)	1618 (75)	3554 (603)
% + ve	3.7	4.4	2.3	4.6	17

[a] Data from original stool examination records at Victoria Hospital.

found at Victoria Hospital, and for most patients data included information on age and area of residence. Analysed, the data confirm the focality of infection, with Castries, Soufriere and nearby Canaries being the only infected areas in the early 1940s; however by the end of the decade infections were reported amongst patients from Vieux Fort and at Babonneau. By the end of the 1950s infections had been reported from all eight of the twelve main areas of the island. By the end of 1961 infections were noted from all areas, and 17% of stools examined were *S. mansoni* positive (Table 2.1). Only since 1955 were children found infected more frequently than adults (Table 2.2) and it seems probable that this could have accelerated the spread and increased transmission of the infection.

The greater number of stools submitted for examination in the 1960s is no doubt an indication of the interest shown in the infection after American tourists were infected at Soufriere (Most & Levine, 1963), and after the results of a stool and skin test survey (Pannikar, 1961) which showed the infection to be in most parts of the island.

It is interesting to speculate that the spread of the infection in the late 1950s was due to the change from a sugar- to a banana-based economy. This change introduced factors beneficial to the snail intermediate host, *B. glabrata*, which are found in the banana drains. The drainage system is a relic of the sugar days and is largely unsuited for bananas which need abundant water at all times (Twyford, 1975). The drains are between alternate rows of trees and take flood water through lateral and collector

Table 2.2. *Age distribution of* S. mansoni *positive patients.*

(*Victoria Hospital data*)[a]

Age group	1940–44		1945–49		1950–54		1955–59		1960–61	
	No. exam.	% +ve	No. exam.	% +ve	No. exam.	% +ve	No. exam.	% +ve	No. exam.	% +ve
0–4	81	2	37	0	297	0	195	8	173	22
5–9	100	4	46	4	148	0	166	11	335	38
10–14	141	4	58	5	137	2	106	5	385	33
15–19	141	4	57	4	250	2	136	4	286	18
20–29	320	5	249	5	307	5	365	4	766	11
30–39	221	1	184	2	213	2	256	2	554	13
40–49	153	3	37	1	194	1	440	1	348	13
50–59	82	2	35	0	161	1	119	0	269	14
60+	82	0	31	0	137	0	116	1	146	5

[a] Difference in numbers compared to Table 2.1 due to incomplete data from some patients.

Fig.2.3. Western end of Cul de Sac valley: banana fields and drainage system. A: road to Castries; B: road to Vieux Fort; C: road to Soufriere; D: Cul de Sac river; E: banana drains; F: collector drains; G: natural water course; H: marsh at base of hillside; I: banana fields. (Photograph by M. A. Prentice & G. Barnish.)

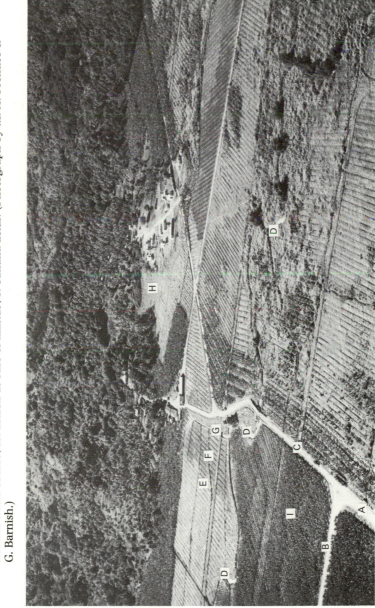

Fig.2.4. Overgrown banana drain. (Photograph by G. Barnish.)

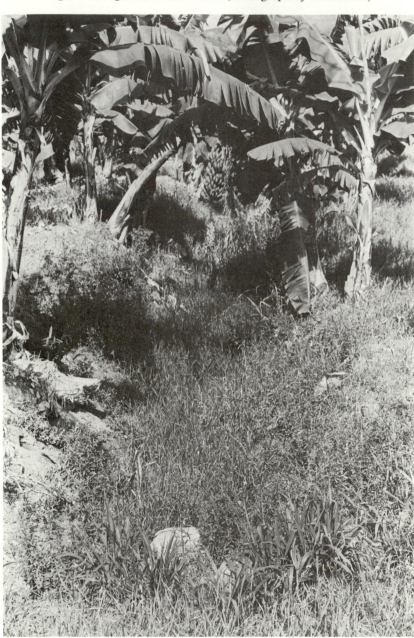

Fig.2.5. Flooded banana drain. (Photograph by G. Barnish).

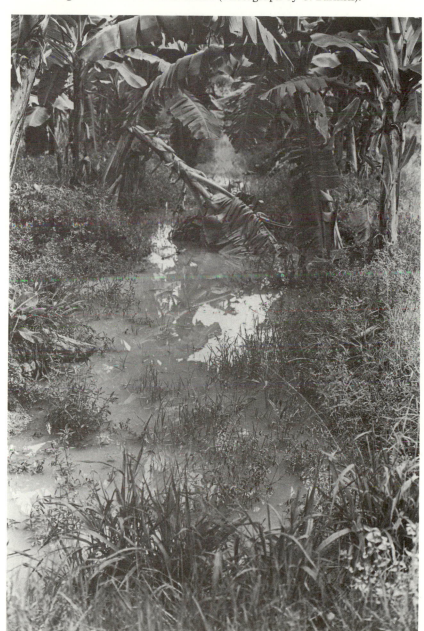

drains to natural water courses. They contain water for variable periods of time, but since they are shaded by the broad banana leaves, evaporation is limited; snails thus survive longer than they would have done when sugar was harvested in the dry season, which left fields exposed to the hot sun so that drying of drains occurred more rapidly. Additionally, year-round harvesting of bananas and the frequent clearing of vegetation from drains necessitates more human involvement in the fields with a greater chance of faecal contamination, infection of snails and subsequent parasite transmission.

Banana cultivation in St Lucia is not, however, without its problems and remedies to cope with them may have some influence on snail colonies. Leaf spot disease is an ever present threat and regular aerial spraying is required to prevent it. A light mineral oil is used and in theory, this could affect snail populations: there could be a direct lethal effect of the oil, or its impurities; a surface film on water could stop oxygen exchange between the water and the air that could be detrimental to snails; or it could minimise evaporation and raise the water temperature to a lethal level. Laboratory investigations, however, using *B. glabrata* and guppies showed no direct toxic effect on the snails or any significant depletion of dissolved oxygen (R. F. Sturrock, unpublished data).

Weeds around banana plants must be controlled and 'Gramoxone' is sprayed regularly. As the chemical is molluscicidal (Webbe & Sturrock, 1964), snail colonies could be affected if it percolates into drainage ditches although detoxification on contact with soil is claimed (Coats, Funderbury, Lawrence & Davis, 1966; Knight & Tomlinson, 1967; Calderbank & Tomlinson, 1968). This was investigated by R. F. Sturrock and G. Barnish (unpublished results): in a standard bench test with *B. glabrata* the LC_{50} and LC_{90} were 3.7 and 10.3 p.p.m. respectively, with a slope value of 1.70 ± 0.24 indicating a molluscicidal effect. Solutions of 2 and 10 p.p.m. were made up and passed through loosely packed columns of clay 0.6 m long and 76 mm in diameter. Groups of 40 *B. glabrata* were exposed to the elutriate for 24 hours and checked for mortality after a 96-hour recovery period. There was no mortality at 24 hours, but at 96 hours, 5% and 55% mortalities occurred with the 2 and 10 p.p.m. solutions respectively. There was no mortality in the controls.

In a second trial similar solutions were run over a mud slope of approximately 0.16 m^2 in area after which snails were exposed to the elutriates. A low mortality of 2.5% was observed at 48 hours in the 10 p.p.m. solution.

The passage of 'Gramoxone' through soil did not entirely eliminate the toxicity to snails but as the concentrations tested were far greater than used for herbicide control the chemical is unlikely to have any profound effect on snail populations in drains, although increasing use is being made of the chemical – from 15 000 kg and 25 000 l in 1977 to 25 000 kg and 80 000 l in 1980 (J. E. Edmunds, personal communication).

Spraying directly into ditches could have some molluscicidal activity, but again, detoxification by suspended silt and muddy substrate would minimise the effect, (G. Barnish & R. F. Sturrock, unpublished data).

Banana crops also require fertiliser and nitrogen, phosphorus and potassium in the ratio 16:3:24 is currently applied to the base of each tree. As it could be washed into banana drains its molluscicidal effect was investigated. Although concentrations of 1200 p.p.m. and 12 000 p.p.m. killed all snails in 24 hours, these concentrations are 8 and 80 times the normal dose if spread evenly over the ground; since only the bases of the trees are treated it is unlikely the chemical would be in sufficient concentration to affect snails in the drains.

Although banana cultivation requires regular aerial spraying, herbicide and fertiliser, it seems likely that the effect on snail populations is minimal.

The change from a sugar to a banana economy may have been partially responsible for the spread of schistosomiasis, but the greater mobility of the population, consequent on improved transport facilities, would also have aided the spread from Castries and Soufriere. Also, the rapidly increasing density of human population (see Fig. 1.7) may have been an important factor. To this day, fires are as common amongst the wooden houses in Castries as they were in the past. Fire virtually destroyed the city in 1948. No one was killed, but many of the population had to seek shelter in the outlying settlements and could have spread the infection at that time. A major fire at Soufriere a few years later (1955) also led to dispersal of the population – again possibly spreading the infection.

3

The strategic plan and methods of investigation

The initial control schemes

The project was not designed as a 15-year programme: this evolved over the years as results of the initial phase became known.

The three approaches to control

These were originally planned in the light of computer predictions of the relative importance in transmission of schistosomiasis, of snail control, chemotherapy, and exposure of humans to infested water (Macdonald, 1965).

Macdonald calculated that even if snail populations or exposure to infection were reduced to $\frac{1}{15}$ of their original level, transmission would decline only slowly and eradication would take 21–23 years. If, however, either of the above factors were reduced by $\frac{1}{3}$ and combined with chemotherapy to reduce egg output by $\frac{1}{5}$, eradication within five years might occur. Macdonald stressed that control campaigns must be intensive.

Three *intensive* experimental programmes, designed for maximum impact, were therefore planned (Fig. 3.1) to compare the effects of:

(1) Snail control: directed against any colony found (area-wide control) in Cul de Sac valley.

(2) Chemotherapy: to reduce contamination of the environment with schistosome ova – treatment offered to all found infected on stool examination at four annual surveys. Initially latrines were planned to reduce contamination further, but as it would have been impossible to differentiate the effect of these from the chemotherapy, they were dropped from the programme. Chemotherapy was originally planned for Roseau valley, but for reasons given later the project was carried out in Marquis valley.

(3) Water supplies: to reduce exposure to infection in rivers and streams piped water was provided to *individual houses* in five villages in the south-west corner of Richefond (Mabouya) valley. In addition communal laundries with shower units, and simple pools (for recreation purposes), were provided.

Results from the different schemes were compared with survey findings from villages on the northern side of Richefond valley where no control was carried out and which thus comprised comparison areas. In all valleys transmission was greater in settlements close to the rivers and streams than in those on the hillsides. Results of control in these 'high' and 'low' transmission areas in Cul de Sac and Marquis valleys are therefore considered separately; those from Richefond cover the five villages combined.

Fig.3.1. Location of control schemes.

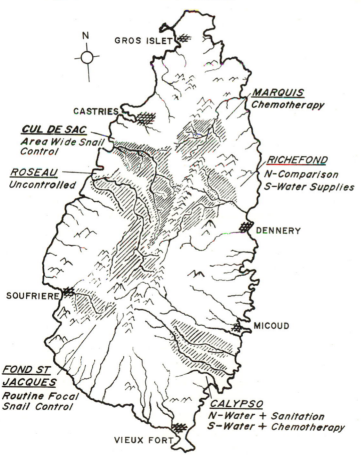

Details of all costs were kept and side benefits, if any, of the schemes were noted.

The valleys chosen for the initial pilot schemes were similar in topography; each with a flat valley floor, utilised for intensive banana cultivation, and steeply rising hillsides. Peak prevalence rates of *S. mansoni* infection were initially similar, but on subsequent surveys incidence of infection was found to be low in Roseau valley and not comparable to that in the other two. On reviewing the initial prevalence data it was apparent that amongst the younger age group prevalence was lower than in Cul de Sac and Mabouya valleys, indicating that transmission in Roseau valley had probably been at a lower level than previously for the past year or two. This, and the fact that doubts had been raised as to the safety of the drug chosen for evaluation as a control tool (hycanthone), led to a delay in the implementation of this pilot scheme and base-line data were, therefore, collected from a further valley, Marquis.

The Richefond valley differs from Cul de Sac and Marquis in that it is Y-shaped with two, instead of one, main streams flowing from the central mountain divide; thus while water supplies were provided for settlements on the stream in the south-west, those on the north side, the comparison settlements, were provided with a Government water supply.

Ideally, comparable biological studies and parasitological surveys should have been carried out in all valleys at the same time, but logistically this was not possible. Detailed investigations into the dynamics of transmission were made in Cul de Sac valley, on the basis of which a suitable snail control strategy was planned; elsewhere limited studies were made.

Cul de Sac valley. Pre-control biological and parasitological studies were made from 1967. Area-wide mollusciciding started in September 1970, the last of the 'pre-control' parasitological surveys being made in early 1971. The time lag was to allow for maturation of schistosome infections acquired immediately prior to control. Parasitological surveys among children were made annually until 1975 when the final evaluation survey included all age groups.

Richefond valley. Once villages to be provided with water had been selected (on the basis of absence of a piped supply and high rates or prevalence of *S. mansoni*) investigations were made for sources of water that could be utilised for piped distribution to settlements. Land surveys were made to collect data esssential for the designing of the water distribution systems and installation commenced in 1968. The first village, Grand Ravine, was supplied with water in 1970, a further three received it by 1971, and the system was completed in 1972. Parasitological surveys were made from 1968 and included adults in 1968, 1970, 1972 and 1975, the final year of evaluation.

Marquis valley. Parasitological surveys were made in 1971, 1972 and 1973, when on the basis of findings at the final survey chemotherapy was offered to all found infected. Treatment was offered after subseqent surveys in 1974, 1975 and 1976. The effect of these four annual treatments was assessed over the next four years until 1980.

Supplementary chemotherapy and consolidation

By 1975 the effects on transmission of the snail control in Cul de Sac and of water supplies in Richefond had been assessed. In both valleys, chemotherapy was offered to persons found infected on stool examinations in 1975 and 1976, and at this time the area-wide snail control strategy (i.e. molluscicide treatment wherever snails were found) was changed to one of focal surveillance control (i.e. treatment of snail colonies only at sites considered important in transmission). In 1977 this was amended to routine focal control (i.e. mollusciciding of transmission sites without prior snail surveys), that could be run by the Ministry of Health. Over the next four years, to 1981, this was assessed as a strategy for a consolidation or maintenance phase of control to keep transmission at a low level after prevalence had been reduced by chemotherapy.

In villages supplied with water, after chemotherapy in 1975 and 1976, treatment was again offered in 1977 to persons known from previous surveys to have been infected but who had not been treated, and over the next four years (to 1981), with no further intervention or control, the use of water in the consolidation or maintenance phase of control was investigated.

By 1975 the Government was introducing laundry and shower units to some of the comparison villages on the northern side of Richefond valley as part of its normal rural development programme: they were, therefore, no longer suitable for comparison purposes. Extra units were provided in three villages to supplement those built by the Government; chemotherapy was offered to those found infected at the 1975 and 1976 surveys and in 1977 to any who had been known to be infected. Over the next four years, to 1981, the use, in the consolidation phase, of a public standpipe water system, supplemented by laundry and shower units, was investigated and results compared with villages on the south of the valley with individual household water supplies.

Thus, after comparing the effects on transmission of snail control, water supplies and reduced contamination (through chemotherapy), the different valleys were used to investigate different consolidation or maintenance phase strategies after therapy:

> In Cul de Sac valley, routine focal snail control.
>
> In Richefond (south), individual household water supplies, laundry and shower units.
>
> In Richefond (north), community household water supplies, laundry and shower units.
>
> In Marquis valley, a Government standpipe water system.

Results of control schemes in these valleys are discussed in Chapters 5, 6 and 7.

Other research control projects.

The initial control project in Cul de Sac valley was designed for maximum effect, with snail colonies found anywhere in the valley being treated with molluscicide. Later, the programme was modified to one of routine focal control. The effect of this as the primary control strategy was investigated in a valley in the south of the island, inland from Soufriere, at Fond St Jacques. Pre-control studies were made from 1974 to 1976 when focal mollusciciding commenced. Parasitological evaluation was made four years later in 1980. Results are described in Chapter 6.

Two further control schemes were initiated in collaboration with the Government. While the Central Water Authority provided water to villages in the Calypso area, between the Troumasse and Canelles rivers in the south-east of the island, the Research and Control Department was responsible for its distribution to individual houses and for constructing laundry and shower units financed by the Rotary Clubs of Castries and Guelf (Canada). With support from the Edna McConnell Clark Foundation latrines were provided to houses on the northern side of the area: chemotherapy was offered in the south, providing a comparison of the effect on transmission of reduced contamination with *S. mansoni* ova through latrines or chemotherapy. Results are described in Chapter 7.

Public health control

As distinct from research control projects, public health control schemes, at times with a limited research objective, were initiated when transmission foci were found in other areas. Such control consisted essentially of chemotherapy, snail control or the repair and improvement of Government water supplies. These projects are described in Chapter 8.

Schistosomiasis treatment

The Research and Control Department was responsible for the treatment of all cases of schistosomiasis on the island and patients were referred to the clinic from hospitals, health centres and private practitioners. Patients living in areas where research control projects were operating received treatment if referred for it, but a note was made in the subject's field records.

Methods of investigation

Parasitological

Household census and parasitological surveys. In each project area a survey team visited houses and recorded the names, sex and age of occupants. In the first surveys some houses were overlooked in dense vegetation, and only became apparent at subsequent surveys when the team became more familiar with the area. Boundaries between villages are ill-defined and there was sometimes confusion as to the name of localities; this also led to difficulties in delineating a village. Occasionally the time involved in reaching some house or a few houses well away from the main village was considered excessive and isolated dwellings were excluded from surveys. Residents of some houses spent more time away than 'at home', leading to difficulty in getting accurate census data. It was also found that mothers would often fail to report the presence of new-born babies until they were about a year old.

In order to check the ages, birth certificates were requested from a number of families after the ages had been given. The sample comprised 1031 children and 290 adults. Amongst the children the stated age was correct in 75% of cases; 21.5% were incorrect by one year and only 1.1% by more than 5 years. Amongst the adults, 45.8% of the stated ages were correct, 28.3% were incorrect by one year, 10.6% by more than 5 years and 1% by more than 10 years. These levels of accuracy were considered sufficient to justify grouping children by 5-year and adults by 10-year age groups.

At subsequent surveys, births and deaths occurring since the last survey were recorded and where possible data on movement of the population were collected – where newcomers were from and where people had moved to, although the latter information was not always available. It was not infrequently found that a house would be completely removed. New houses were numbered and details of occupants were obtained.

In general neighbours were loath to give information about each other. Thus, if a house were empty, it was often difficult to find out where the occupants had moved to. Too much questioning suggested enquiries for tax or some other unpopular purpose!

The first survey of each valley took longer than others owing to the need to explain the programme and to collect census data from each household, so that there was a variable time between first and second surveys in some areas. Later, however, surveys were carried out as nearly as possible at 12-monthly intervals.

In addition to annual surveys in the three initial pilot control areas, surveys were made amongst school children in different localities of the island to detect spontaneous changes in transmission. These surveys were gradually stopped as areas where they were being made were brought into subsequent control programmes.

Stool collections. Although the prevalence of infection with *S. mansoni* was known to vary considerably in different parts of the island, the extent of the variation was unknown and this, combined with unknown variations in settlement size, made the design of a sampling technique difficult. It was further appreciated that, although the rate of response to the initial request for faecal samples might be good, repeated requests for further samples in order to determine changes in the indices of infection might prove less productive, with an inadequate number being obtained. A total population stool survey was therefore attempted to provide base-line data on *S. mansoni* prevalence and intensity of infection. At subseqent surveys stools were requested from children to the age of 7 years (later extended to 14); the effects on transmission of control strategies were assessed from the results of examining these stools. Surveys of all age groups were made for the final assessment of control.

Table 3.1. *Prevalence of* S. mansoni *amongst persons providing stools readily and amongst less co-operative individuals*

| | Age in years | | | | | |
| | 0–14 | | 15–39 | | 40+ | |
Prevalence	No. exam.	% +ve	No. exam.	% +ve	No. exam.	% +ve
High						
Responsive	1097	39	479	61	318	53
Unresponsive	179	34	159	50	82	35
Low						
Responsive	1685	5	825	20	543	9
Unresponsive	248	7	222	25	93	13

Stool containers, individually labelled, were left at each house. The containers were collected the following day from many houses, but two or three return visits were necessary to retrieve as many as possible. It is recognised that some containers probably held a stool specimen from a person other than the one named on the label, containers may have been accidentally mixed, or persons may have 'shared' a stool. It is thought, however, that such cases occurred infrequently. Generally over 75% of the children provided stool specimens at each survey. Adults were less responsive, particularly males between the ages of 15 and 30 years, and, in general, compliance became less as more surveys were made.

In an attempt to determine how representative of the whole population were those who provided stools, prevalence amongst groups who freely gave stools was compared with prevalence amongst groups who gave specimens only after considerable persuasion. Groups investigated were from different endemic areas. Overall, prevalence was similar in the two groups, but amongst persons from high prevalence areas those who gave stools readily were more frequently *S. mansoni* positive than those less co-operative. In settlements with low rates of prevalence the reverse was found, i.e. the less responsive had higher rates of infection. In both groups the difference was significant at the 0.1% level (Table 3.1).

Parasitological techniques. For determining the prevalence of infection, stools were examined qualitatively by a formalin–glycerine sedimentation method, up to three slide preparations being examined for *S. mansoni* ova (Appendix 1). The presence of other helminth ova, hookworm, *Ascaris lumbricoides*, *Trichuris trichuria*, and larvae of *Strongyloides stercoralis* were noted. Stools qualitatively positive for *S. mansoni* were examined quantitatively by the filtration-staining method (Bell, 1963). Since in this technique, egg output is based on volume, rather than weight of stool, results are expressed in terms of eggs per ml (e.p.ml) faeces. If the quantitative technique failed to show *S. mansoni* eggs (although qualitatively the stool was positive) the egg output was considered 10 eggs per ml faeces, the lowest level detectable by the technique. If there was insufficient stool for the above quantitative evaluation, a modification of the Kato method was used. Using this technique, Martin & Beaver (1968) had shown that eggs of *S. mansoni* are distributed randomly in faeces; this was confirmed using the filtration-staining quantitative method (Woodstock, Cook, Peters & Warren, 1971).

Indices of infection. The following indices of infection were calculated:

Prevalence: The percentage of persons found infected at a given time; calculated for specific age or sex groups or overall.

Intensity of infection: The mean egg output *of those infected*, calculated for specific age or sex groups or overall. For most purposes the geometric mean was calculated because of the lognormal distribution of output in a community (the majority of egg counts being low with only a few high ones).

Index of potential contamination (IPC): The sum of the product of prevalence and intensity of infection for each age group gives a 'crude' index. This can be adjusted ('corrected') when the proportional contribution of each age group to the total population is considered (Farooq & Samaan, 1967). The Egyptian workers also made allowance for the hatchability of eggs from people of different ages. Although they found differences in hatchability to be minimal, in St Lucia such differences were directly related to intensity of infection and decreased in older patients (Upatham, Sturrock & Cook, 1976).

Relative IPC: Denotes the contribution of different age groups to the total level of potential contamination (Jordan, 1963).

Incidence (of new infection): This is the only measure of the level of transmission in an area over a given period and shows the *percentage* of children who are negative at one survey but are infected at a subsequent survey. It is usually calculated over 12 months, but if used over a shorter period results can indicate seasonal changes in transmission.

Conversions: The *number* of children negative at one survey who subsequently become infected (i.e. convert from being negative to positive).

Reversions: The *number* of children who are positive at one survey who are subsequently found to have apparently *spontaneously* lost their infection (i.e. revert from positive to negative).

Conversion/Reversion ratio (C/R ratio): In areas where there is active transmission, there are more conversions that reversions amongst children, so the ratio is greater than 1 (usually 3 or more) (Table 3.2). As control becomes effective the ratio declines, and when less than one, effective control is indicated. If this level is maintained the parasite will gradually die out.

Owing to the declining prevalence in the older age groups, even in areas of active transmission, there are usually more lost than acquired infections so the ratio is less than one.

Change in the status of infection: In longitudinal studies the re-examination of the same group of people after a few years (cohort study) enables the conversions and reversions to be calculated. From these data the change in status of *S. mansoni* in the community can be derived.

In areas where there is a high level of population movement the 'change in status' of infection amongst the stable population provides a more accurate indication of transmission than would be indicated by cross-sectional prevalence studies. These could be affected by population movement, whereas cohort studies should involve only persons resident in the area between surveys.

Maintenance of standard of stool examination. Since the results of large scale parasitological studies, such as described here, depend on the competence of microscopists carrying out a monotonous and boring task, a system of checking at least 10% of the negative slides was introduced. The percentage of negative slides found positive on checking is shown in Table 3.3 together with the calculated false negative rate (FNR). The FNR is a more realistic measure for the maintenance of examination standards than the percentage reported falsely negative, as it takes into account variations in the

Table 3.2. *Change in* S. mansoni *status: calculations from a cohort study (1970–74).*

(*Data from high transmission comparison area (6 settlements in the northern side of Richefond valley)*

Age at 1970	No. in cohort	1970		Conv.[a]	Rev.[b]	1974	
		No. +ve	% +ve			No. +ve	% +ve
0–4	204	27	13.2	95	10	112	54.9
5–9	246	91	37.0	99	19	171	69.5
10–14	103	77	74.8	22	9	90	87.4
15–19	34	31	91.2	2	7	26	76.5
20–29	41	34	82.9	2	5	31	75.6
30–39	61	44	72.1	8	18	34	55.7
40–49	62	44	71.0	6	12	38	61.3
50–59	48	27	56.2	11	7	31	64.6
60+	42	21	50.0	10	8	23	54.8
0–14	553	195	35.3	216[c]	38[c]	373	67.5
15+	288	201	69.8	39[c]	57[c]	183	63.5

[a] Conversions: negative in 1970, positive in 1974.
[b] Reversions: positive in 1970, negative in 1974.
[c] Note the conversion/reversion (C/R) ratio amongst children: $216:38 = 5.68$; amongst adults $39:57 = 0.68$.

prevalence of infection in the population being examined (Jordan, Wood-stock, Unrau & Cook, 1975).

This is illustrated in Table 3.3, showing figures from the last pre-control survey (1970) of the villages to be supplied with water and those of the 1975 survey. Although 13.0% and 3.4% of the checked slides were found positive before and after control respectively, suggesting a change in the standard of microscopy, the FNR at the two surveys (44/328 or 13.4% and 18/210 or 8.5%) are not significantly different. The standard of microscopy therefore was comparable.

In 1974 the existing system of quality control of the stool examinations was refined and expanded to show graphically the competence of each microscopist (Bartholomew & Goddard, 1978). This served a dual function in allowing rapid assessment of each new staff member *versus* experienced staff, together with an easily understood presentation of individual technician's accuracy; updated weekly it allowed staff to monitor their own progress. This latter facility led to some spirit of competition which offset the inevitable tedium of large scale microscopy.

The system required all 'sets' of slides (a set comprised three preparations of sedimented stool deposit), found apparently negative, to be placed in racks labelled with the relevant microscopist's name, and passed immediately to the supervisor. From each microscopist approximately 10% of 'negatives' were randomly selected for re-examination by the supervisor, any found to be positive were noted and the microscopist at fault was called in to confirm her error.

Table 3.3. *Calculation of false negative rate in 1970 survey in settlements to be supplied with water and in 1975 after settlements had water for 3–5 years*

	1970	1975
No. stools examined	621	713
No. *S. mansoni* positive	284	192
Prevalence (%)	45.7	26.9
No. *S. mansoni* negative	337	521
No. re-examined	208	116
No. positive on re-examination	27 (13.0%)	4 (3.4%)
Calculated missed positives	13.0% of	3.4% of
	337 = 44	521 = 18
Calculated total number of	284 + 44	192 + 18
positives (and corrected prevalence)	= 328 (52.8%)	= 210 (29.5%)
False negative rate	44/328 = 0.134	18/210 = 0.085

From Jordan *et al.*, 1975.

In addition, other species of helminths present were recorded and provided a further check on staff. This was of particular importance in surveys of villages with low *S. mansoni* prevalence, although stools from such areas were sometimes 'seeded' with known *S. mansoni* positive stools to maintain interest and alertness amongst staff (Bartholomew & Jordan, 1978).

Performance graphs were, however, restricted to missed schistosomiasis positives, and a standard level of such errors was set at one missed positive in every 30 sets of slides (i.e. 90 slides examined) pronounced negative on initial examination.

Fig. 3.2 shows the record of a good reliable microscopist whose cumulated errors were consistently below the standard. A second line indicates three standard deviations above this level and was the upper level of acceptability that was of particular value during the training of new staff. The level was calculated using the normal approximation to the binomial, and the equation

$$R_L = Np + d\sqrt{Np(1-p)}$$

where R_L is the upper limit of acceptability, N the number of checks made, p the standard error rate of one in 30 and d the standard deviation.

In practice microscopists generally rapidly attained proficiency within the 1 in 30 limit, and some achieved overall missed positive rates of only one error in every several hundred slides examined.

A composite chart was kept of all slides re-examined with total slides found positive, plotted by week, allowing immediate visual assessment of overall laboratory performance.

Fig.3.2. Quality control: cumulative errors found by laboratory supervisor on re-examining stools found *S. mansoni* negative by technician. (Adapted from Bartholomew & Goddard, 1978.)

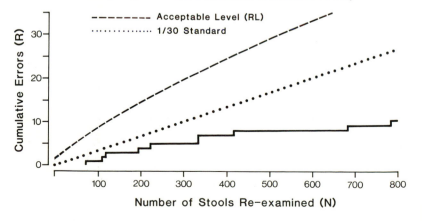

By the conclusion of the project in 1981, 12 255 apparently negative stools had been re-examined by the laboratory supervisor and 262 found positive. Invariably positives were low intensity infections with usually only a single egg found in all three slides from that patient.

Accuracy of a single stool examination. Apart from the possibility of microscopists missing *S. mansoni* ova, it was recognised that with the examination of a single stool some infected persons excreting low numbers of eggs would be undetected. Ideally further stool specimens should have been asked for from those negative on examination, but this would have received little support and logistically would have been difficult. Since more cases are likely to go undetected in areas of low prevalence compared with areas where prevalence is high (and therefore with high intensities of infection), three stool specimens were examined from children in eight settlements with different prevalence rates. Results are shown in Fig. 3.3.

The relationship between the single stool and the three stools examined could be expressed by the formula:

$$y = 4.987 + 1.72754x - 0.0077x^2$$

where y = prevalence on three stools and x = prevalence on a single stool.

Comparison of parasitological techniques. As the Kato method, or a modification of it, is now generally regarded as the stool examination technique of choice

Fig. 3.3. *S. mansoni* prevalence amongst school children based only on a single stool examination compared with results from examining three specimens.

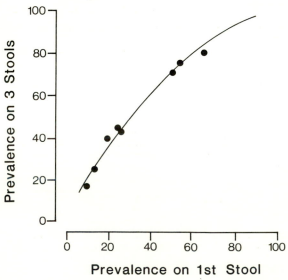

in field operations for qualitative and quantitative purposes, it was necessary to compare it with methods used in the St Lucia programme, quantitatively with the filtration-straining (Bell) method, and qualitatively with the sedimentation method.

The quantitative comparison was made during a community based epidemiological study in the village of La Caye in the south-east of Richefond valley where no control had been introduced: few, if any, patients had been referred to the department for treatment and it was thought there was little infection there. Stools were collected in the usual way by house to house visits, and processed for the filtration-staining (Bell) method by microscopists at the Research and Control laboratories, who also examined them. Three filter papers were used. Two Kato preparations were made and examined by Mr P A Peters of Case Western Reserve University, Cleveland, Ohio (Jordan, Bartholomew & Peters, 1981). Results of 351 paired examinations are shown in Table 3.4.

The Kato method gave higher counts than obtained by the Bell method but the difference between the two varied with intensity of infection (Fig. 3.4). With light infections (under 25 e.p.ml by Bell) the mean Kato count was 17 times greater, but with Bell counts between 201 and 600 e.p.ml the ratio was 6.1 with a mean for all intensities of 8.2. In other studies the mean Kato:Bell ratio was found to be 7.1 (Chaia *et al.*, 1968), 2.8 (Terpstra, van Helden & Eyakuze, 1975), and 2.2 (Sleigh *et al.*, 1982).

Results of this study were also used qualitatively to compare the prevalence of *S. mansoni* infection as assessed by the Bell and Kato techniques, and, among the same persons, by serodiagnosis by ELISA and radioimmunoassay (RIA) using sera obtained from bloodspots on Whatman No. 3 filter paper (Long *et al.*, 1981*b*). Results are shown in Fig. 3.5.

Table 3.4. *Relationship of intensity of infection as indicated by the Bell and Kato methods*

Egg load (Bell)	Egg load (Kato)							
	0	1–50	51–250	251–500	501–1000	1001–3000	3000+	Total
0	90	19	11	1	—	—	—	121
1–50	43	27	50	22	10	2	1	155
51–250	2	1	12	15	16	17	2	65
251–500	—	—	—	—	1	6	1	8
501+	—	—	—	—	—	1	1	2
Total	135	47	73	38	27	26	5	351

From Jordan *et al.*, 1981.

Not unexpectedly the lowest level of prevalence, 44% was obtained from a single Bell filter paper; three papers, 65% and the Kato preparations, 63%, gave similar results as did the two serodiagnostic tests – RIA, 73%, and ELISA, 71%.

The Bell method is not normally used for qualitative investigations but a comparative study with the sedimentation technique was made during a routine survey of Fond St Jacques. Three slide and filter paper preparations for the sedimentation and Bell methods respectively were made and examined. Comparative results are shown in Table 3.5. It is apparent that results from three slides prepared by the sedimentation method are equivalent to a single filter paper preparation. The insensitivity of the sedimentation method has been referred to above and a correction factor established. When this factor was used as a basis for 'correcting' the

Fig. 3.4. Relationship of the Kato:Bell ratio (●--○) with different egg load groups (● Kato: ○ Bell). (Adapted from Jordan *et al.*, 1981.)

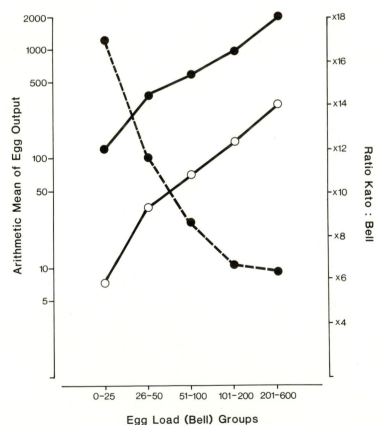

insensitivity of a single Bell paper, the calculated rate of 33.2% was found to be similar to the 31.1% found positive on three papers.

When this correction factor was applied to the results from a single filter paper preparation in the La Caye study a prevalence curve similar to that obtained by examining three papers was obtained (Fig. 3.5).

Table 3.5. *Results of comparative study of sedimentation and Bell stool examination methods*

Village	No. exam.	Sedimentation technique (3 slides)	Bell technique		
			Filter papers examined		
			(1)	(2)	(3)
Ravine Claire	95	9.4	4.2	17.8	20.0
Migny	238	9.6	10.0	16.3	20.0
Ti Bourg	157	21.0	27.3	34.3	40.1
St Phillip/Esperance	126	34.9	28.5	42.0	49.2
Overall	616	17.6	17.3	26.4	31.1

% stools +ve by

Fig.3.5. La Caye: *S. mansoni* prevalence by age in a community-wide survey determined by parasitological and serodiagnostic techniques. ◆ calculated from results of one Bell filter paper. (For clarity, close points in some age groups separated on horizontal scale.) (Adapted from Long *et al.*, 1981.)

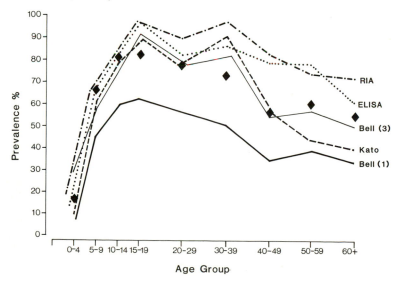

Biological studies

Sampling of snail population. Quantitative studies on snail populations were made by sampling at selected index sites at fortnightly intervals – the technique of sampling depending on the type of habitat.

> *Ponds and streams* – one man using a standard scoop searched a fixed area of bank for a pre-determined time (Webbe, 1962 a, b).

> *Marshes* – 1 m² quadrats were sampled at 6–8 fixed stations using the standard scoop except during dry conditions when snails were hand collected.

> *Banana drains* – a mud-corer technique (Crossland, 1962) was used at each of four stations 5–10 metres apart with central and marginal samples being taken.

To increase the sensitivity of these methods as transmission was reduced, supplementary qualitative collections of snails were made around the routine sampling sites.

When necessary, samples were sieved, washed and sorted. In early work when snail population dynamics were being investigated, snails were measured across the maximum diameter using a Vernier caliper and individually examined for cercarial shedding in the laboratory (Webbe 1962*a*), after which they were returned to their original habitat. The technique for assessing snail infections was used until 1978, but then it was then found that some infected snails failed to shed cercariae. This was overcome by setting up tubes in the field and leaving snails exposed to sunlight for one hour (M. A. Prentice, unpublished data).

Cercariometry. Information on the density of cercariae in natural waters is important epidemiologically and can be of value in planning control by defining transmission sites for mollusciciding. In addition, cercariometry is a useful tool for assessing the effect of chemotherapy in control when findings can supplement infection rate data from field snail collections. Also, if snails are sparse some of the many cercariae shed by an infected snail may be detected and indicate the need for a more intense search for the snail colony.

In the early years of the project attempts were made to detect cercariae in natural habitats by exposing sentinel mice: 20–30 two-month old male animals were floated in individual wire cages supported by a cork for one hour between 10 a.m. and midday (the time of maximum cercarial shedding) (Webbe and Jordan, 1966). Seven weeks later the animals were killed and perfused (Radke, Berrios-Duran and Moran, 1961) and the number of male and female adult worms determined.

Although the animal immersion technique has been used successfully elsewhere, in St Lucia the number of infected animals was disappointingly low. Thus, in 1969, only 12 infections were found in the 7594 mice which survived out of nearly 9000 animals exposed. As the cost of maintaining the colony was nearly $10 000 (US) *per annum* it was considered inappropriate to continue with this technique. Apart from the high cost of holding the animals for seven weeks, there are disadvantages with this method of detecting cercariae, particularly the delayed result following exposure and the mortality during the holding period. In the St Lucia work the technique failed to detect infected snail colonies not already found.

In view of these poor results, experiments were made to develop an alternative technique for detecting cercariae and to compare it with others (Sandt, 1973*a*) As a result of these studies a modification of the Rowan vacuum paper filtration method (Rowan, 1965) was devised and evaluated (Sandt, 1973*b*). The technique was suitable for St. Lucia (although at times turbid water made detection of cercariae on filters difficult); if used in Africa the differentiation of *S. mansoni* from *S. haematobium* and bovine schistosome cercariae would be an additional problem.

Detection of miracidia. The first attempt at exposing caged laboratory-bred snails to miracidia in natural waters was reported by McClelland (1965) from Mwanza, Tanzania. the technique was subsequently developed in St Lucia by Upatham (1972*a*) and, after evaluating different types of cage, exposure of sentinel snails became a routine research tool for epidemiological investigations and for assessing results of control. The technique was later successfully introduced into the WHO/UNDP/World Bank programme on lake Volta in Ghana (Chu, Vanderburg & Klumpp, 1981).

The cage selected for routine use consisted of a fibre-glass mosquito gauze envelope 10×15 cm supported by a 1.25 cm diameter plexiglass rod along two sides and one end (Fig. 3.6). Cages containing snails were placed at the margins of water habitats for 24 hours, and subseqently maintained in the laboratory for 12 days before being crushed and examined for daughter sporocysts (Chernin & Dunavan, 1962) (Fig. 3.7).

Later a miracidial trap for use in flowing water was devised. In comparative trials this gave a higher infection rate, 3.7%, compared with the 0.5% obtained in the routinely used fibre-glass mosquito net cages. The trap was a length of rectangular section PVC pipe, in which water entered through a mosquito screen over one end and left through a screened tube

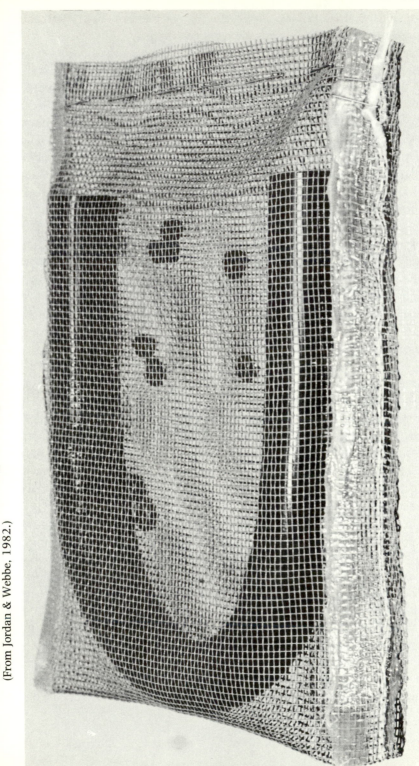

Fig. 3.6. Sentinel snails, *B. glabrata*, in cage made of glass-reinforced plastic mosquito screen over a PVC electricity conduit. (From Jordan & Webbe, 1982.)

projecting inward from the opposite end. The entrance screen was fastened by a rubber band and was removable for inserting sentinel snails (Prentice, Christie & Barnish, 1981).

Chemical analysis of water. A Hack chemical analysis kit was used for the analysis of water from different types of snail habitat.

Water velocity. The velocity of flowing water was measured by an Ott flow meter.

Fig.3.7. Sporocysts in the head-foot region of B. *glabrata* 12 days after exposure as a sentinel snail. (From Jordan & Webbe, 1982.)

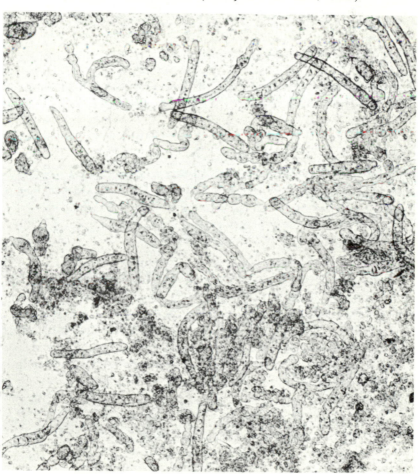

Costing procedures

In calculating the cost of the different projects, no overhead costs for maintenance of offices, laboratories, equipment, microscopes etc. (except vehicles) are included, neither are salaries of senior staff.

Chemotherapy programmes

Case detection. Stools were collected during different surveys by three men. A note was kept as to the hours they spent actually collecting specimens and the cost was based on their average hourly salary (i.e. monthly salary divided by 22 working days divided by $6\frac{1}{2}$ working hours per day). The time taken in travelling from the main laboratory to the valley being surveyed was determined from vehicle trip records and the cost calculated on a similar basis and combined with the actual collection costs.

The cost of examining stools was calculated on the basis of an average qualitative examination (including preparation) taking 20 minutes. The average salary per hour was calculated as for stool collectors.

Treatment. The cost of treatment included nurses' time (costs calculated as above) and costs of drugs, syringes, spirit, cotton wool, pregnancy test kits etc. based on storekeeper and accountant records. Working and travelling times were recorded by the nursing team which usually included a Ward Sister or Staff nurse and two junior nurses.

The services of the Health Educator were sometimes used when prospective patients were disinclined to co-operate. In these cases his salary and transportation costs were included in the cost of the campaign.

Mollusciciding

Records were kept of the actual hours worked and the cost per man-hour was calculated on the same lines as for stool collecting. A cook was employed in the field to provide lunch for the field teams. A proportion of her salary, based on the number of weeks meals were provided for the mollusciciding team, was counted in the cost of control. The cost of spray and spare parts was included in the original mollusciciding programme: no replacements were required, so later no equipment costs were included. The cost of materials covers molluscicide, acetone and alcohol for cleaning sprayers, protective clothing and other expendable items. Relevant information was obtained from storekeeper and accountant records.

Transportation costs were calculated in terms of vehicle costs per mile and travelling time.

Table 3.6. *St Lucia Government salaries and wages that applied to staff in the Research and Control Department.* (Eastern Caribbean Currency)

Classification	1966	1971 Revised scales	1976/1978 COL[a]	1980 Revised scales	1981 COL[a]
Laboratory:					
Microscopists	$1848–2400	$2400–3420		$3840–6240	
Lab. attendant	$1200–1440	$1620–1920	$1400–$2880 plus 30%	$3120–4320	
Clinic:					
Ward Sister	$2352–3092	$3840–4800		$8856–10 056	
Staff Nurse	$1872–2208	$2400–3600		Post abolished	
Nursing assistant	$1620–1872	$2040–2880	$3060–6000 plus 25%	$4668–6348	
Hospital aide	$900–1560	$1440–1560		Post abolished	50% for all grades
Biology staff:					
Field technician	$1848–2400	$2400–3420	$6300–18 000 plus 20%	$3840–6240	
Field attendant	$1200–1440	$1620–1920		$3120–4320	
Driver	$1560–2280	$2040–2880	In 1978 the allowances were increased to: 70%, 60%, 50%	$5352–6312	
Medical survey:					
Field technician	$1848–2400	$2400–3420		$3840–6240	
Water Project:					
Field technician	$1848–2400	$2400–3420		$3840–6240	
Field attendant	$1200–1440	$1620–1920		$3120–4320	

Labourers:	1970	1973	1974/75	1976/77	1977/78	1978/79	1979/80
Male	0.46[b]–0.50	0.56–0.63	0.59–0.65	0.71–0.78	0.78–0.86	1.12–1.25	1.28–1.42
Female	0.34–0.38	0.44–0.48	0.46–0.49	0.55–0.59	0.61–0.65	0.88–0.94	1.01–1.07
Semi-skilled	0.50–0.60	0.63–0.75	0.65–0.78	0.78–0.94	0.86–1.03	1.25–1.48	1.42–1.70

[a] COL: Cost of living allowance.
[b] $ per hour.

Experimental water supplies

All equipment originally purchased was included in the capital cost of installing the water supply system. All material had to be imported into St Lucia and was allowed in duty-free. After installation was completed the cost of tools and other items (cement, lumber, chlorine for pools, paint, pipes, junctions, unions etc.) necessary for maintenance were noted. Electricity costs for pumping water were based on the electricity company's billing. Maintenance and repair work was carried out by a staff of three plus an hourly paid labourer. Pool maintenance (cleaning and chlorination) took 100 hours *per annum*. When work above normal maintenance was required (as a result of excessive rain or landslides) a contract was made with a local worker for the work to be done.

Details of the cost of control projects have little meaning and are of limited value to workers in other endemic areas unless an indication is given of salaries, cost of petrol, cement and other commodities essential for the work. Table 3.6 shows salaries of the different St Lucian personnel employed and Table 3.7 gives the cost of a selection of items used in the different projects. The tables also reflect the rapid increase in the cost of living over the last 10 years of the project. This is also shown in Fig. 3.8 which shows changes in the official Cost of Living Index published monthly in the Government Gazette (cost of living at April 1964 is taken as base 100).

For comparing schemes which were not running concurrently costs were adjusted to allow for variation with time in costs of different items. Apart from escalating prices a further complication to comparative studies was the change in the value of the currency – $1 US being equivalent to $2.00 ECC when it was tied to sterling, but from 1976 equivalent to $2.70 when tied to the dollar.

Records and analyses

In any longitudinal study record keeping is of prime importance. Results of stool examinations were recorded on 'Household Cards' which gave the name, sex and age of all persons in each numbered house. Data relating to deaths, births and immigration or emigration were also noted at each survey. From the Household Cards analyses of results of different surveys could readily be made for different sex and age groups and, as results of all surveys were available on the same card, it was a simple matter to record changes in infection for the calculation of incidence and the rate of reversion. These calculations could be made for consecutive years or to determine changes between surveys two or more years apart.

Towards the end of the scheme all results were put on tape for computer analysis, some of which were used in the work described in this volume.

Table 3.7. *Examples of rising cost of common commodities purchased in St Lucia.*

(Eastern Caribbean Currency)

Commodity	1970 ($)	1974 ($)	1978 ($)	1981 ($)
Molluscicide: per litre	6.12	13.60	45.50	—
Cement: per bag	2.20	4.45	9.30	12.05
Gasolene: per gallon (duty-free)	0.52	1.22	1.75	4.21
Electricity: per unit	0.067	0.137	0.178	0.155
Surcharge: per unit			0.09	0.254
Tyres: size E.70 × 14		72.00	138.37	—
recapped			86.00	126.00
Paint: per gallon white emulsion	13.00	22.00	28.70	46.10
Lumber 1 × 10 × 16 pitch pine	6.24	10.00	20.80	28.00

Fig. 3.8. Increasing Cost of Living Index in St Lucia (COLI) (baseline 100 in 1964). Data from Government Gazette.

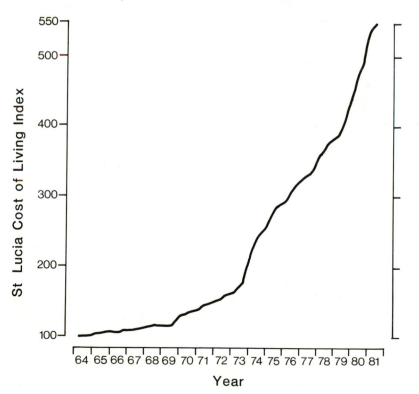

Water contact studies

Preliminary surveys were made to identify the most common water contact sites. In a major study in the experimental water area of Richefond valley 15 sites were selected and, in order to avoid seasonal bias, water contact patterns were observed over a 15-month period. The sites were arranged in a balanced incomplete block of 7 (days) × 15 (months), or 105 observation days. Each site was observed on each of 7 days of the week. In each month observations were conducted for 7 days (one for each day of the week), and the design was balanced so that any two sites were observed during the same week of observations three times in the 15 months (Appendix 2) (Dalton, 1976).

In a less detailed study on the northern side of the valley seven sites were selected. Observations were made every fourth week for seven months, each site being observed on a different day of each week. Except for a few observation days in the first study the same observer carried out both series of investigations.

For each individual observed, the following data were collected: name, age, sex, time of arrival and departure from river, extent of body surface exposed and type of activity. The weather conditions and the state of the river were also noted.

For investigating the relative risk of infection associated with different activities involving contact with water the total surface area of the body was calculated from the mean height and weight of different age groups by the formula:

$$\text{Log } S = \text{Log } W \times 0.425 + \text{Log } H \times 0.725 + 1.8564$$

where S = surface area in cm²; W = weight in kg, and H = height in cm (Diem & Lentner 1970).

The proportion of the total surface area of different parts of the body that might be in contact with water are:

Both ankles	7%	Both wrists	6%
to knees	19%	to elbows	12%
to thighs	39%	to shoulders	20%
to waist	42%	to neck	88%

Assessment of control

Each of the initial three projects had one primary objective: either to reduce snail populations, or to reduce exposure (entry) to potentially cercarial infested water, or to reduce contamination of water with *S. mansoni* eggs. If these primary objectives were attained the secondary but more important effect should be reduced transmission as shown by lower indices of infection in the population.

Assessment of primary objectives

In Cul de Sac, the immediate effect of snail control was obtained by searching index sites for snails. These were selected to represent the most difficult areas for control.

In Richefond valley, water contact studies were carried out after the household water supplies had been installed and compared with previous water contact observations.

In Marquis valley, the immediate effect of chemotherapy on the level of contamination was assessed by the use of sentinel snails, reduced infection rates indicating less contamination of the water with *S. mansoni* ova.

Success in achieving the primary objective led to changes in indices of human infection.

Changes in indices of human infection

Initially, incidence amongst a cohort of 0–7-year-old children (being 1–8 years old at the second survey) were to be the index group: this was later extended to the 0–11-year age group.

Before control, the age distribution of uninfected 0–11-year-old children is skewed, with many young children and few older ones. As control becomes effective, the age distribution of uninfected 0–11-year-old children changes and includes more older children than before. As incidence varies within this age range, a suitable statistical method to allow for differences in age structure must be used in the comparison of pre- and post-control data (see below).

With reduced transmission, brought about by control of snail populations or entry to water, the incidence of new infections among children falls, leading to a lowering of prevalence and intensity of infection. These indices of infection also decline in the older age groups as the worm population dies and is not replaced.

Annual incidence data from children provided information on changing levels of transmission, but from cohort studies of all age groups (ie examination of the same infected and uninfected individuals at 1-, 2- or more year intervals) the effect on prevalence of changes in transmission can be calculated. Cohort studies provide a more accurate indication of changing prevalence rates than do cross-sectional studies which may be affected by emigration or immigration patterns.

Statistical methods

Prevalence and incidence. For comparison of prevalence and incidence data from different areas, between sexes or at different times, Cochran's method for combining 2×2 tables was used (Snedecor & Cochran, 1967).

Cohort studies. The significance of the changes in the percentage infected at different surveys was analysed by comparing the difference between the numbers of conversions and reversions by the sign test.

Quantitative data. For comparison of the geometric means of egg counts of different age groups with data from different areas, between sexes, or at different times, the individual differences were weighted by the reciprocal of the variance. The weighted mean differences was regarded as normally distributed and having, under the null hypothesis, a mean of zero and a variance of the reciprocal of the sum of the weights. Accordingly, to test whether the mean difference differed from 0, a normal approximation was taken of $Z = \bar{d}/SE\,\bar{d}$ (method proposed by C. White, personal communication, 1973).

4

Untreated comparison areas

To demonstrate convincingly that a decline in indices of infection in the human population is due to control methods applied requires evidence that the changes in transmission are unlikely to have taken place spontaneously. Such evidence, however, derived from comparison areas or pre-control studies, can only be circumstantial. The use of untreated areas for parasitological study in parallel with those in nearby intervention or control areas assumes that natural changes that might influence transmission would affect the two areas similarly. Comparison areas have been studied in parallel with the control area in a number of research schemes, but not in all (Table 4.1). However, while use of comparison areas may increase the validity of decreased transmission in control areas being due to intervention, it may be difficult to find two areas alike in terms of human infection rates, human population density, snail densities, rainfall, immigration, treatment facilities and the many other factors that can influence transmission; in addition although at the commencement of control prevalence in the two areas may be similar (indicating transmission patterns had probably been similar in the recent past), it does not follow that they will be similar in future. Climatic changes are most likely to affect the pattern, as in Nigeria where drought conditions resulted in a drastic reduction in transmission without control (Pugh & Gilles, 1978), but while such gross changes in the ecology will be apparent, others may not be. As more results of longitudinal studies are reported it is being realised not only that transmission may vary considerably from year to year, but also that changes occurring in one village may not parallel those in others nearby. Furthermore, different age groups and the two sexes may be affected differentially.

Spontaneous reductions in prevalence were noted over five years in the comparison area in Ethiopia (Lemma, Goll, Duncan & Mazengia, 1978),

Table 4.1. *Summary of various pilot control schemes with particular reference to duration and assessment*

Country	Control strategy	Duration	Pre-control data	Assessment	Age	Comparison area studies	Comment	Author
Philippines (Leyte)	Environmental snail control	1957–59	1954	Prevalence	To 30 years	1954, 1959 Children 0–9	Pre-control data collected 3 years before control	Pesigan & Hariston, 1961
South Africa	Water supplies pools, reduced contact	1959–68	—	Prevalence	5–19 years	—	—	Pitchford, 1970
Egypt (49)[a]	Mollusciciding (niclosamide)	1963–65	1962 and 63 1962/63	Prevalence Incidence	0–6 years 0–6 years	In parallel	—	Farooq et al., 1966a
Brazil (Pontezhina)	Water sanitation Health education	1964–68	1951 1961	Prevalence	0–14 years	1963 and 69	Prevalence in 2 of 3 comparison villages fell	Barbosa et al., 1971
Egypt	Chemotherapy (Astiban)	1964–68	1964	Prevalence	All ages	—	—	Sherif et al., 1970
Rhodesia	Mollusciciding (niclosamide) (some chemotherapy)	1968–71	—	Incidence	0–6 years	In parallel	Mollusciciding from 1960	Shiff 1973; Shiff et al., 1973
Brazil (North-east)	Mollusciciding (niclosamide)	1968–74	1966 and 68 1966 and 68 1966/69	Prevalence Intensity Incidence	1–14 years	In parallel	All indices fell in comparison area	Barbosa & Costa, 1981
Ghana (Wa)[a]	Mollusciciding	1969–71	1969 1969 1968/69 1968/69	Prevalence Intensity Incidence Reversions	5–14 years	In parallel (2 areas)	Marked fall in incidence in both comparison areas	Lyons, 1974
Ethiopa	Mollusciciding (Endod)	1969–74	1969	Prevalence	All ages	In parallel	Fall in comparison area	Lemma et al., 1978
Tanzania (2101)[a]	Chemotherapy (niridazole) Mollusciciding (niclosamide)	1970–72	1968–70	Prevalence Intensity (% reduction) Incidence	2–9 years	In parallel	Little change in comparison area	Eyakuze, 1974 McCullough, 1973
Sudan (Gezira)	Mollusciciding (triphenmorph)	1973–76	1973 1973	Prevalence Intensity Incidence Reversions	Pre-school and school children	In parallel	Prevalence fell in 2 of 4 comparison villages: intensity increased in all	Amin et al., 1982

[a] Designation of WHO assisted schemes.

and over six years in two of three comparison villages in the environmental control scheme in Brazil (Barbosa *et al.*, 1971). Prevalence, intensity and incidence declined over a 6-year period in another comparison area in Brazil (Barbosa & Costa, 1981), and in northern Ghana over a 2-year period, incidence, but not apparently prevalence, fell markedly in two comparison areas (Lyons, 1974). Even in the Sudan where climatic conditions are stable and transmission is associated with irrigation (rather than natural water habitats), prevalence fell in two of the four comparison areas (Amin *et al.*, 1982).

Such spontaneous changes complicate the interpretation of intervention measures, but in most cases these produced greater declines in indices of infection. The spontaneous changes do, however, emphasise the need for some biological and water contact studies in comparison areas to detect variations in snail populations or habits of the population that may account for such changes.

The use of comparison areas raises ethical questions in that persons with diagnosed infections are left untreated. Although there may be a promise of eventual treatment it is not certain that untreated subjects will not be harmed by their infection. Repeated examination of the comparison area population without any positive 'input' into the community can be difficult, co-operation may be lacking and treatment may be sought elsewhere by infected individuals.

An alternative to the use of comparison areas is the collection, in the control area, of base-line parasitological data for a year or two prior to intervention. Such pre-control data in relation to snail population dynamics is frequently needed for the planning of effective molluscicide control, and parasitological data collected over a 2-year period will provide two measures of incidence and three of prevalence and intensity of infection. The use of such data as a base-line for comparing with post-control findings assumes steady transmission and that any post-control decline in indices of infection is due to intervention or control strategies. Declining indices may, however, be spontaneous as transmission can be subject to short or long term variation, often dependent on climate. The collection of pre-control data extends the duration and cost of a project, and while this may be acceptable in a research orientated scheme it is less likely to be so in a public health programme, though evidence of the effectiveness of the measures may be required to justify continued expenditure on control. In Puerto Rico, such evidence was obtained from the annual examination of 6-year-old children amongst whom prevalence gradually fell (Ferguson *et al.*, 1968; Palmer *et al.*, 1969; Jobin, Ferguson & Palmer, 1970).

In spite of the limitations of pre-control and comparison area data, such studies are probably necessary and in St Lucia settlements were designated for comparison purposes and, in addition, pre-control data were collected. In some areas prevalence dropped after the first survey, possibly due to the effect of the survey teams having to explain what was being done. The awareness of the community to schistosomiasis was thus increased, as the community was exposed to a limited form of health education.

Conventionally, a change in the prevalence of infection is the index of infection most widely used to show reduced transmission, but changes in the incidence of new infections are being used more frequently, as the limitations of prevalence, particularly in areas of high population move-ment, are realised (Shiff, 1973). With chemotherapy playing an increasing role in control programmes, incidence, the only true measure of trans-mission over a given period of time, assumes greater importance as therapy has a direct effect on prevalence and intensity of infection in those treated. In addition, in view of the concept of disease control as opposed to transmission control, our better understanding of the aetiology of schisto-somal disease and its dependence on worm load, and the development of better quantitative techniques, intensity of infection is now being investigated.

In assessing results of the St Lucia experiments, in most areas incidence, prevalence, intensity of infection and the level of potential contamination are all considered pre- and post-control in the comparison and intervention areas. In cohort studies, the ratio between conversions and reversions has been calculated.

Water contact studies were not made in the untreated areas, but limited biological studies were. In view of events described below these should probably, however, have been on a larger scale.

Untreated areas

Two areas in St Lucia were untreated: parasitological studies were made regularly in one that was designated for comparison purposes and which showed a marked *increase* in transmission (the northern side of Richefond valley), and less regularly in the other (Roseau valley), where transmission spontaneously *declined*.

Survey and parasitological methods used were the same as those used in the experimental valleys. High and low transmission areas of the Richefond settlements were used for comparing results from high and low transmission areas in the chemotherapy control (Marquis) and snail control (Cul de Sac) valleys. Changes in the high transmission areas were also compared with those where water supplies were provided in Richefond south.

Roseau valley

The study area

Roseau valley, on the west side of St Lucia, is dog-legged in shape, with the main river rising in the foothills on the northern side of Mount Gimie, flowing in a northerly direction on the western side of the Barre de L'Isle before turning west into the Caribbean. The inhabited part of the valley is about 12 miles long and less than a mile wide. The valley floor

Fig.4.1. Roseau valley: map of the study area.

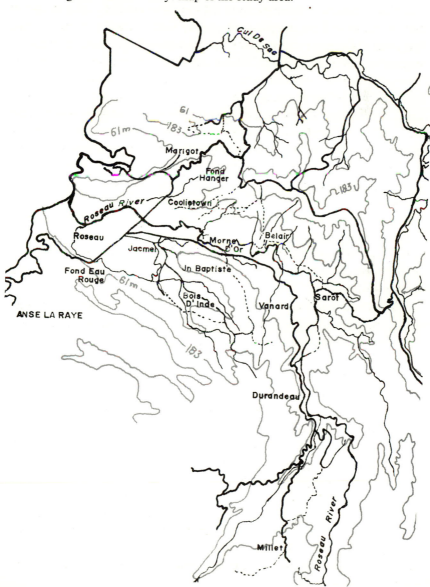

is flat and bounded on the northern side by 250 m hills that separate it from Cul de Sac valley and to the south by uninhabited hills rising to over 300 m (Fig. 4.1).

The single road up the valley terminates at Millet, in the hills near the centre of the island. A road was recently constructed linking the valley with Cul de Sac, to the north, through the village of Sarot.

The valley was an important sugar growing area in the past but today bananas are the main crop.

The population of approximately 4000 live in relative isolation in the typical wood-built houses found elsewhere in the island. Within the last few years a standpipe water system has been provided in most settlements, but there are no laundry and shower units.

Parasitological surveys

A household census and the first parasitological survey were made in 1967. Overall prevalence in the 14 villages ranged from 10% to 69%. In general, rates were lower than in Cul de Sac valley, but the peak of the age prevalence curve was only minimally less, and it appeared that as transmission was likely to have been similar in the two valleys in the recent past they would be suitable for comparative evaluation of different control measures. Snail control was planned for Cul de Sac and chemotherapy for Roseau valley, after a 4-year period of detailed study in each.

Subsequent surveys were made among children only, in 1969 and 1970, and amongst all age groups in what was planned as the final pre-control survey of 1971.

The pattern of change between 1967 and 1971 was complex (Fig. 4.2).

Fig.4.2. Roseau valley: changes in *S. mansoni* prevalence between 1967 and 1971.

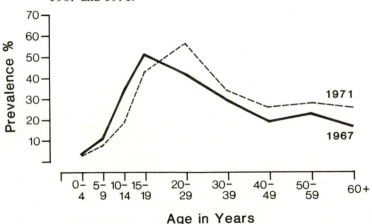

Age in Years

In the valley as a whole, prevalence was lower in 1971 among children ($Z = 4.66$ significant at the 0.1 % level), but in age groups greater than 20 prevalence was higher than in 1967 ($Z = 2.72$ significant at the 1 % level); the two sexes were similarly affected. This pattern was found in most villages, but in two at the top of the valley (Millet and Durandeau) prevalence had increased in children as well as in adults.

The variation in pattern of transmission was reflected in cohort studies which showed high C/R ratios in children and adults in Millet and Durandeau and low ratios in 12 other settlements (Table 4.2).

The measurement of incidence of new infections amongst children is of prime importance is assessing the effect on transmission of chemotherapy (originally planned for the valley). However, as in the 4-year period incidence in the 0–14-year age group in Millet and Durandeau (where

Table 4.2. *Roseau valley; results of a 1967–71 cohort study in Millet and Durandeau and the other villages showing a different transmission pattern*

Age group		Millet and Durandeau			12 other villages	
		0–14	15+		0–14	15+
No. examined		201	120		355	278
No. +ve (%)	1967	10 (5)	28 (23)	1967	59 (17)	85 (31)
Conversions		27*	24*		12*	30**
Reversions		5*	6*		32*	40**
C/R ratio		5.4	4.0		0.38	0.75
No. +ve (%)	1971	32 (15)	46 (38)	1971	41 (12)	77 (28)

* Difference between Conversions and Reversions significant at 0.1 % level.
** Difference not significant.

Table 4.3. *Roseau valley: change in overall prevalence of S. mansoni in five villages*

Year of survey	Belair		Vanard		Durandeau		Millet		Jacmel	
	No. exam.	% +ve	No. exam.	% +ve	No. exam.	% +ve	No. exam.	% +ve	No. exam.	% +ve
1967	105	33	236	29	229	23	505	13	145	10
1971	83	11	262	26	191	28	673	23	217	18
1977	77	3	252	12	172	8	555	8	223	9
1981	32	3	206	9	98	14	459	4	186	2

Table 4.4. *Roseau valley: spontaneous changes in prevalence and intensity of S. mansoni, by age, in five settlements*

Age group	1967			1971			1977			1981		
	No. exam.	% +ve	GM[a]	No. exam.	% +ve	GM	No. exam.	% +ve	GM	No. exam.	% +ve	GM
0–4	250	4	13	268	5	12	175	1	15	106	0	Mean
5–9	237	8	28	308	11	16	274	2	15	210	2	for
10–14	162	31	32	240	20	18	263	4	15	201	3	all
15–19	94	51	34	106	43	22	127	9	18	97	4	groups
20–29	135	42	36	126	56	20	100	28	19	95	11	12
30–39	99	23	25	103	33	17	108	19	16	80	19	
40–49	93	23	22	109	35	22	91	19	14	81	15	
50–59	79	28	14	79	22	19	71	18	12	58	7	
60+	71	21	15	87	29	23	70	11	12	56	5	
0–14	649	12	27	816	12	16	712	2	15	517	2	
15+	571	32	28	610	32	21	567	17	16	467	10	
Crude IPC[b]	6250			5018			1702			988		
Reduction				20%			66%			42%		
Cumulative reduction				20%			73%			84%		

[a] Geometric mean of egg output.
[b] Sum of product of prevalence and GM for each age group.

prevalence increased) was only 13.4% (27 of 201 subjects), the valley was considered unsuitable for the proposed chemotherapy control programme.

An alternative intervention area was proposed (Marquis valley) but periodical surveys continued to monitor the situation in the valley. Changes in the overall prevalence in five communities in different parts of the valley are shown in Tables 4.3, 4.4 and 4.5. Although findings from Millet and Durandeau indicated continuing transmission, this later declined and a steady spontaneous fall in prevalence, intensity of infection and the crude IPC occurred in all areas.

Biological studies

Detailed studies were not undertaken, but two sites (one swamp and one ravine) were routinely sampled along with sites in other valleys to confirm that the same trends in snail population occurred as in Cul de Sac valley where snail control was planned.

Sampling began in April 1967; habitats examined were in the Vanard area in the middle of the valley and results confirmed that snail population changes in Roseau, Richefond and Cul de Sac were similar. Infected snails were found occasionally. Sampling ceased in 1971 when it was apparent that the area was unsuitable for the proposed chemotherapy programme. Later, in view of proposals for impounding the Roseau river, studies were initiated at sites in the Millet and Vanard areas in 1976. Between 1976

Table 4.5. *Roseau valley: results of a 1971–81 cohort study showing change in status of* S. mansoni *in five villages*

| Age at 1971 | No. in cohort | 1971 | | | | 1981 | | Age at 1981 |
		No. +ve	% +ve	Con.[a]	Rev.[b]	No. +ve	% +ve	
(Unborn)	316					4	1	0–9
0–9	190	8	4	5	7	6	3	10–19
10–19	49	10	20	3	8	5	10	20–29
20–29	29	13	45	2	9	6	21	30–39
30–39	47	12	26	1	8	5	11	40–49
40–49	34	10	29	0	8	2	6	50–59
50+	34	7	21	0	5	2	16	60+
All ages	383	60	16	11[c]	45[c]	26	8	

[a] Conversions.
[b] Reversions.
[c] C/R ratio 0.24.

and 1981 snail populations at Millet were diminishing and, after 1978, none was found infected. Surveys in the rest of the valley showed few snails were present (Table 4.6).

In 1976 a small dam was constructed across the Roseau river near Sarot to supplement the Castries water supply. A pool 300 m long was created, and although there were several areas with emergent aquatic vegetation, and apparently ideal for *B. glabrata*, none was found.

A dam was also built for irrigation purposes in the Jacmel area. Although it became choked with vegetation, no snails were found.

Future development and recommendations

As Roseau river rises in the foothills of the highest mountain in St Lucia, (Mount Gimie, 950 m), it provides one of the most reliable sources of ground water in the island. For many years there had been talk of a large dam in the valley to provide for increasing water needs for the north-west of the island, and two possible sites were surveyed. One would involve the main river at Durandeau, the other a ravine nearby.

Although there appeared to be little risk of an *S. mansoni* problem developing, a reservoir of infection existed around the upper reaches of the river and *B. glabrata* were consistently found in the area of one of the proposed dam sites. Ecological changes resulting from such construction work cannot be predicted, but changes – above and below the dam – may favour *B. glabrata* and the spread of *S. mansoni*. Careful monitoring of the situation from the biological and human aspects was recommended as well as the inclusion, *at the planning stage*, of measures to reduce the risk of renewed transmission. It was further recommended that the cost of such measures should be included in the overall cost of the development.

Table 4.6. *Roseau valley: numbers of* B. glabrata *collected by routine quantitative sampling and number infected*

Year	Vanard ditch	Vanard dasheen marsh	Lower Millet ravine	Upper Millet ravine	Roseau river	Total	% infected
1976 (3 months)	41	103	119	102 (1)	0	365 (1)	0.27
1977	380	166	184	530 (2)	0	1260 (2)	0.16
1978	356	439	0	407 (2)	0	1292 (2)	0.17
1979	409	653	0	118	0	1180	0.00
1980	382	288	0	131	0	801	0.00
1981 (6 months)	170	142	0	96	0	408	0.00

Richefond valley (north)

The study area

Richefond valley is on the Atlantic side of St Lucia, with the main river, the Mabouya, flowing easterly into it. The valley is Y-shaped and

Fig. 4.3. Richefond valley north: the study area (LS units constructed 1975).

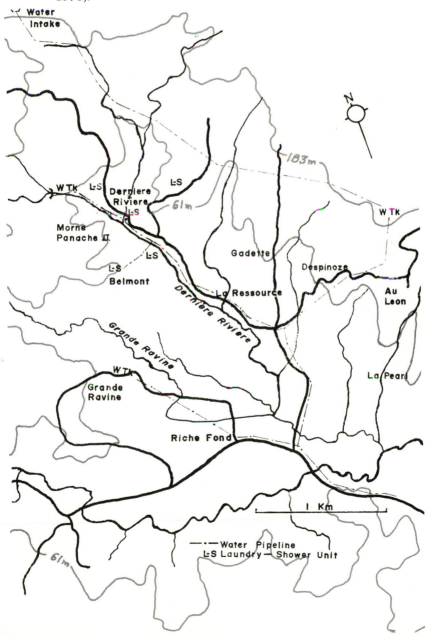

narrower toward the sea, with villages on the southern arm being provided with water as a control against schistosomiasis while those on the northern arm were designated comparison settlements. (For a fuller description of the valley see Chapter 7). The area involved on the northern side of the valley included 9 villages, with a population of approximately 3000 persons. The settlements of Belmont, Morne Panache II, Derniere Riviere, La Ressource and La Pearl are situated close to a main tributary of the Mabouya river – the Derniere Riviere; Richefond lies towards the southern side of the valley floor. Despinose, Gadette and Au Leon are located on the hillside of the northern boundary of the valley (Fig. 4.3).

The villages were served by a gravity-fed community standpipe water supply, installed by the Central Water Authority in 1969. However, although water was pumped to the hillside villages, water storage facilities were inadequate and the supply was, therefore, sporadic. Although no control scheme was operating, treatment for *S. mansoni* was available for any of the population who needed it.

Parasitological findings

Surveys were made at regular intervals between 1968 and 1975. At the first survey of 1968 the prevalence of *S. mansoni* was found to vary

Table 4.7. *Richefond valley north – comparison settlements: overall prevalence by settlement in 1968, and subsequent incidence amongst children aged 0–7 years*

Villages in order of incidence between 1969 and 1970

| Village | Overall prevalence (%) 1968 | 1968–69[a] | | 1969–70 | | Overall prevalence (%) 1970 |
		No. neg.[b]	% inc.[c]	No. neg.	% inc.	
Richefond	50	27	29.6	35	28.6	57
La Pearl	35	15	6.6	22	22.7	43
Derniere Riviere	37	120	10.0	159	20.1	46
Belmont	55	33	18.1	63	19.0	56
Morne Panache II	30	28	25.0	32	15.6	51
La Ressource	39	38	7.8	53	15.1	49
Gadette	22	51	1.9	63	11.1	36
Au Leon	8	110	1.8	105	6.7	25
Despinose	17	19	0	26	3.8	22

[a] Approximately 18 months between surveys (% incidence *not* adjusted to 12 month rate).
[b] Number negative at first of two surveys.
[c] Percentage positive at second survey (% incidence).

considerably from village to village. Based on subsequent incidence data, settlements were categorised as in high or low transmission areas if the incidence of new infections amongst 0–7-year old children was above or below 15% between 1969 and 1970. (This basis was generally used for categorising settlements in other valleys). Results are shown in Table 4.7. The 1969–70 incidence rates were generally (but not consistently) higher than 1968–69, and in all settlements prevalence was higher in 1970 than in 1968.

High transmission villages were on the valley floor or close to the main streams, while others were on the northern wall of the valley.

Prevalence and intensity of infection by sex in the two areas are shown in Table 4.8. Prevalence was generally higher amongst females than males

Table 4.8. *Richefond valley north – comparison settlements: prevalence and intensity of infection by age and sex in 1968*

Age in years	Males			Females			Total		
	No. exam.	% +ve	GM[a]	No. exam.	% +ve	GM	No. exam.	% +ve	GM
High transmission areas									
0–4	130	5	29	122	10	26	252	8	27
5–9	138	38	50	153	43	49	291	41	50
10–14	109	57	48	101	71	67	210	64	58
15–19	49	71	46	71	75	92	120	73	68
20–29	53	51	41	90	57	38	143	55	39
30–39	33	42	41	66	41	61	99	41	53
40–49	51	31	36	61	44	42	112	38	40
50–59	34	47	39	40	40	31	74	43	35
60+	44	27	43	60	32	44	104	30	44
0–14	377	32	48	376	40	56	753	36	52
15+	264	45	42	388	50	52	652	48	47
Low transmission areas									
0–4	105	2	27[b]	115	0	41[b]	220	1	23[b]
5–9	114	4	27[b]	115	6	41[b]	229	5	23[b]
10–14	82	16	27[b]	64	15	41[b]	146	16	35
15–19	42	33	43	56	36	41[b]	98	35	33
20–29	28	11	43[b]	79	29	31[b]	107	24	39
30–39	29	17	43[b]	32	22	31[b]	61	20	17[b]
40–49	25	4	43[b]	36	14	31[b]	61	10	17[b]
50–59	14	14	43[b]	22	18	31[b]	36	17	17[b]
60+	12	0	43[b]	32	16	31[b]	44	11	17[b]
0–14	301	7	27	294	6	41	595	6	34
15+	150	17	43	257	25	32	407	22	34

[a] Geometric mean of egg output.
[b] Mean of age groups indicated.

Table 4.9. *Richefond valley north – comparison settlements: annual incidence of new S. mansoni infections*

Age in years[b]	1968–69[a]		1969–70		1970–71		1971–72		1972–73		1973–74		1974–75	
	No. neg.[c]	% inc.[d]	No. neg.	% inc.	No. neg.	% inc.	No. neg.	% inc.	No. neg.	% inc.	No. neg.	% inc.	No. neg.	% inc.
High transmission areas														
0 & 1	41	9.8	77	7.8	48	8.3	40	17.5	58	20.7	49	16.3	38	5.3
2 & 3	81	13.6	106	15.1	66	12.1	66	28.8	54	25.9	54	25.9	51	17.6
4 & 5	90	17.8	102	24.5	81	13.6	91	36.3	56	23.2	47	23.4	47	17.0
6 & 7	49	12.2	79	31.6	86	32.6	87	50.6	65	33.8	53	37.7	50	30.0
8 & 9	40	37.5	48	37.5	38	42.1	51	56.9	44	38.6	44	38.6	41	19.5
10 & 11					28	71.4	13	53.8	19	42.1	28	32.1	33	36.4
0–9	301	17.3	412	21.8	319	21.0	335	39.4	277	28.2	247	28.3	227	18.5
0–11					347	25.1	348	39.9	296	29.1	275	28.4	260	20.8
Low transmission areas														
0 & 1	29	0	31	3.2	28	3.6	31	3.2	46	6.5	39	7.7	38	0
2 & 3	44	0	46	6.5	33	0	59	8.5	62	8.1	52	9.6	53	1.9
4 & 5	54	1.9	52	7.7	55	5.5	59	6.8	61	4.9	62	4.8	57	7.0
6 & 7	53	3.8	65	10.8	46	2.2	64	7.8	80	15.0	59	6.8	70	4.3
8 & 9	36	16.7	45	20.0	37	27.0	54	16.7	64	29.7	50	10.0	62	14.5
10 & 11					23	34.8	30	33.3	45	31.1	39	12.9	43	25.6
0–9	216	4.2	239	10.0	199	7.5	267	9.0	313	13.4	262	7.6	280	6.1
0–11					222	10.4	297	11.4	358	15.6	301	8.3	323	8.7

[a] Approximately 18 months between surveys
[b] Age at first of two surveys.
[c] Number negative at first of two surveys.
[d] Percentage positive at second survey (% incidence).

in the high transmission areas and amongst adult females in the low transmission areas; intensity tended to be higher among females than males.

Changes in incidence over the years 1968–1975 (i.e. during pre-control and control studies in Cul de Sac valley and in the experimental water supply (EWS) settlements on the south side of Richefond valley) are shown in Table 4.9. Incidence increased steadily from 17.3% (1968–69) to peak at 39.4% (among 0–9 year olds) in the high transmission areas, and from 4.2% to 13.4% in the low transmission villages: transmission then declined to near the original levels – 18.5% and 6.1% respectively. Peak incidence occurred in 1971–1972 in the higher transmission areas, and in the following year elsewhere.

The fluctuating incidence led to changes in prevalence, and by 1975 it was markedly higher than in 1968 in both the high and the low transmission areas, with significant increases among adults (at 0.1% level) and children (at 1% level) in both areas (Fig. 4.4). Males showed greater changes than females.

Amongst females below the age of 14, prevalence increased slightly in both areas although the change was not significant, but a significant increase at the 0.1% level was noted amongst older women in both areas ($Z = 4.01$ and 3.61 in high and low transmission areas respectively). Amongst males below the age of 14, the increase was significant at the

Fig.4.4. Richefond valley north: changes in *S. mansoni* prevalence in high and low transmission areas between 1968 and 1975.

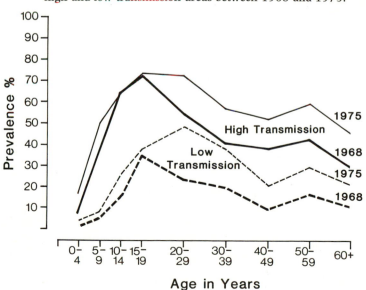

1% level (Z = 2.64) in the high transmission areas and at the 5% level
(Z = 2.51) in the low transmission areas. Among older males the increase
was significant at the 1% and 0.1% level in the high and low transmission
areas respectively (Z = 2.61 and 3.32).

Further analysis of data showed that the pattern of change was not
consistent in all villages (Fig. 4.5). Thus, while in three high transmission
settlements, Belmont, Morne Panache II, Derniere Riviere (designated
Group I settlements), and the low transmission settlements, Despinose,
Gadette, Au Leon (Group III), overall prevalence at 1975 was higher than
in 1968, it was lower in Group II villages (the remaining three high

Fig.4.5. Richefond valley north: changes in prevalence at surveys
between 1968 and 1975 in three groups of villages. A: The horizontal
rule cutting the columns shows the overall prevalence. Children are
represented by the white column, adults by the black column. B:
White columns, males; black columns, females.

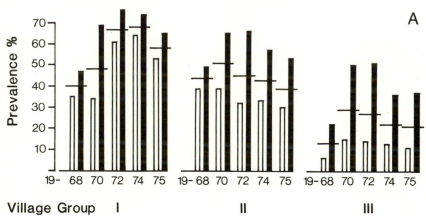

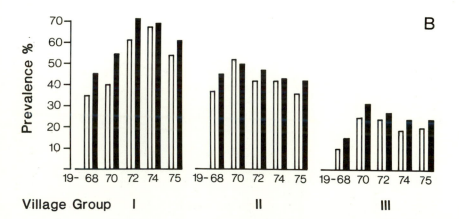

Table 4.10 Richefond valley north – comparison settlements: results of cohort studies[a]

Age group		1968–70			1970–72			1972–75	
		0–14	15+		0–14	15+		0–14	15+
Group I villages									
No. examined	1968	343	223	1970	430	256	1972	394	250
No. +ve (%)		111 (32.4)	108 (48.4)		145 (33.7)	170 (66.4)		288 (73.1)	208 (83.2)
Conversions		70	67		169	39		70	11
Reversions		22	15		20	17		57	63
C/R ratio		3.5	4.5		8.5	2.3		1.2	0.2
No. +ve (%)	1970	159 (46.4)	160 (71.7)	1972	294 (68.4)	192 (75.0)	1975	301 (76.4)	156 (62.4)
Group II villages									
No. examined	1968	161	109	1970	184	103	1972	169	92
No. +ve (%)		53 (32.9)	57 (52.3)		67 (36.4)	64 (62.1)		55 (32.5)	68 (73.9)
Conversions		38	22		29	13		25	6
Reversions		11	6		17	13		18	32
C/R ratio		3.5	3.7		1.7	1.0		1.4	0.2
No. +ve (%)	1970	80 (49.7)	73 (67.0)	1972	79 (42.9)	64 (62.1)	1975	62 (36.7)	42 (46.7)
Group III villages									
No. examined	1968	264	141	1970	357	187	1972	416	207
No. +ve (%)		7 (2.7)	34 (24.1)		54 (15.1)	94 (50.3)		61 (14.7)	109 (52.7)
Conversions		42	39		46	21		51	19
Reversions		3	3		22	21		33	48
C/R ratio		14.0	13.0		2.1	1.0		1.5	0.4
No. +ve (%)	1970	46 (17.4)	70 (49.6)	1972	78 (21.8)	94 (50.3)	1975	79 (19.0)	80 (38.6)

[a] The different time periods relate to pre-control studies (1968–70) in the water supply settlements; the period (1970–72) when water was available in some villages; and 1972–75 when all five villages had water (cf. Table 7.6).

transmission settlements, La Ressource, La Pearl and Richefond). However, in this group, prevalence had increased between the years in adults but not in children. In Group I settlements overall prevalence increased in 1972–74 but dropped in 1975; in Groups II and III there was a steady decline from a peak in 1970. Although the pattern of change amongst children and adults differed, among males and females the pattern was similar in the three village groups (Fig. 4.5).

Results of cohort studies in the three village groups are shown in Table 4.10. The very high C/R ratio in children and adults between 1968 and

Table 4.11. *Richefond valley north – comparison settlements: prevalence, intensity of infection and crude IPC in high and low transmission areas*

Age group	1968			1970			1975		
	No. exam.	% +ve	GM	No. exam.	% +ve	GM	No. exam.	% +ve	GM
High transmission areas									
0–4	252	8	27	319	11	19	244	17	17
5–9	291	41	50	393	37	24	366	50	25
10–14	210	64	58	238	67	42	354	64	27
15–19	120	73	68	141	81	42	144	73	29
20–29	143	55	39	136	78	34	136	73	24
30–39	99	41	53	102	68	27	101	57	19
40–49	112	38	40	113	67	25	105	53	17
50–59	74	43	35	94	56	24	84	60	20
60+	104	30	44	94	47	19	90	46	22
0–14	753	35	52	950	36	31	964	47	25
15+	652	48	47	680	68	30	650	63	23
Crude IPC[a]		19 605			15 713			11 332	
Low transmission areas									
–4	220	1	23	179	5	13	187	4	14
5–9	229	5	23	222	10	13	258	8	14
10–14	146	16	35	121	39	22	195	26	18
15–19	98	35	33	58	60	30	82	38	17
20–29	107	24	39	77	68	31	97	49	18
30–39	61	20	17	57	42	22	82	38	13
40–49	61	10	17	47	49	21	52	21	16
50–59	36	17	17	46	41	24	55	40	11
60+	44	11	17	47	26	15	45	22	11
0–14	595	6	34	522	15	18	640	12	16
15+	407	22	34	332	52	25	413	37	15
Crude IPC[a]		3775			8288			3676	

[a] Crude index of potential contamination – based on the sum of the product of prevalence and geometric mean (GM) of egg output (e.p.ml faeces) for all age groups.

1970 in Group III villages is noteworthy and the declining ratios in later periods are consistent with transmission falling, probably due to reduced snail populations (see below).

Prevalence and intensity of infection in the high and low transmission areas in 1968, 1970 and 1975, corresponding to the pre- and post-control periods in other valleys, where snail and environmental control were evaluated, are shown in Table 4.11. Between 1970 and 1975 in the high transmission comparison areas, prevalence in children of both sexes increased from 36% to 47% (Z = 3.01 significant at the 1% level), whereas it decreased in adults, 68% to 63% (Z = 2.48 significant at the 5% level). This pattern differed from that in the low transmission areas where a decline in prevalence was noted in children as well as adults (Z = 3.98 significant at the 0.01% level). In general, intensity of infection tended to be lower in both areas although among children in the Group I villages where sentinel snail exposures were made it increased from 1971 to 1974 (see below).

The change in status of *S. mansoni* in the high and low transmission areas between 1970 and 1975 were similar (Table 4.12). The cohort prevalence increased among children but fell amongst adults; the difference between conversions and reversions being significant in both areas and both age groups

By 1975, Government development in the area included two laundry and shower units (although water was often inadequate) so that villages were less suitable than previously for comparison purposes. It was also considered expedient to start control in the area, particularly in view of the increased transmission in some villages. This work is described in Chapter 7.

Table 4.12. *Richefond valley north – comparison settlements: results of a 1970–75 cohort study showing change in status of* S. mansoni

		High transmission		Low transmission	
		0–14	15+	0–14	15+
No. exam.	1970	603	345	275	180
No. +ve (%)		212 (35)	248 (72)	35 (13)	100 (56)
Conversions		222**	31**	54**	15**
Reversions		56**	90**	16**	43**
C/R ratio		3.96	0.34	3.38	0.35
No. +ve (%)	1975	378 (63)	189 (55)	73 (27)	72 (40)

** Difference between conversions and reversions significant at 1% level

Biological studies

As indicated elsewhere, biological studies were concentrated on Cul de Sac valley, but in view of the increased transmission in Richefond north it is now apparent that interesting biological data were missed with only the limited studies that were made.

Sentinel snail exposures started in streams in the Derniere Riviere area in 1971 and continued to 1981. Results during the non-intervention period, 1971–75, are shown in Table 4.13. Snail infection rates in the area of Group I villages increased in parallel with the level of contamination, both peaking in 1974. The lower rate of snail infections in 1975 coincided with a fall in contamination.

From 1973 index sites in Derniere Riviere were examined. At that time snails were frequently found and 31 of 3268 (0.95%) were infected, but numbers rapidly declined and in 1974 only 1344 were found of which 4 (0.30%) were infected. In 1975 none of 244 was infected, and in 1975 no snails were found. Other habitats were searched but failed to reveal any substantial numbers and none was infected.

The drop in snail numbers may be due to a number of reasons: there had been a combination of severe drought and torrential rain that wiped out snail colonies and, as feeder marshes were fewer than in other valleys, snail colonies from them were not available to reseed the streams. Such marshes as were present had dried up, been modified for cultivation, or were remote and not planted with dasheen.

There is the possibility that the increase in transmission in the early

Table 4.13. *Richefond valley north: results of sentinel snail exposures 1971–75 'comparison phase', with human data and index of potential contamination from 0–14 year olds.*

(*For data to 1981 see Table 7.26*)

| Year | Sentinel snails | | | Human infections | | |
	No. examined	No. infected	% infected	Prevalence %	Intensity GM	IPC[a] (% × GM)
1971	1869	4	0.21	37.2	30	1116
1972	1777	6	0.34	52.4	31	1624
1973	2076	11	0.53	55.1	46	2535
1974	2521	18	0.71	54.3	52	2824
1975	2723	1	0.04	47.0	25	1175

[a] Crude Index of Potential Contamination – based on product of prevalence and geometric mean of egg output (e.p.ml faeces) of 0–14 year old children.

1970s was due to greatly increased snail populations following five years of high rainfall, and that the lower populations in the mid-1970s were due to low rainfall at this time. (Fig. 1.4), but the longitudinal parasitological studies confirm that spontaneous changes, with increasing and later decreasing transmission, can occur within a comparatively short period of time.

The results from these two valleys emphasise that variations in transmissions of schistosomiasis can occur spontaneously and can differentially affect indices of infection in different age groups, sexes and communities in adjacent villages. Thus in Roseau valley, while prevalence declined among children it increased among adults, and while in Richefond valley it increased in children the change was initially much greater in adults. In the same valley, overall prevalence was similar in Group II villages in 1968 and 1975, but it increased in Groups I and III villages.

It is apparent that while pre-control and comparison area data may add validity to results from intervention areas, these should be interpreted with caution, particularly if they are from short term observations from children only and not backed up by biological and, possibly, water contact studies to monitor any change in snail populations or exposure patterns.

5

Chemotherapy in control

The toxicity of antimonial drugs, and the need for systemic delivery, precluded their widespread use in control schemes. This situation was minimally changed with the introduction of lucanthone hydrochloride (Kikuth, Gönnert & Mauss, 1946); although given orally, up to 7-day courses of treatment were required and side effects were unpleasant and frequent. These were less severe with niridazole ('Ambilhar'), introduced in the early 1960s (Lambert, 1964), but the treatment regime of several days made large scale administration of the drug generally impracticable.

The single dose treatment of hycanthone mesylate ('Etrenol'), an active metabolite of lucanthone (Rosi *et al.*, 1965), raised hopes of a breakthrough in treatment and control of schistosomiasis in spite of necessary intra-muscular injections. However, although low dose regimes were suggested (Warren & Mahmoud, 1976), fears regarding its toxicity (acute hepatic necrosis; Andrade, Santos, Borojevic & Grimaud, 1974), and doubts regarding mutagenicity in submammalian test systems (Hartman, Levine, Hartman & Berger, 1971), but not in mammals in (Russell, 1975), as well as teratogenicity in mice and rabbits (Moore, 1972; Sieber & Adamson, 1975), led to its being replaced by the more costly, orally administered oxamniquine as the drug of choice for *S. mansoni* in community-based chemotherapy programmes. (Praziquantel was later favoured in some areas.) Thus, in the St Lucia control project hycanthone was used initially but later oxamniquine was given in the evaluation of chemotherapy as a single intervention method of transmission control.

Treatment was given to infected persons found on four annual stool surveys (selective population chemotherapy – SPC). Thereafter trans-mission was monitored for a further four years. It was originally planned to implement the programme in Roseau valley, south of and adjacent to Cul de Sac valley, but in the course of pre-control studies it was evident that transmission of *S. mansoni* was spontaneously declining (Chapter 4). Pre-control data were therefore collected in Marquis valley where the project was carried out between 1971 and 1980.

The study area

Marquis valley lies to the north-east of St Lucia. It is separated from Richefond valley by sparsely populated hills rising over 350 m. The valley extends in a north-easterly direction towards the Atlantic Ocean into which the main river flows (Fig. 5.1). The walls and floor of the valley are less distinct than those of Cul de Sac or Richefond, the sides being gently sloping, so that streams are less precipitous and water-flow more gentle.

Over 3000 people live in nine settlements in the valley in conditions typical of other areas in the island. Houses are small and built of wood, though around Babonneau, the main settlement of the valley with the church and Health Centre, there are a number of stone built houses. This village is only a few miles from Castries and many residents of the area work in the capital, but farming is the main occupation. Sanitation is generally poor: in the low transmission settlements (see below) 8% of

Fig.5.1. Marquis valley: map of the study area.

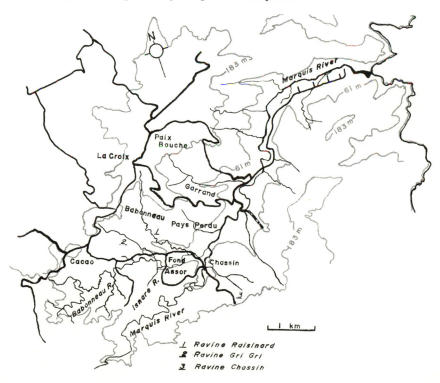

houses had septic tanks, 80% pit latrines and 12% had no latrines; corresponding figures for the high transmission areas were 5%, 94% and 1%. A community water supply with standpipes approximately every 300 m along the roads existed in the area before the study commenced. The water was used mainly for domestic purposes but rivers or streams were used for washing and bathing purposes. One settlement (Babonneau) had a laundry and shower unit and two were built by the Government during the course of the programme; one was in the high transmission area. Maintenance of the water supply left much to be desired; the water was available sporadically and taps were often leaking or broken.

Treatment campaigns

After pre-control surveys from 1971 to 1973, treatment was offered to all found infected during four stool surveys from 1973 to 1976 (Cook, Jordan & Bartholomew, 1977; Jordan, Bartholomew, Grist & Auguste, 1982).

Persons were notified in writing 24 to 48 h prior to treatment to attend the Health Centre (situated at Babonneau) at a specific time on selected days. Undelivered notices were retained for record purposes.

Prior to treatment sessions, treatment cards were completed for each patient. Cards gave identification data – obtained from survey records – showing name, sex, age, villiage of residence and house number. On reporting for treatment patients were first seen by a nurse who recorded the patient's temperature, weight, present or past illness (particularly liver disease and epilepsy), and the calculated drug dose, from prepared weight/dose charts, to be given. When hycanthone was to be given a urine specimen was obtained from non-menstruating female patients between 14 and 44 years of age, and a pregnancy test (immunologic urinary chorionic gonadotropin slide test) was carried out by a physician. An abdominal examination, and any other required by the history, was made, and the physician then checked the weight and drug dose (2.5 mg/kg body weight), reconstituted the hycanthone in sterile water, and injected it into the gluteus minimus using a $2\frac{1}{2}$ inch 22 gauge needle from a disposable syringe. The same pretreatment routine was carried out when oral oxamniquine (15 mg/kg body weight) was given.

Pregnant patients were not treated until after delivery; patients with organomegaly, very old patients, or those with other diseases were referred to the research ward for treatment. Children under 3 years of age or weighing less than 15 kg were given a 7-day course of niridazole or prolonged treatment with low dose hycanthone hydrochloride.

Post-treatment, patients were visited daily by field team staff until all side effects (recorded daily) had ceased. This routine was followed initially when oxamniquine was used in the third treatment campaign, but with increased experience with the drug the checking of side effects was discontinued.

In the hycanthone campaigns no side effects were noted in 43% of persons treated but 22% experienced vomiting. In the majority of cases this lasted only 24 hours and only one or two episodes were reported. Females tended to suffer more than males, but all age groups were similarly affected. Pain at the site of the injection was reported by 29%, but in spite of this, the vomiting, and occasional complaints of abdominal pain, nausea, malaise, fever, dizziness and 'weakness' (a common complaint amongst St Lucians), patients were not deterred and the compliance rate at the second campaign was similar to the first.

Side effects were less frequent with oxamniquine and 80% had no complaints, but mild dizziness (14%), abdominal pain (42%), headache (2%) and vomiting (1%) were reported.

A total of 998 persons were treated in the four field campaigns or in the research ward. 23 received two treatments. The acceptance rate was similar in both sexes (males 93%, females 95%) but males in the 10–19-year age group were least co-operative, with 10%, not being treated. Due to pregnancies in the age group 20–29 years, 10% of infected women were not treated, though many received treatment after delivery. The compliance rate did not differ significantly in the high (94%) and low (97%) transmission areas. The original plan was to observe the effect of chemotherapy on transmission for four years after the 1976 treatment. However, as the Department was to close in 1981, when there was a resurgence of transmission in two villages in 1979 their populations were re-surveyed and treatment offered; routine focal mollusciciding was started the following year.

A final chemotherapy campaign was launched for all areas after the last evaluation survey of 1980 in order to leave as small a reservoir of infection in the valley as possible: 86% of detected cases (124 persons) were treated, but only two-thirds of the population had submitted a stool for examination. In addition 49 persons who had been found infected at any time during the programme but had not previously been treated accepted therapy, bringing to 1250 the number treated. Of these, 58 had two, and six had three, treatments.

Parasitological findings
Pre-treatment

A house to house census and stool survey was started at the end of 1971. Subsequent surveys followed annually until 1973 when the first treatment campaign was launched. Parasitological data existing prior to control thus comprised two rates of annual incidence and three of prevalence and intensity of infection.

In the pre-treatment period the prevalence and incidence of new infections varied and on the basis of incidence between 1972–73 settlements were categorised as having high or low transmission according to rates being above or below 15% among children to the age of 11 years (Table 5.1). Although incidence was higher in 1972–73 than in 1971–72, prevalence was lower in 1973 than in 1971. The decline affected children and adults of both sexes in the high and low transmission areas.

At the survey in 1973 83% of 1670 males and 87% of 1708 females submitted stools for examination. The prevalence and intensity of infection, with corrected index of contamination, are shown in Table 5.2. The 5–19-year age groups were responsible for only 43% and 41% of potential contamination in the high and low transmission areas respectively.

Post-treatment

The first three chemotherapy campaigns (after surveys in 1973, 1974 and 1975) had a rapid effect and reduced the incidence of new *S. mansoni* infections from the 1972–73 level of 22.2% to 6.6% and to 3.9% in 1975–76 in the high transmission areas. In the low transmission areas incidence fell from 5.1 to 0.4% after the third treatment (Table 5.3).

Table 5.1. *Marquis valley: overall prevalence by settlement at 1971 and 1973 surveys and incidence between surveys amongst children aged 0–11 years*

Villages in order of incidence between 1972–73

Settlement	1971 Overall prevalence (%)	1971–72 No. neg.[a]	% inc.[b]	1972–73 No. neg.	% inc.	1973 Overall prevalence (%)
Fond Assau	56	69	23.2	94	28.7	47
Paix Bouche	57	44	11.4	62	27.4	40
Talvern	42	82	15.9	104	17.3	39
Garrand	38	58	6.9	64	15.6	33
Pays Perdu	36	84	9.5	93	10.8	29
La Croix	25	84	3.6	95	10.5	15
Cacao	13	111	4.5	149	3.3	8
Barbonneau	11	128	5.4	147	2.7	11
Chassin	14	87	5.7	108	0.9	7

[a] Number negative at first of two surveys.
[b] Percentage positive at second survey.

Table 5.2. *Marquis valley: 1973 prevalence and intensity of S. mansoni infection by age and sex, and combined with corrected index of potential contamination (IPC)*

Age in years	Males			Females			Total			Corrected IPC[b]	Relative IPC (%)[c]
	No. exam.	% +ve	GM[a]	No. exam.	% +ve	GM	% pop. (1)	% +ve (2)	GM (3)		
High transmission areas											
0–4	99	12	18	84	15	21	17.2	14	20	48	6
5–9	118	26	21	134	33	17	20.2	30	19	115	14
10–14	104	52	16	96	57	22	14.7	55	18	146	18
15–19	62	55	16	62	56	21	10.0	56	19	106	13
20–29	57	51	19	85	58	27	12.0	55	23	152	19
30–39	42	45	23	56	52	18	8.2	49	20	80	10
40–49	43	37	20	45	36	20	7.0	36	20	50	6
50–59	35	46	29	41	59	22	5.3	53	25	70	8
60+	26	42	21	42	50	20	5.4	47	21	53	6
0–14	321	28	17	314	36	20	(100)	32	19	(820)	(100)
15+	265	47	20	331	53	22		50	21		
Low transmission areas											
0–4	165	2	18[d]	130	4	15[d]	17.2	3	16[d]	8	3
5–9	188	6	18[d]	154	10	15[d]	20.2	8	16[d]	26	10
10–14	133	17	25	136	15	18	14.7	16	21	49	18
15–19	75	19	21	89	31	15	10.0	26	17	44	17
20–29	72	31	18	109	23	21	12.0	26	20	62	23
30–39	52	25	27	74	18	27	8.2	21	27	46	17
40–49	49	12	19	58	7	12[d]	7.0	9	13[d]	8	3
50–59	37	8	14	46	22	12[d]	5.3	16	13[d]	11	4
60+	37	14	15	43	23	12[d]	5.4	18	13[d]	13	5
0–14	486	8	21	420	9	17	(100)	8	18	(267)	(100)
15+	322	20	20	419	21	17		21	17		

[a] Geometric mean of egg output of infected persons.
[c] IPC of each age group expressed as percentage of total

[b] Product of (1) × (2) × (3)/100 for each age group.
[d] Based on GM on 0–9 and 40+ age groups owing to few infected persons.

Table 5.3. *Marquis valley: annual incidence of new S. mansoni infections amongst children prior to chemotherapy 1971–73, and after four annual chemotherapy campaigns – 1973–76*

Age in years[a]	1971–72		1972/73		1973/74		1974/75		1975–76		1976–77	
	No. neg.[b]	% inc.[c]	No. neg.	% inc.	No. neg.	% inc.	No. neg.	% inc.	No. neg.	% inc.	No. neg.	% inc.
High transmission												
0 & 1	50	0.0	58	12.1	33	0.0	32	0.0	35	0.0	18	0.0
2 & 3	51	2.0	57	17.5	51	0.0	50	2.0	52	3.8	52	5.8
4 & 5	54	14.8	76	15.8	72	5.6	47	0.0	56	1.8	58	12.1
6 & 7	38	23.7	54	20.4	66	7.6	74	2.7	61	3.3	48	6.3
8 & 9	41	34.1	40	37.5	46	8.7	82	9.8	67	3.0	66	7.6
10 & 11	19	31.6	39	43.6	37	18.9	57	3.5	66	9.1	65	13.8
0–11	253	14.6	324	22.2	305	6.6	342	3.8	337	3.9	307	8.8
Low transmission												
0 & 1	68	2.9	65	0.0	42	0.0	36	0.0	35	0.0	27	0.0
2 & 3	85	0.0	102	3.9	79	1.3	58	0.0	55	0.0	51	2.0
4 & 5	99	1.0	133	3.8	115	0.9	89	2.2	88	0.0	71	1.4
6 & 7	95	3.2	118	5.9	108	3.7	114	2.6	101	1.0	83	2.4
8 & 9	72	6.9	96	6.3	111	1.8	100	3.0	100	0.0	106	1.9
10 & 11	73	23.3	79	10.1	81	3.7	86	7.0	96	1.0	76	2.6
0–11	492	5.6	593	5.1	536	2.1	483	2.9	475	0.4	414	1.9

[a] Age at first of two surveys.
[b] Number negative at first of two surveys.
[c] Percentage positive at second survey.

Table 5.4. *Marquis valley: annual incidence of new* S. mansoni *infections amongst 0–11-year-old children by settlement, before, during and after four annual chemotherapy campaigns 1973–76*

High transmission

	Whole area		Fond Assau		Talvern		Paix Bouche		Garrand	
	No. neg.	% inc.	No. neg.	% inc.	No. neg.	% inc.	No. neg.	% inc.	No. neg.	% inc.
1971–72	253	14.6	69	23.2	82	15.9	44	11.4	58	6.9
1972–73	324	22.6	94	28.7	104	17.3	62	27.4	64	15.6
1973–74	305	6.6	94	4.3	95	8.4	63	11.1	53	1.9
1974–75	342	3.8	105	4.8	105	6.7	77	1.3	55	0.0
1975–76	337	3.9	88	4.5	116	4.3	94	0.0	39	7.7
1976–77	307	8.8	78	17.9	95	12.6	105	1.0	29	0.0
1977–78	261	5.4	62	8.1	87	8.0	75	1.3	37	2.7
1978–79	270	10.7	68	19.1[a]	97	16.5[a]	66	0.0	39	0.0
1979–80	232	10.3	49	14.3	93	13.8	63	6.3	26	0.0

Low transmission

	Whole area		Pays Perdu		La Croix		Cacao		Babonneau		Chassin	
	No. neg.	% inc.	No. neg.	% inc.	No. neg.	% inc.	No. neg.	% inc.	No. neg.	% inc.	No. neg.	% inc.
1971–72	492	5.6	82	7.3	84	3.6	111	4.5	128	5.5	87	5.7
1972–73	593	5.1	93	10.8	95	10.5	149	3.3	147	2.7	109	0.9
1973–74	536	2.1	84	3.6	96	3.1	132	1.5	124	0.6	100	2.0
1974–75	483	2.9	83	2.4	94	4.3	120	2.5	97	4.1	89	1.1
1975–76	475	0.4	87	0.0	76	0.0	124	0.0	100	1.0	88	1.1
1976–77	414	1.9	69	1.4	60	5.0	113	0.9	97	0.0	75	4.0
1977–78	298	1.0	51	0.0	43	0.0	83	0.0	61	0.0	60	5.0
1978–79	235	4.7	48	6.3	28	0.0	60	5.0	41	0.0	58	8.6
1979–80	257	4.3	50	10.0	29	6.9	70	5.7	61	0.0	47	0.0

[a] Treatment offered after 1979 survey.

Table 5.5. *Marquis valley: prevalence and intensity of infection before chemotherapy, after two and three treatments and in 1980*

Age group	1973 No. exam.	% +ve	GM[a]	1975 No. exam.	% +ve	GM	1976 No. exam.	% +ve	GM	1980 No. exam.	% +ve	GM
High transmission												
0–4	183	14	20	153	1	Mean	163	1	Mean	88	5	Mean
5–9	252	30	19	197	5	for	199	6	for	174	13	for
10–14	200	55	18	189	4	all	190	6	all	136	4	all
15–19	124	56	19	118	7	groups	117	4	groups	101	9	groups
20–29	142	55	23	109	10		108	5		94	7	
30–39	98	50	20	83	7	13	89	2	14	65	11	21
40–49	88	36	20	72	3		69	3		58	3	
50–59	76	53	25	70	3		73	3		59	5	
60+	68	47	21	46	7		59	3		58	2	
0–14	635	31	19	539	3	13	539	5	14	398	8	26
15+	596	50	21	498	6	13	498	3	14	435	7	15
Crude IPC[b]	8201			611			462			1239		
Reduction by phase				93%			24%			Increase		
Cumulative change				93%			94%			85%		

Low transmission

Age	GM[a]			GM[a]		Mean for all groups	GM[a]		Mean for all groups	GM[a]		Mean for all groups
0–4	295	3	16	147	0		181	1		131	2	
5–9	342	8	16	277	3		316	<1		218	6	
10–14	269	16	21	210	5		276	2		220	9	
15–19	164	26	17	132	5		159	4		124	6	
10–29	181	26	20	113	9		155	8		124	4	
30–39	126	21	27	74	4	12	105	1	15	93	9	19
40–49	107	9	13	68	3		84	1		78	5	
50–59	83	16	13	68	6		86	2		63	2	
60+	80	19	13	44	2		81	4		72	1	
0–14	906	8	19	634	3	12	773	1	15	569	6	24
15+	741	21	18	499	4	12	670	4	15	554	5	14
Crude IPC[b]	2613			444			360			798		
Reduction by phase	83%					19%			Increase			
Cumulative change				83%			86%			69%		

[a] Geometric mean of e.p.ml faeces.
[b] Sum of product of prevalence and GM for each age group.

Table 5.6. *Marquis valley: changes in prevalence after the 1976 chemotherapy campaign in different village groups according to mean incidence (MI) between 1976 and 1980*

| | Fond Assau and Talvern: MI > 5% | | | | Chassin, La Croix, Pays Perdu and Cacao: MI = 3–5% | | | | Barbonneau, Paix Bouche and Garrand: MI < 3% | | | |
| | 1976 | | 1979[a] | | 1976 | | 1980 | | 1976 | | 1980 | |
Age group	No. exam.	% +ve	No. exam.	% +ve	No. exam.	% +ve	No. exam.	% +ve	No. exam.	% +ve	No. exam.	% +ve
0–4	87	0	77	7	135	1	97	2	113	1	62	2
5–9	119	8	111	23	243	1	164	7	132	1	59	5
10–14	108	8	114	29	214	1	173	11	129	3	81	5
15–19	63	6	67	13	118	3	97	8	89	2	67	4
20–29	70	4	64	6	124	8	99	5	71	7	57	4
30–39	52	4	51	14	84	1	70	10	52	0	44	5
40–49	44	2	46	4	65	2	55	5	41	7	38	3
50–59	39	3	34	3	68	1	52	2	47	2	27	7
60+	30	3	31	7	59	3	57	2	50	2	43	2
0–14	314	6	302	21	594	1	434	8	374	1	202	4
15+	298	4	293	9	518	4	430	6	350	3	276	4

[a] Treatment offered after 1979 survey.

In spite of additional chemotherapy in 1975, incidence was not reduced further, and increased from 3.9 to 8.8% and from 0.4 to 1.9% in the two areas.

A more detailed analysis (Table 5.4) showed that in Fond Assau and Talvern, after the third treatment, there was a rapid increase in transmission and thereafter incidence was only a little lower than before chemotherapy. In Paix Bouche and Garrand incidence remained low but results from Paix Bouche in 1979–80 suggested transmission was occurring at a low level. In three of the five low transmission settlements, also, incidence was as high in 1979–80 as pre-intervention.

The changes in incidence were reflected in changes in prevalence and intensity of infection (Table 5.5). Both indices declined with 94% and 86% reductions in the level of potential contamination in the high and low transmission areas respectively at the time of the third treatment. However, in the next few years both indices increased and prevalence in Fond Assau and Talvern reached 29% among 10–14-year-old children three years after the 1976 treatment (Table 5.6). In view of this, a survey of all age groups was carried out in the two villages in 1979 and all found infected were offered treatment with oxamniquine. Although 178 of 595 stools (30%) were *S. mansoni* positive, only 37% of those infected accepted treatment; the effect on incidence was, therefore, minimal (Table 5.4). By 1980, high and low transmission villages showed an increase in prevalence and intensity of infection (Table 5.5), but the levels of potential contamination were 85% and 69% less than at the start of control.

When the villages were regrouped according to the mean incidence between 1976 and 1980 (Table 5.6), there was evidence that prevalence had increased even when the incidence was less than 3% and a communal standpipe water supply and limited laundry shower units were available.

Population response

The importance of population participation in stool surveys in selective population chemotherapy (SPC) treatment campaigns cannot be overstressed. In the present study it varied considerably from year to year, with area, and with sex and age. The response was best at the survey of 1973 when there was the promise of treatment; it dropped the following years (particularly among males), but improved in 1976 when the last of the four treatments was offered (Table 5.7).

The response varied, being generally lowest in the low transmission areas and best in the high transmission villages of Fond Assau and Talvern, suggesting the populations there were not feeling their best and offered stools to ensure treatment if they were infected. Other evidence supports this – when those found infected at the 1973 survey were offered treatment there were requests, by those who had not given stools, for a further chance to be examined, and many additional stools were submitted. Amongst those from the high transmission areas 40% were *S. mansoni* positive compared with 47% at the regular survey, but in the low transmission areas prevalence was a little higher among the less responsive (Table 5.7).

Males were generally less co-operative, with the 20–29-year age group being consistently the least responsive. Amongst females the 15–19-year age group was least co-operative.

The reservoir of infection

After chemotherapy campaigns the reservoir of infection remaining, and available for continuing transmission, is dependent on a number of factors. When the basis of treatment is an infected stool, the co-operation of the population in submitting a specimen for examination is a prime factor in the success of a scheme; while there was a good response in the first survey to be followed by treatment, interest in the campaign declined thereafter so that some infected persons would not have been detected.

The choice of the stool examination technique is also important. The sedimentation concentration technique for examining stools would not have detected all infections at the 1973 survey, but with three subsequent surveys additional infections were detected and treated. In Table 5.8, the more likely 1973 prevalence – calculated on the basis of infections found in 1971 and 1972 (but who were 'negative' in 1973) – is shown (column 2) and compared with the 'true' 1973 prevalence, calculated by the formula given in Chapter 3 for positives missed on a single stool examination (column 3). The total infections found at the three surveys is not unlike

Table 5.7. *Marquis valley: mean per cent response to different stool surveys by sex and area*

	Males					Females				
	1973	1974	1975	1976	1980	1973	1974	1975	1976	1980
Fond Assau/ Talvern	93	80	69	76	68	95	83	84	80	78
Paix Bouche/ Garrand	85	77	66	72	58	96	82	74	81	70
Low transmission	90	69	59	71	53	96	81	71	81	69

From Jordan *et al.*, 1982.

Table 5.8. *Marquis valley: 1973 prevalence of S. mansoni compared with prevalence based on three surveys (1971/2/3) and 1973 data re-calculated for positives missed on a single stool examination*

	High transmission areas			Low transmission areas		
	at 1973 survey[a] (1)	% Prevalence: based on 1971/2/3 surveys (2)	calculated from 1973 data (3)	at 1973 survey[a] (1)	% Prevalence: based on 1971/2/3 surveys[a] (2)	calculated from 1973 data (3)
Age group						
0–4	16.3	27.4	31.1	2.7	5.1	9.6
5–9	38.8	64.3	60.4	7.9	18.1	18.2
10–14	53.9	77.2	75.7	16.0	32.3	30.7
15–19	58.8	71.1	79.9	25.6	35.4	44.2
20–29	61.7	77.7	82.3	26.0	38.7	44.7
30–39	49.4	70.1	71.5	20.6	27.8	37.3
40–49	33.3	53.1	53.9	9.3	21.5	20.4
50–59	58.3	76.7	79.5	15.7	27.7	30.2
60+	45.8	61.0	65.0	17.5	27.5	32.9
Overall	43.0	62.0	65.0	13.7	27.2	27.2

[a] Computer analysis of data.

the calculated prevalence, and in spite of the lack of sensitivity of the sedimentation technique, few infections were probably not detected in the surveys prior to the four treatment campaigns. It is likely that few, if any, additional cases would have been found if the Kato technique (insensitive at low levels of infection) had been used on a single stool in 1973.

A further source of a reservoir of infection is from 'failed' treatments. While it is unreliable to assess results of treatment from a single stool examined a year after therapy, there was evidence that the oxamniquine treatments were less satisfactory than hycanthone (see below).

Immigration of infected persons can be a problem in chemotherapy control schemes – it is less important where control is directed against the snails or when control is by the provision of water. In the four years of the treatment campaign, 69 infected immigrants (8.4% of 309 males: 13% of 320 females) were detected, and 59 were treated, but the rest had moved on before treatment could be given. In the last years of the scheme (1977–80), 205 male immigrants (15 infected: 7.3%) and 228 females (18 infected: 7.9%) were documented. While there is no 'mass' movement of population, the steady influx of infected persons could be a cause of continued transmission in the absence of a consolidation phase control strategy.

The rapid increase in incidence in the Fond Assau and Talvern areas, from 5% to 15%, in the year after the last of the four annual treatments, is not easy to explain, particularly when it had been at a low level for the preceding years. It is unlikely to have been the result of undetected cases, due to misdiagnosis, failed treatments or immigrants, but the presence in the area of an unrecorded, heavily infected person, even temporarily, cannot be excluded as the source of the infection.

Hycanthone *versus* oxamniquine

A computer analysis was made of the long term results of treatments with hycanthone and oxamniquine. Results of 687 hycanthone- (2.5 mg/kg body weight) and 84 oxamniquine- (15 mg/kg body weight) treated subjects who were re-examined sometime after therapy are shown in Table 5.9. The greater mean number of stools examined from the hycanthone-treated patients is due to the longer follow-up after treatments in 1973 and 1974 compared with the 1975 and 1976 oxamniquine campaigns, but in spite of this there was a marked difference between the infection rates after the two drugs.

Although transmission increased rapidly in the Fond Assau and Talvern areas, this did not account for the difference in the two treatments (Table 5.10) as oxamniquine was less effective in all areas.

A comparison was made of the infection rates between 1977 and 1980 amongst persons who had received hycanthone, oxamniquine, or both drugs (16 patients), and those who were negative at the time of the treatment campaigns and who, therefore, had no treatment. Results are shown in Table 5.11.

The infection rates for hycanthone-treated cases and those who had not been treated were similar for 5–14 year olds and adults, suggesting that any immunity the treated group of patients may have had at the time of treatment was destroyed by chemotherapy. The higher infection rates among the oxamniquine-treated cases is likely to be a reflection of the lower 'cure' rate rather than any increased susceptibility to re-infection.

Although there were 16 patients (12 children, 4 adults) who were treated with oxamniquine after hycanthone had failed to 'cure' them, and the 5–14-year-old group showed a high positivity rate (27.3%), suggesting decreased susceptibility to chemotherapy, the possibility that the children were exposed more frequently to infection (and therefore required a second treatment) cannot be excluded.

The intensity of infection at 1980 in those who had been treated between 1973 and 1976 was compared with those negative during the treatment campaigns but positive in 1980. Although intensity was a little higher in those treated, the difference was not significant at the 5% level ($Z = 1.87$; Table 5.12).

Table 5.9. *Marquis valley: comparison of long term effect of hycanthone and oxamniquine.*

(*Computer analysis*)

Age at treatment	No. re-examined[a]	Total stools examined	Stools/ person	No. persons +ve	% persons +ve
Hycanthone					
0–14	276	838	3.0	37	13.4
15+	411	1058	2.6	15	3.6
Oxamniquine					
0–14	41	91	2.2	14	34.1
15+	43	62	1.4	3	7.0

[a] Includes 16 persons treated with hycanthone and later oxamniquine.

Table 5.10. *Marquis valley: long term effects of hycanthone and oxamniquine in patients from different areas.*

(Computer analysis)

Location	No. re-examined	Total stools examined	Stools/persons	No. persons +ve	% persons +ve
Hycanthone					
Paix Bouche and Garrand	188	453	2.4	5	2.6
Fond Assau and Talvern[a]	288	978	3.4	41	14.2
Low transmission	211	465	2.2	6	2.8
Oxamniquine					
Paix Bouche and Garrand	13	22	1.7	2	15.4
Fond Assau and Talvern[a]	37	87	2.4	11	29.7
Low transmission	34	44	1.3	4	30.8

[a] Greater numbers of stools examined due to total population survey in 1979.

Table 5.11. *Marquis valley: comparison of infection rates 1977–80 among those treated and those negative 1973–76 and not treated.*

(*Computer analysis*)

Age[a]	Hycanthone 5–14 No. exam.	5–14 No. +ve	15+ No. exam.	15+ No. +ve	Oxamniquine 5–14 No. exam.	5–14 No. +ve	15+ No. exam.	15+ No. +ve	Both drugs 5–14 No. exam.	5–14 No. +ve	15+ No. exam.	15+ No. +ve	No treatment 5–14 No. exam.	5–14 No. +ve	15+ No. exam.	15+ No. +ve
1977	88[b]	5	146	1	27	4	10	0	10	4	1	0	603	29	109	2
1978	67	3	2	0	15	1	1	1	4	0			494	26	2	0
1979	54	2	143	12	12	0	10	0	4	0	1	0	392	36	83	2
1980	70	7	253	7	16	3	36	2	4	2	2	0	465	47	454	21
Total	279	17	544	20	70	8	57	3	22	6	0		1954	138	648	25
% +ve	6.1		3.8		11.4		5.2		27.3		0.0		7.1		3.9	

[a] Age as at 1977.
[b] Persons positive one year were not counted in subsequent years if they were re-examined and found positive.

Cost analysis

The total cost of the four chemotherapy campaigns was $11 904: an analysis is shown in Table 5.13.

The rising cost per stool examined reflects the steadily rising cost of living as salaries of the microscopists and members of the survey team increased. the cost of stool containers had also increased from 7.5 cents to 13 cents each. Although attempts were made to collect unused containers, this was generally not feasible as they were considered too useful in the home.

The overall cost per person protected did not decline (except after the first treatment when drug costs were high), due to the continuing need for case detection, the cost of which steadily formed an increasing proportion of total costs (46% to 85.6%) as fewer people needed treatment, leading to the gradually falling proportion spent on actual therapy (54% to 14.4%).

The cost of drugs per person treated increased from an average of $1.59 with hycanthone to $4.05 with oxamniquine. This was partly offset later when it was considered follow-up was not needed with oxamniquine and nursing staff could dispense it in place of the physician considered necessary for the hycanthone treatments. (Physicians' time has not been included in the cost analysis.)

The cost of drugs in the four campaigns amounted to 16% of the overall total. If oxamniquine had been used from the start the proportion would have been 25%, but it is clear that drugs, involving foreign exchange for their purchase, may represent a comparatively small proportion of a chemotherapy control scheme.

The sedimentation stool examination technique used throughout the whole programme is recognised as less sensitive than the recently introduced Kato technique. It is probable that if this had been used, a far greater number of infected persons would have been detected at the time of the first

Table 5.12. *Marquis valley: comparison of intensity of infection at 1980 among those who had been treated between 1973 and 1976 and those who had been negative at that time.*

(*Computer analysis*)

Age at 1980	Not treated				Treated			
	No.	GM	Mean log	SD	No.	GM	Mean log	SD
10–14	32	16.86	1.2270	0.4548	12	25.89	1.4131	0.3403
15+	29	12.57	1.0994	0.1739	13	18.84	1.2751	0.5158

Table 5.13. *Marquis valley: cost analysis of four annual chemotherapy campaigns (following survey at end of previous year)*

	1974			1975			1976			1977		
	Comment	Cost ($US)	% of total	Comment	Cost ($US)	% of total	Comment	Cost ($US)	% of total	Comment	Cost ($US)	% of total
Case detection												
Stool collection:												
No. specimens	2911			2523			2170			2510		
Survey team (man hours)	690	748		624	690		573	601		506	734	
Transportation (miles)	899	120		599	124		773	198[a]		516	93[b]	
Stool containers	3805[c]	285	27.3	2909	314	44.3	3142	289	44.0	3172	412	46.6
Stool examination (man hours)	879	792	18.7	748	722	28.4	723	719	29.1	837	1038	39.0
No. positive	734			164			96			78		
Therapy												
No. treated	688			159			96			78		
Nursing team (man hours)	312	252		82	79		41	45		33	42	
Transportation (miles)	243	48	7.1	128	31	4.3	72	17	2.5	59	14	2.1
Drugs and materials:												
Hycanthone	438 vials @ $2.25	986		91 vials @ $2.25	205			389			316	
Oxamniquine		32										
Alternative drug		112										
Pregnancy tests												
Syringes, treatment cards, etc.		104	29.2	31	22	10.2	12	7	16.5		7	12.3
Follow-up (man hours)	537	497		276	191		123	123			3	
Transportation (miles)	861	251	17.6	723	136	12.8	383	73	7.9		—	
											—	
Total		4227			2545			2473			2659	
Cost per: Stool examined		0.67			0.73			0.83			0.91	
Case detected		2.65			11.28			18.82			29.19	
Person treated		6.14			16.00			25.76			34.09	
Person protected		1.36			0.82			0.80			0.86	

[a] This high transportation cost was due to repair bills for an old vehicle.
[b] Low transportation cost due to new vehicle.
[c] High number of stool containers due to 'additional' specimens at time of chemotherapy: cost of containers increased with each survey.

treatment, leading to a more rapid reduction in the reservoir of infection; almost certainly the last two chemotherapy campaigns would then have been unnecessary. As case detection (stool collection and examination) accounted for 66% of the overall cost of the programme, it is apparent that the best use should be made of stools collected and that a sensitive parasitological technique be used in schemes to control transmission. In view of the high cost of detecting infected persons, all found should be treated although this may increase the drug costs slightly. The final result could now be achieved at a much lower cost than in the present programme by using a more sensitive examination technique (Kato) and fewer surveys.

Biological findings

The main interest in biological findings in the chemotherapy programme was to investigate changes in infection rates in field *B. glabrata* and sentinel snails after treatment, indicative of an immediate effect on transmission of the control strategy.

Eleven index sites were chosen amongst flowing and static habitats in the vicinity of Paix Bouche and Fond Assau – settlements with high human incidence rates of *S. mansoni* infections. Routine sampling started in May 1972; uninfected snails were returned to their habitat. Surveys showed that rainfall had a marked effect on snail populations which were high in the dry season (January to June) in flowing habitats, and decreased with the onset of the rains. In static habitats snail numbers similarly increased initially in the dry season, but subsequently decreased as the habitats dried.

Before the first chemotherapy campaign, 117 infected *B. glabrata* were found amongst more than 10 000 snails examined (1.09%): 113 were from a stream site at Fond Assau and 4 from a static site at Paix Bouche. Among the 54 000 snails from index sites examined after the first chemotherapy campaign to 1980, not one was found infected. Regular sampling indicated that while snail populations were reasonably constant in the first few years of chemotherapy (Christie & Upatham, 1977), they were declining over the period 1976 to 1980 (Fig. 5.2).

Sentinel snails were exposed in four flowing water habitats at Fond Assau and Paix Bouche. Over 3700 snails were examined in the pre-control period – 1.4% were infected. Infections were found throughout the year and similar rates were obtained at Fond Assau (1.4%) and Paix Bouche (1.6%). After chemotherapy no infections were found amongst over 3000 exposed snails. Sentinel snail studies were discontinued in October 1977 as no infections had been found since March 1974.

When it was apparent that transmission was increasing in Talvern and Fond Assau additional snail surveys were made in the area, and fresh index sites identified in the Isnare River, a marsh complex flowing into it, and three streams. Intermittent sampling of the streams began in April 1976 and from early in 1978 all sites were sampled routinely at fortnightly intervals (Prentice & Barnish, 1981).

Infected snails were found regularly in the Talvern Ravine (67 of 6888: 0.97%) and less regularly in the Ravine Raison (8 of 4723: 0.17%) and the Isnare River (14 of 3320: 0.42%). No infected snails were found in one ravine near the marsh. The transmission pattern – principally in the dry season January to June – followed the general pattern in St Lucia where infections occur in streams when snail colonies can become established (Fig. 5.3). A marked reduction in the number of snails was noted in the middle of 1979 after unseasonal rains in March and June, and they only returned to some sites – thus the effect on snail infection rates of the treatment given in Fond Assau and Talvern at the end of 1979 could not be determined.

Owing to the potential risk of transmission recurring in these sites and the imminent closure of the Department, routine focal mollusciciding in selected sites was introduced in March 1980. As the heavy rains in the middle of 1979 had flushed most sites clear of snails there were only a few

Fig.5.2. Marquis valley: (*a*) monthly rainfall, and numbers of *B. glabrata* from index sites in (*b*) flowing and (*c*) static water habitats. Shaded areas represent the approximate 'wet season' – July to December. Note declining number of snails. (From Barnish, 1982.)

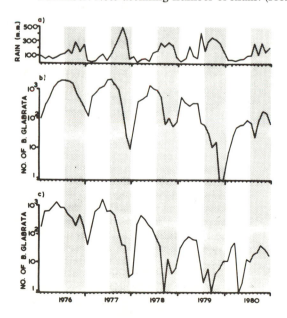

sites to be controlled. This appeared to have been successful as only Ravine Talvern was found re-infected on one occasion after mollusciciding started and the Department closed at the end of 1981.

The Isnare marsh complex was treated with niclosamide granules

Fig.5.3. Marquis valley: monthly rainfall and numbers of infected and uninfected *B. glabrata* from 'additional' index sites in three Fond Assau streams and the Isnare river and marsh. (From Barnish, 1982.)

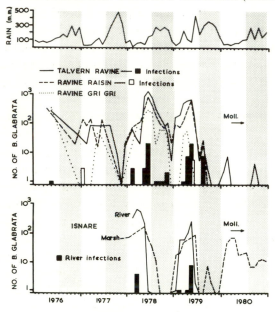

Fig. 5.4. Marquis valley: summary of sentinel and field snail findings and prevalence of *S. mansoni* in Fond Assau and Talvern.

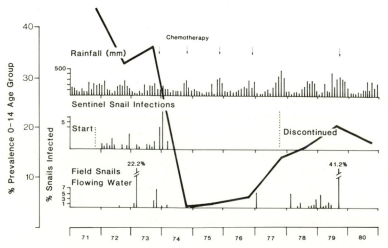

(Prentice & Barnish, 1980). Although snails were not eliminated, a ten-fold decrease in numbers was achieved under difficult conditions.

No infected snails were found in the last 12 months of the programme.

The total cost of the ten-month mollusciciding (March–December 1980) was $641, 76% being for molluscicide.

In the course of routine surveys *Thiara granifera* were found in Ravine Gri Gri in November 1979 and in May the following year large numbers were collected in the Isnare River from 200 m upstream of the Gri Gri/Isnare junction. This appears to have been a natural introduction of the snail into the watershed but may be important in future control of *B. glabrata* (see Chapter 12). Fig. 5.4. summarises the sentinel and field snail data in relation to prevalence of *S. mansoni* in Fond Assau and Talvern.

Summary and recommendations

The Marquis valley project was to evaluate the effect on transmission of four selective population chemotherapy campaigns.

Pre-control studies were made between 1971 and 1973 after which the first of two hycanthone treatments was given. These resulted in a rapid fall in transmission, prevalence and intensity of infection in the human population and in infection rates in sentinel and field-collected *B. glabrata*. After a third treatment (the first of two with oxamniquine) there was evidence of a resurgence of transmission in two high transmission areas and three years after the final treatment incidence of new infections was only a little lower than pre-intervention levels; infected *B. glabrata* were found in field collections. Treatment was offered to the population in these two settlements in 1979 and again in 1980 when all areas were re-surveyed and re-treated. At this survey there was evidence of a low level of transmission in a further four settlements and focal mollusciciding was started at potential transmission sites although *Thiara (Tenebia)* was found in the watershed.

The results of the project show that with chemotherapy all indices of infection in the human population are rapidly reduced, but it is more difficult to reduce further a low prevalence and, in the absence of a consolidation phase strategy of control, transmission recurs and further treatment is necessary. The timing of this probably depends, among other factors, on local epidemiological conditions, and may be after three to four years. At the doses used hycanthone was the more effective drug.

It was recommended that focal mollusciciding be continued, that water supplies be improved and more laundry and shower units be constructed, particularly in high transmission areas.

6

Control of the intermediate snail host

Since the early days of schistosomiasis control, the snail intermediate host has been considered the 'weak link' in the life cycle of the parasite and various chemicals have been used in efforts to break the cycle. None of the molluscicides used is specific for freshwater snails and all forms of aquatic biota suffer as a result.

The Japanese were the first to attempt snail control using calcium cyanamide, calcium oxide, and chlorinated lime. In 1920 copper sulphate was shown to be lethal to the intermediate snail hosts in Egypt, and the chemical was used in many countries including Zimbabwe (then Rhodesia), Egypt, Venezuela, Japan and Sudan. As a result of extensive investigations into the mollusciciding effect of numerous chemicals (McMullen, 1952) sodium pentachlorophenate was field tested in many endemic areas; however since 1959 niclosamide has been the chemical of choice though triphenmorph had limited use in the late 1960s and early 1970s.

Snail control through weed control was advocated by Barlow (1937). This was an important aspect of the Lake Volta control project in Ghana and is currently applied in the Sudan. The grass-eating carp, *Ctenopharyngodon idella*, has been suggested for trial (Kilgen & Smitherman, 1971).

Owing to the increasing costs of molluscicide and the concern of conservationists, other biological methods of snail control have been investigated. Amongst these are the use of snail-eating fish *Tilapia melanopluera*, *Serranochromis* spp., *Astatoreochromis alluadi*, *Clarisa* spp., *Gambusia* spp., and *Lepomis microlophus* (Ferguson & Ruiz-Tibén, 1971; McMahon, Highton & Marshall, 1977), but there are no reports of transmission having been reduced by their use.

Aquatic larvae of sciomyzid flies have been shown to feed on medically important molluscs (Berg, 1964) and shrimps in St Lucia were found to attack *B. glabrata* in natural stream situations and in the laboratory (Barnish & Prentice, 1982).

Various pathological agents have been investigated (reviewed by Jordan, Christie & Unrau, 1980*a*), but none was found suitable for extensive use; the efficacy of echinostome antagonism toward schistosome sporocysts has been studied in the laboratory and field but no control schemes have been developed (Lie, Kwo & Owyang, 1970, 1971; Lim and Heyneman, 1972). *Ribeiroia marini guadeloupensis* has, however, been used successfully in Guadeloupe (Pointier *et al.*, 1981).

The ampullarid snail *Marisa cornuarietis* has been an integral part of the schistosomiasis control in Puerto Rico (Jobin, Brown, Vélez & Ferguson, 1977); there, and in St Lucia (Prentice, 1983a), *Thiara (Tarebia) granifera* has been noted to reduce *B. glabrata* populations. In St Lucia *Helisoma duryi* was also shown to limited snail populations (Christie *et al.*, 1981). In laboratory tests in Brazil, *Pomacea australis* was shown to destroy *B. glabrata* (Paulinyi & Paulini, 1972), but in field trials in St Lucia *P. glauca* failed to reduce numbers of *B. glabrata* (M. A. Prentice, unpublished). Thus, although extensive studies have been made into biological methods of snail control, none (with the possible exception of *Marisa* and *Thiara (Tarebia)*) has been developed to the stage of its being of proven use in the field.

Engineering methods of snail control may be suitable in a few circumstances – elimination of ponds or marshes being the most effective. Drainage of swamps can lead to collector drains which are more amenable to treatment with molluscicide than the source of water. Swamps can sometimes be dried by the planting of trees; water from springs that cause small seepage areas inhabited by snails can be 'protected' and the seepage area controlled, and changes to increase the flow of streams and rivers may facilitate flushing out of snails. Such changes may be simple to accomplish, i.e. removal of vegetation, fallen trees etc., or more complicated canalation, deepening of marginal areas and elimination of contiguous pools. However, while in general velocity may be high, micro-habitats with lower velocities may remain where snails are found.

In limited areas control of snail populations can be achieved by methods other than molluscicides but their use was virtually synonymous with schistosomiasis control. Snail control was considered to offer the most effective and rapid means of reducing transmission (Farooq *et al.*, 1966*a*), although this opinion was based as much on theoretical considerations and the failure of other methods as on demonstrated success.

It was thought, therefore, that if snail control were to be effective in St Lucia it would have to be thorough and intensive. It was thought by some that in an island situation eradication of the snail might be possible and an attempt at area-wide snail control (i.e. attacking them wherever they were found) was planned and executed in Cul de Sac valley. Elsewhere, at Fond St Jacques, a modified snail control project, focal snail control, was initiated where molluscicide was applied only in those situations where human water-contact was thought to be associated with transmission of schistosomiasis.

After the area-wide snail control had been evaluated, chemotherapy was introduced and a snail control programme, suitable for the Government to operate, was developed and tested as a consolidation phase strategy.

PART 1: CUL DE SAC VALLEY

The work in this valley can be divided into three phases:

    (i) Area-wide snail control – pre-control studies (1967–1970), control and evaluation (1970–75)

   (ii) Focal surveillance/mollusciciding control plus chemotherapy (1975–77)

  (iii) Consolidation – routine focal mollusciciding and evaluation (1977–81).

(i)   Area-wide snail control
The study area

Cul de Sac is one of the large alluvial valleys in St Lucia, surrounded by hills rising to 275 m (Fig. 6.1) It is dog-legged in shape, the main river rising near the centre of the island on the central mountain ridge, the Barre de L'Isle, down which it flows in a north-westerly direction to the valley proper. Downstream it turns towards the west coast, entering the Caribbean sea in Cul de Sac Bay. A number of streams, locally known as ravines, flow down the valley walls to the valley floor, across which they flow to join the main river. Where the hillsides join the valley floor marshy areas are common.

Cul de Sac was originally one of the principal sugar growing areas of St Lucia. Most of the valley floor is now taken over for the commercial production of bananas, with small holders growing the fruit on the hillsides and towards the head of the valley. The valley floor is traversed by an extensive root-drainage system, a remnant of the sugar days, and calculated to total more than 1000 km in length.

Rainfall is greater at the top of the valley than near the sea (Fig. 1.2). As indicated in Chapter 1, although the early months of the year are generally comparatively dry, heavy rains can occur. Similarly, low rainfall has been recorded in the so-called wetter months of the year (Fig. 1.3).

At the first survey in 1967, 17 settlements of varying size were recorded. They were situated on the floor of the valley and on the surrounding hillsides, but in two, situated on the northern rim, very low rates of prevalence were found (Forestiere 3.2%; Victoria Road 0.9%), and these were dropped from further study. The population of the valley was approximately 5000.

Ribbon development has taken place along the main road which runs

Fig. 6.1. Cul de Sac valley: map of the study area.

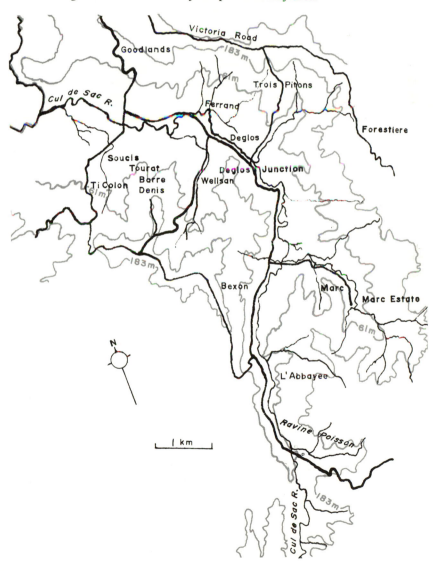

roughly parallel to the river. In other settlements on the hillsides houses are generally more widely dispersed. Housing is typical of the island, the majority being small wooden buildings with some newer brick constructions.

Apart from two communal laundry units, both in a state of disrepair during much of the period of control, springs, ravines and the river were the only sources of water in most areas, until the early 1970s when a few standpipes were erected. In 1978 a household survey was made of water (Table 6.1) and sanitary facilities (Table 6.2). As water was distributed by gravity, supplies were better in settlements on the valley floor than in those on hillsides.

Even when piped water was available the supply was inadequate and infrequent and households needed an alternative source. Thus, while the river was infrequently the main source of water, it was inevitably the secondary source in 89% of hillside houses and 62% of those on the valley floor. By 1981 there were 26 standpipes (6 were broken); 26 laundry tubs had been provided but 12 were non-functional, as were 6 of 14 showers and 4 of the 6 public toilets. Regrettably distribution of standpipes and

Table 6.1. *Cul de Sac valley: showing main source of water in Cul de Sac in 1978*

	Houses surveyed	Water to house (%)	Standpipe (%)	Cistern[a] (%)	River (%)
Hillside houses	405	2.7	45.2	51.6	0.3
Valley floor houses	463	6.7	73.2	18.1	1.9

[a] Cistern – water collected from roof into small storage tank – invariably an old oil drum.

Table 6.2. *Cul de Sac valley: type of latrine in hillside and valley floor houses*

	Houses surveyed	Septic tank (%)	Pit latrine (%)	Open pit (%)	Nil (%)
Hillside houses	405	2	89	9	—
Valley floor houses	463	4	80	15	1

laundry and shower units were rarely in those places at high risk of schistosomiasis.

During the period covered by the programme (1967–81), development in the valley was inevitable and changes were particularly marked near the mouth of the river and in Cul de Sac Bay. On the south side a supertanker wharf was built as part of an oil storage facility and on the eastern side a wharf for a nearby rum distillery was planned.

These changes resulted in considerable population movement with the original community of Soucis settling elsewhere in the valley. The population of another small community, Ferrands, also dispersed when the estate on which they worked ceased dairy farming.

Biological studies

Qualitative snail surveys

Between August 1966 and July 1967 qualitative surveys were carried out in Cul de Sac and other valleys; snails found were sent for identification and results are given in Appendix 3. In view of the presence of *B. straminea* in neighbouring Martinique it is noteworthy that none was found in St Lucia.

From these surveys it was possible to identify the characteristics of potential habitats for *B. glabrata*.

'*Static*' *habitats*: with little or no water flow, mainly natural but sometimes subject to human interference. They included the following:

(a) small pools, rarely more than 10 m² in area and 0.6 m in depth, found either in the hills at the head of water courses or at the edge of the valley floor.

(b) Larger, deeper pools on the valley floor near the river mouth – probably ox-bows.

(c) Marshy, swampy areas either at the head of water courses where they rarely exceeded an acre in extent or at the base of valley walls where they were larger. Some of these were covered in thick, matted aquatic vegetation which defied penetration. Neither contained significant areas of open water surface.

(d) Banana drains – these were mainly on the valley floor and were intended to take surface water from the roots of the trees. Lateral drains, approximately 0.6 m wide and 0.6 m deep were spaced 6 m apart in the banana fields, with two rows of trees between adjacent drains. They carried excess water into collector drains which were man-made and approximately 1.3 m wide by 1.3 m deep, or canalised natural courses. These led to larger drainage courses or into the river (Fig. 2.3). Drains were cleared of silt and vegetation two or three times a year. *Lymnaea*, the intermediate host of *Fasciola hepatica*, was common in banana drains.

'*Flowing*' *habitats*: these were natural water courses generally with a substantial, but highly variable, flow of water. They could be subdivided into the following:

(a) The 'torrent stage' down the valley walls, as ravines, which sometimes dried out.

(b) Slower streams, usually permanent, flowing across the valley floor: some collector drains were included in this category.

(c) The permanent, main river.

The qualitative findings from Cul de Sac suggested that stable colonies of *B. glabrata* occurred primarily in pools high up on the sides of the valley, with less stable colonies occurring in the marshy areas there, and at the base of the valley walls. There was little flow in these sites which were not subject to much scouring, but the marsh sites were likely to dry up. Colonies were found in the slow flowing streams and, rarely, in protected pools in the ravines, probably seeded from the high level pool and marsh sites, and were relatively unstable. Snail colonies were not found in the main river, although they had been observed there in the past. Scouring during rains, particularly in the main river and in the ravines, and the drying up of the ravines in the drought, tended to reduce or minimise snail populations.

Fig.6.2. Cul de Sac valley: isometric projection showing topography, hydrology and general location of *B. glabrata* habitats. (From Sturrock, 1973a.)

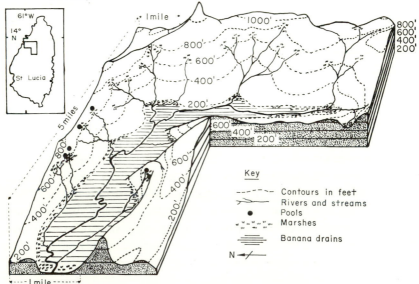

Apart from these natural sites, colonies were also found in many banana drains on the valley floor, which reproduced small pool, marsh or slow flowing stream sites. Infected snails were recovered from some sites in all the habitat types except the high level pools where human contact was minimal. An isometric projection of the valley is shown in Fig. 6.2.

In the course of the qualitative survey some areas free of *B. glabrata* were found. Reasons for this are obscure, but a further qualitative survey of the valley in 1969 confirmed these areas to be snail free. Although during this second qualitative survey some additional colonies of *B. glabrata* were found, they were all in areas previously known to have been infested.

Quantitative snail surveys

Based on findings from the qualitative surveys, a number of index sites, 4 pools and 5 marshes ('static sites'), 13 banana drains and 5 river/stream ('flowing sites'), were selected for quantitive study to enable the *S. mansoni* transmission pattern to be determined and to identify the most important habitats.

Quantitative studies and sentinel mouse exposures, using the techniques described in Chapter 3, were carried out from February 1967 until July 1969.

During the last 12 months of the investigation supplementary qualitative collections of snails were made around the routine sampling sites to check on the pattern of transmission suggested by the first 18 months of observation.

Results of these studies showed the pattern of *S. mansoni* transmission and how it was influenced by rainfall. Snail densities, and cercarial infection rates in *B. glabrata* in the different types of habitat, are shown in Fig. 6.3. As the data from ponds and marshes were similar, findings from these habitats were combined.

Snail populations in the streams built up rapidly when rainfall and water velocity were low; at this time infected snails and sentinel mice were frequently found. The snail populations were, however, drastically reduced when scouring by heavy rains occurred, notably in September 1967, when the island was severely affected by Hurricane Beulah. Snail populations recovered slowly thereafter, possibly restrained until the general ecology of the various habitats, especially the vegetation, recovered from the traumatic effects of the hurricane. The original levels were only just being approached when the mollusciciding programme began in 1970 and at the time of a supplementary study in November 1970 large snail populations with up to 6% infected were found. These studies also showed that in prolonged dry periods streams may dry entirely, with cessation of transmission.

Snail populations in the banana drains did not show such a clear pattern, but it seemed that some collector drains might act as streams and harbour increased snail populations in the early part of the dry season. Lateral drains followed the pattern of ponds and marshes with reduced populations

Fig.6.3. Cul de Sac valley: transmission data from 1967–69 showing the number of snails collected from the routine sampling sites (where less than 10 snails were collected the number is given in brackets), and their infection rates (solid histogram); the infection rates in additional samples from around the routine sites (the number of snails examined is given above the stippled histogram); the presence (solid circle) or absence (clear circle) of cercariae in certain sites as indicated by mouse exposure; and the rainfall pattern (the number of days per fortnight when more than 1 in of rain fell). (From Sturrock, 1973a.)

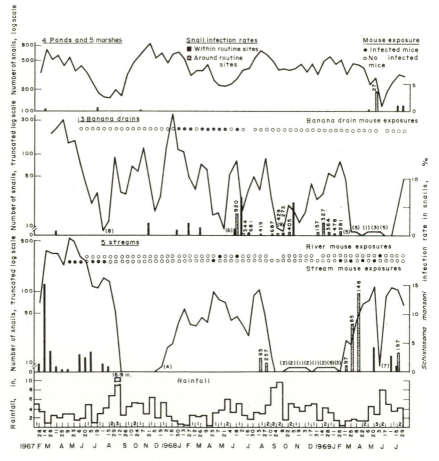

when rainfall dropped below 60–80 mm a fortnight and sites began to dry. With increased rainfall the populations rapidly recovered except during excessive rainfall.

Infected snails were rarely found in these sites, an indication of the limited contact the human population had with them, but sporadic infections were found, indicative of human activity in the banana fields. It was believed, however, that the stream sites formed the main transmission foci of *S. mansoni*, since more persistently infected snail colonies were found in them and they were also centres of human contact for washing clothes, bathing, playing and other activities.

Similar patterns of changing snail densities in different habitats in relation to rainfall were found in parallel quantitative studies at selected index sites in Castries, Richefond and Roseau valleys.

Non-human cercariae found in snails

During the course of the qualitative and quantitative surveys in Cul de Sac, cercariae other than of *S. mansoni* were found to be shed by *B. glabrata*.

One, shed at night, was identified as *Ribeiroia marini*. The infected snails were from banana drains where, in different collections, 27 of 478 (5.6%) and 31 of 745 (4.2%) *B. glabrata* were infected. Guppies, *Poecilia* (*Lebistes*) sp., from banana drains were found infected with metacercariae and *R. marini* were found in immature Little Blue Heron, *Florida caerulea*, which had fed on fish from the banana drains. Six Green Herons, *Butorides virescens*, a bird known to be infected in Puerto Rico, were uninfected (Basch & Sturrock, 1969).

Two other species of cercariae were seen rarely. They were furcocercous; one with eye spots (probably cercariae of striegids found in herons), and the other with long fin-like furci, and readily differentiated from *S. mansoni*.

S. mansoni *and other helminths in wild and domestic animals*

S. mansoni has been found in a number of animals in different endemic areas (reviewed by Jordan & Webbe, 1982). In Africa and the New World primates were found infected, various rats in Africa, South America and Guadeloupe harboured the parasite, as did cattle in Brazil. A limited survey of potential animal reservoirs in St Lucia was therefore made by Dr Harry Huizinga. Most of the animals were obtained in Cul de Sac Valley.

Five mammals are known on the island, the mongoose (*Herpestes auropunctatus*), the brown rat (*Rattus rattus*), the opossum or manicou (*Didelphys marsupialis insularis*), the house mouse (*Mus musculis*) and *Agouti*. Specimens were trapped and examined for helminths. None was found infected with *S. mansoni*, but in the laboratory 3 of 9 opossums, 7 of 10 brown rats and 2 cats exposed to *S. mansoni* cercariae became infected. Other helminths were frequently found (Appendix 4). None of the parasites found would complicate biological studies in the field but it is amongst birds that such parasites would more likely be found.

The finding of *R. marini* in the Little Blue Heron is referred to above; other parasites of interest from the herons were the striegids, the cercariae of which could cause confusion in cercariometric techniques unless the eye spot could be identified. *Clinostomum* spp. from the Little Blue Heron could cause the same problem. As no bird schistosomes were detected it is unlikely that immuno-diagnostic tests would be affected by cross-reactions with *S. mansoni* antigens.

Faecal samples of 71 domestic animals (cattle, pig, horse) slaughtered at the Castries abattoir were examined; no *S. mansoni* ova were found, but 31 of 61 cows were infected with *F. hepatica*. *Dicrocoelium* sp. eggs were found in one faecal sample, but as some cows are imported this record does not imply the parasite is endemic on the island.

The high prevalence of *F. hepatica* in cattle on the island results in the condemnation of a considerable amount of liver each year, which, in view of the short supply of locally produced protein, the island can ill afford.

Later in the programme of the Research and Control Department, *Lymnaea cubensis* from many parts of the island were examined for *F. hepatica*. Infections were found in most low level areas with 25% of nearly 200 snails being infected at Jacmel in the Roseau valley and 14% around the mouth of the Cul de Sac river (Barnish, Prentice & Harris, 1980).

Although *Lymnaea* sp. is susceptible to mollusciciding and might therefore be controlled in a programme directed against *B. glabrata* in general they were not found in the main *S. mansoni* transmission foci so the effect of the mollusciciding is likely to have been minimal.

Control of *B. glabrata*
Strategy

As a result of the pre-control investigations the *S. mansoni* transmission pattern became clear: it is shown schematically in Fig. 6.4.

Based on this the following points were considered in the design of the mollusciciding programme:

(a) The most intense period of transmission coincided with the dry season and involved snail colonies in flowing water habitats. Some sporadic transmission occurred among snail populations in static water habitats, generally in the wetter months of the year.

Fig.6.4. Long term snail population changes and *S. mansoni* transmission patterns in relation to weather conditions for *B. glabrata* colonies in static and flowing water bodies. (From Sturrock, 1973*b*.)

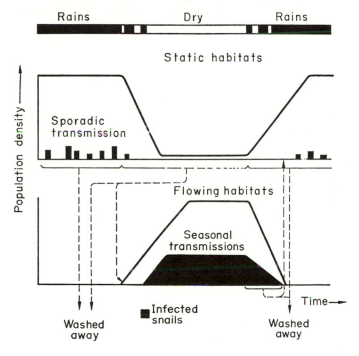

Fig.6.5. Ideal strategy for controlling *S. mansoni* transmission with a single molluscicide application killing 100 per cent of the snails. (From Sturrock, 1973*b*.)

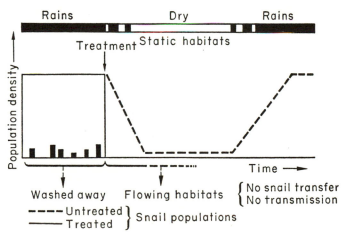

(b) Snail populations in marshes, ponds and banana drains (i.e. static habitat) appeared to be necessary to seed the flowing stream habitats.

(c) The colonies in flowing waters built up during the dry season but were subsequently dislodged by the next heavy rains.

(d) Re-invasion of low level sites cleared by molluscicides was likely if high level sites were not treated.

An ideal strategy was designed (Fig. 6.5) so that maximum snail kills coincided with adverse ecological factors. Survivors of the chemical treatment then faced an immediate further hazard, thus minimising the risk of re-population.

In practice, most adverse factors, being climatic, were predictable in only the most general terms. Further, such factors could themselves interfere with the efficacy of the molluscicide; heavy rain not only dislodged snails but both diluted and washed away the chemical. Droughts kill snails by desiccation but aestivating snails would not be exposed to a water-borne chemical. Finally, it was logistically impossible in a large area to apply the chemical in a sufficiently short time to get the maximum benefit from many ecological factors. A practical strategy was therefore devised to utilise adverse ecological conditions where possible (Fig. 6.6).

Pre-control molluscicide trials

Choice of molluscicide. Two molluscicides were available: niclosamide (niclosamide-2'5-dichloro-4'-nitro salicylanilide) produced by Bayer

Fig.6.6. Practical strategy for controlling *S. mansoni* transmission with molluscicide. (It is assumed that the molluscicide will give a 90 per cent kill.) (From Sturrock, 1973*b*.)

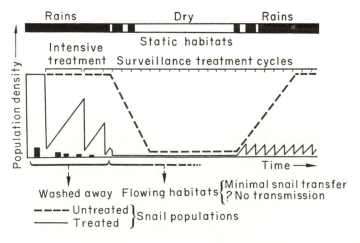

AG under the registered names Bayluscide® and Clonitralide®; and tri-phenmorph, (*N*-tritylmorpholine) marketed by Shell as Frescon®. The former chemical kills eggs as well as snails, the latter only snails.

Trials were made to compare the susceptibility of St Lucian *B. glabrata* to the two chemicals. Two formulations of each were investigated in the laboratory:

> Niclosamide as Bayer 6076, the emulsifiable concentrate, containing 25% weight to volume of active ingredient, and Bayer 73, a wettable powder containing 70% W/W active ingredient.
>
> Trityl morpholine as FX 28, an emulsifiable concentrate containing 16.5% W/V active ingredient and FX 1300 as a water dispersable liquid containing 50% W/V active ingredient.

As the chemical composition of water, and particularly its pH, can affect the activity of trifenmorph, which is hydrolysed to inactive triphenylcarbinol in an acidic environment, water for the trials was made up with 0.26 g magnesium sulphate with 0.10 g calcium chloride in 1 000 ml distilled water; unbuffered this had a pH of 5.9–6.1 which remained unchanged for 24 hours in the presence of snails. Phosphate buffers were used to obtain other pH values. Standard calibration curves were prepared using a Bausch and Lomb Spectronic 20 colorimeter and regression lines were fitted to the data from four runs with each of the four formulations being investigated. Tests followed the standard WHO procedures using groups of 40–50 snails exposed for 24 h to the solutions and allowed to recover

Table 6.3. *Bench trials of susceptibility of* B. glabrata *to candidate molluscicides*

Chemical	Slope (SE)	LC_{50} with 95% confidence limits (p.p.m.)	LC_{90} (p.p.m.)
pH 5.9–6.1 Tritylmorpholine			
FX 28	41.76 (5.63)	0.363 (0.357–0.365)	0.389
FX 1300	9.61 (1.59)	0.227 (0.209–0.245)	0.300
Niclosamide			
Bayer 73	2.81 (2.81)	0.19 (0.018–0.019)	0.053
Bayer 6076	6.97 (0.94)	0.19 (0.018–0.019)	0.029
pH 6.9–7.1 Tritylmorpholine			
FX 28	5.85 (1.00)	0.042 (0.041–0.043)	0.070
FX 1300	6.64 (0.99)	0.035 (0.032–0.039)	0.054
Niclosamide			
Bayer 73	7.88 (1.14)	0.032 (0.031–0.033)	0.046
Bayer 6076	14.62 (4.00)	0.045 (0.043–0.049)	0.055

for 48 h. Snails were collected in the field and held for two days in laboratory ponds before use. Results are shown in Table 6.3.

The adverse effect of an acid pH was not excessive with either chemical but it was more marked with tritylmorpholine.

Degradation of molluscicides. The persistence of niclosamide and triphenmorph was investigated in four laboratory ponds and in flowing water.

The ponds were filled with 200 l of freshly collected spring water; Bayer 6076 and FX 28 were then each added to two ponds to give concentrations of 0.25–0.50 p.p.m. One pond of each molluscicide was left exposed to sunlight, the other being kept in shade. Water samples for analysis were taken at intervals commencing at 8.30 a.m.

The standard laboratory technique for triphenmorph analysis does not differentiate it from its hydrolysis product, triphenylcarbinol, which is molluscicidally inert. The technique of Meyling & Meyling (1969) was therefore used to remove the triphenylcarbinol on an alumina sorption column. By a process of differential analysis the concentration of the two compounds was determined. Niclosamide determinations were made by the method described by Strufe (1963). Results are shown in Table 6.4.

Triphenmorph was virtually inactivated within 2 and 7 hours in the sun and shaded ponds respectively. The loss of niclosamide exposed to the sun was due to ultra-violet irradiation and was not excessive.

Toxicity of niclosamide and triphenmorph to bananas. With the economy of the island being dependent on bananas, it was essential that any chemical used in the plantations be harmless to the plant, and that it did not concentrate

Table 6.4. *Degradation of molluscicides in sunlight and shade at pH 6.9–7.1*

		Hours after application					
Condition	Chemical	0	1	2	3.5	7	24
Shade	FX 28 – morpholine	0.26	0.24	0.23	0.22	0.04	0.03
	– carbinol	0.00	0.04	0.02	0.01	0.15	0.13
	Total as morpholine	0.26	0.28	0.26	0.24	0.23	0.18
Sun	FX 28 – morpholine	0.25	0.19	0.03	0.04	0.04	0.01
	– carbinol	0.02	0.03	0.19	0.16	0.14	0.11
	Total as morpholine	0.27	0.23	0.27	0.23	0.23	0.15
Shade	Bayer 6076	0.48	0.47	0.45	0.48	0.53	0.46
Sun	Bayer 6076	0.39	0.38	0.37	0.39	0.47	0.33

in the fruit which could not only affect its quality but could lead to rejection by the importing country.

Tests were made at the Windward Island Banana Research Centre (WINBAN) in Roseau Valley with the assistance of the Director, Mr Ian Twyford, and Mr J. Seeyave, agronomist. Although molluscicide would normally be applied only to the banana drains, in this test it was watered directly onto the bed around the base of the plants; the test was therefore more stringent than would be expected during a control programme, except for occasional accidental spillage (Sturrock, Barnish & Seeyave, 1974a).

It was assumed that each plant stood in 5 m² of soil on which there would be 75 mm of water. Molluscicide was added to give concentrations of 0.125 and 1.25 p.p.m of active ingredient – 6 and 60 times the dose plants could receive if only adjacent drains were sprayed. The chemicals were applied to six plants at each of two dose levels; an additional six plants were untreated controls. No immediate (1–3 days) or long term (3 months) phytotoxic effects were noted. Samples of fruit were sent to Shell Research Ltd at Woodstock, England for analysis for triphenmorph and to the Tropical Products Institute, London for niclosamide analysis. As no residues of either chemical were detectable it was assumed they were safe to use in banana fields in St Lucia.

As a result of these tests, niclosamide was chosen as the chemical of choice in St Lucia principally because a survey of different natural waters in Cul de Sac valley showed acid waters to be common (Table 6.5).

Owing to possible problems with clogging of sprays with the wettable powder formulation, the emulsifiable concentrate was selected for use.

Carriage of molluscicide. Trials were made in flowing water habitats to which niclosamide was applied for 1 h to give a concentration of 1 p.p.m. In a

Table 6.5. *Results of a pH survey of 129 water samples*

Habitat	Altitude	Number examined	Mean pH	Range of values
River	Low	5	8.10	7.1–8.6
Stream	Low	13	7.70	6.5–8.9
Pond	Low	6	7.14	6.5–8.1
	High	17	6.90	6.3–7.5
Marsh	Low	11	6.68	5.6–8.1
	High	5	7.00	6.4–8.2
Banana drains				
Collector	Low	34	7.20	6.5–8.1
Subsidiary	Low	32	7.20	6.2–8.1

large, clear stream, with a flow of 150 l/s, the molluscicide was detectable by chemical analysis and bio-assay 1.6 km below the dosing point within 4.5 h; in a small stream with dense vegetation and a flow of 3 l/s no chemical was detected beyond 0.16 km (Sturrock, Barnish & Upatham, 1976).

Re-population studies. The duration of effect of mollusciciding was studied in three habitats (a pond, a marsh and a stream) outside the control area. Pre-mollusciciding data on snail densities were obtained and at fortnightly intervals thereafter. Results are shown in Fig. 6.7. The stream was treated early in the dry season, the pond and marsh in the wet season.

Snails were found 12 weeks after treatment in the stream and marsh sites and after 18 weeks in the pond. Populations appeared to be stabilised 32 weeks after mollusciciding but at levels lower than before treatment (Sturrock *et al*, 1974b).

Application of molluscicide
Equipment. With the need to treat many different types of snail habitat, different types of equipment were necessary.

For flowing water sites drip-feed dispensers (Crossland, 1967) were made out of 20-litre polythene bottles using perspex and rubber for the other

Fig.6.7. Re-population by *B. glabrata* after treatment with niclosamide in three habitats. (From Sturrock *et al.*, 1974b.)

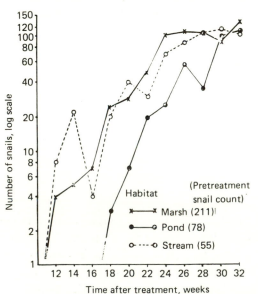

components. They were light to carry and easy to repair. Each one incorporated a constant-head device so that, with minor adjustments, it would empty at a steady rate over one hour. Two dispensers were used alternatively to give continuous treatment for six hours. The molluscicide was diluted at the application point with strained field water.

For marshes, ponds and banana drains standard Hudson X-Pert sprayers were used. Charged with 11.4 litres of solution, the sprayers were pumped by hand to 55 psi (pounds per square inch). The pressure dropped when the chemical was discharged but, between 25 and 55 psi, the application rate was uniform and controlled. They were carried fairly easily, although the weight when full was about 25–30 kg.

Fine 65° fan-jet nozzles were used for low volume spraying when the charge would last approximately one hour. For use with these fine nozzles, water was taken from the laboratory to the field – field water led to clogging even when filtered. Later designs of the sprayers included a filter as an integral part of the apparatus, so that field water could be used. Larger 80° nozzles were used for bigger drains. For impenetrable marshes a commercially produced S60 Kindelder Knapsac sprayer was used. A petrol two-stroke engine worked a fan to give a jet of air through a 76.2 mm diameter spray lance. The chemical solution was drawn from a 13.5 l reservoir into the lance, fine spray penetrated 4–6 m through vegetation. The sprayer was fitted with shoulder straps for carrying in the field. Normally the wettable powder was used with strained field water.

In some situations the emulsifiable concentrate was soaked onto commercial mouse food pellets which were then broadcast by hand to areas beyond the range of power sprayers.

Organisation and training. The organisation of teams was as follows:

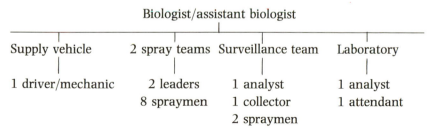

	Biologist/assistant biologist		
Supply vehicle	2 spray teams	Surveillance team	Laboratory
1 driver/mechanic	2 leaders	1 analyst	1 analyst
	8 spraymen	1 collector	1 attendant
		2 spraymen	

In August 1970 a full training programme was organised to familiarise everyone with apparatus and their role within the programme. Preliminary team training for treating banana drains and marshes was given in simulated drains and marshes on flat ground adjoining the laboratory. The open condition allowed mistakes to be seen and rectified easily. When proficient, the teams were moved to natural, snail-free habitats in the valley to experience field conditions. Training in the use of dispensers was given at a nearby stream. Finally, a series of dress rehearsals was held in the valley to eliminate any organisational problems before the programme started. Particular attention was paid to developing versatility in switching from one type of habitat to another. Potassium permanganate was used instead of molluscicide during training.

The supply vehicle transported most of the equipment, the chemical and 1363 l of clean water for the pressure sprayers from the laboratory to the field. The driver prepared the chemical for the sprayers and carried out repairs to any equipment.

The leaders of the spray teams were responsible for getting their spraymen to the field with all their equipment, food, supplies and protective clothing; for controlling the teams in the field and for making the appropriate records of their progress. In addition, the leaders were able to use the power sprayer and drip-feed dispensers. The spraymen were trained to use both the handsprayers and the dispensers.

The analyst controlled the surveillance team, carried out a field analysis of niclosamide concentration in water samples, and returned the rest of the sample for a more sophisticated laboratory analysis.

The collector in the surveillance team collected water samples from areas treated by each of the spraymen and at the same site placed bioassay snails for retrieving the following day. The surveillance spraymen treated any main drains and searched previously treated areas for living snails, re-treating any area where they were discovered.

The attendant maintained the snails required for bioassay before and after exposure in the field, and cleaned the field equipment at the end of each day.

Procedures for treating different habitats. Ponds: Four spraymen discharged the molluscicide from a hand sprayer into the pond. Usually the ponds were overdosed to give a yellow coloration even after stirring.

Rivers and streams: The calculated amount of chemical was applied with two constant-head dispensers over a six-hour period. One man carried the dispensers, chemical and accessories to the application sites and tended them during the application. Periodic checks were necessary to ensure steady flow rates.

Banana drains: Hand sprayers were used. The four spraymen were lined up in numerical order at the head of four consecutive drains. When the spraymen were ready to start, the team leader set the pace and moved up the drain at about 1 m per 4 seconds. He checked that spraying was carried out correctly with the spray fan across the drain, and cleared obstructions ahead of the team, if necessary stopping the whole team to clear major obstructions. The number of strokes required by each sprayman to pump his sprayer to 55 psi was recorded and teams were lined up in the same order on the next set of drains. The procedure was then repeated. The two teams worked together or separately as conditions demanded. Main drains and cross drains were sprayed by the surveillance team spraymen working independently.

It was estimated that the three teams should be able to spray about 40 km of banana drains a day, i.e. about 30 acres. The work of each sprayman was checked by chemical and bio-assay in treated drains besides the pumpstroke records and periodical checks by his team leader and the biologist or assistant biologist.

Marshes: Where possible these were treated in the same way as the banana drains except that the spraymen lined up shoulder to shoulder at one side of the marsh, and crossed then re-crossed it spraying successive swathes. Numbered posts were set up opposite each man to help him to keep on course. It was later found that this was only partly successful and involved considerable delays as the team turned round each time. Human markers were later found to be more effective.

For impenetrable marshes the team leader, assisted by one sprayman, operated the power sprayer for 15 seconds from successive points four paces apart around the margin of the marsh. This covered a series of overlapping quadrants to a distance of 4–6 m into the marsh. Simultaneously, two spraymen sprayed the margin with handsprayers by circling the marsh in opposite directions at the normal pace, passing each other *en route*. The last sprayman set his handsprayers to empty into the inlet to the marsh, and then broadcast mouse pellets soaked in molluscicide into the centre, beyond the range of the power sprayer.

Implementation of the scheme. All areas of Cul de Sac valley where *B. glabrata* had been found pre-control were given an intensive blanket treatment with molluscicide during a 6-week period in September and October 1970. Particular care was taken to locate and treat snail colonies high on the hillsides. Incomplete kills and therefore re-population were anticipated in the static water habitats where, post-treatment, conditions for the snail would be favourable.

Mollusciciding started at the head of the valley with treatment of infested areas down to and including Deglos. Subsequently high level sites on the north and south walls were treated, followed by treatment of all banana drain and marsh sites on the valley floor from Ferrands to the sea. Flowing streams in that area were then located and treated from sites above the valley floor and finally the main Cul de Sac river was treated at sites at Ravine Poisson and Deglos.

During this intensive treatment campaign biological and chemical assays were made at sites to assess the molluscicide concentration in different habitats. In bio-assays, 10 laboratory-bred snails were placed in fibre-glass gauze cages and exposed in water after the treatment teams had passed. Ten cages were lost in a flash flood. Mortality of snails was complete in 228 of the remaining 233 cages; the 5 in which some snails survived came from sites flushed with heavy rain immediately after treatment. Results of laboratory chemical analyses were generally lower than those obtained in the field – 80.3% of the former and 20.6% of the latter showing concentrations over one mg/l.

Owing to the probable inaccuracies of the chemical analyses (possibly as a result of turbidity of water), their high cost, and the satisfactory results of the bio-assays, such assays were discontinued.

After the intensive treatment, and following the November rains, all areas were re-examined and re-treated where necessary.

Once the dry season started in early 1971, the re-treatment cycles were rationalised into a systematic programme of surveillance and treatment. The valley was divided into 45 banana blocks (about 10–14 acres each), 28 streams and 47 marshes. All the marshes and streams were sampled at fortnightly intervals and the banana fields at 3–4 weekly intervals. If live snails were found the area was re-treated with molluscicide. Another examination was made of the areas previously 'snail free'. Treatment was required only at one pond where a few snails were found. A similar survey in October 1971, after the rains resumed, located snails in one banana drain. In 1971, after the rains resumed in August, rapid expansion of the static habitat colonies might have been expected and the critical question was whether, if it occurred, it could be contained by the surveillance-treatment programme. If it could not be, a repeat of the 1970 'blanket' treatment would be required. In the event, snail populations were under control although more frequent treatments were necessary in four sections in the central and lower parts of the valley. These sections included low-lying marshes and banana fields which had remained relatively damp throughout the dry season, providing particularly favourable conditions for snails. They tended to have a dense overgrowth of vegetation which sheltered aestivating snails when surface water dried up. The vegetation also hampered surveillance and the application of molluscicide. An intensive treatment was therefore applied to all potential snail habitats in these four sections in November, 1971: surveillance-treatment was suspended temporarily elsewhere in the valley during this period. In addition, most of the marshes outside these four sections were given a complete treatment. An attempt was made also to treat the large valley-mouth marsh by the aerial application of molluscicide (see below). The surveillance-treatment programme was resumed in December and continued to April 1975.

In 1973 the cultivation of bananas in 220 acres at the mouth of the valley was discontinued. The banana drains became overgrown to such an extent that searching for snails was impossible. Although *B. glabrata* were known to be present, in the absence of human contact they were left untreated.

Aerial treatment of the valley-mouth marsh. An area of 20 to 30 acres of marshy pasture at the mouth of Cul de Sac valley was known to harbour *B. glabrata*, but it was not treated in the initial spraying programme as it was considered to be of little significance in the transmission of the parasite. Further, there were considerable technical difficulties in treatment of such a large and remote area. However, it was included in the surveillance-treatment programme established at the start of the 1971 dry season. Isolated snail colonies were located and treated. Such colonies were detected more frequently after the rains resumed in August 1971. Complete treatment of the area by the field teams was not feasible in wet season conditions – it was estimated that it would occupy the entire biology section for at least a week, which seemed excessive for an area of dubious importance in transmission, but an attempt was made to spray the area from the air.

As there would inevitably be a hazard of drift of the chemical from the target area to surrounding banana crops, the effect of this was investigated in the laboratory grounds. A 2% solution of niclosamide in water was applied with a motorised power sprayer to several plants at a rate of about 1 l per banana plant – far in excess of what might be expected from an aerial treatment. There were no immediate phytotoxic effects, but pinpoint burns were detected after several days. The effect on the plants was minimal and leaves unfolding after treatment were unaffected and subsequently plants bore normal fruit.

A Thrush Commander S2R aircraft fitted with a Micronair spraying system used by the St Lucia Banana Growers' Association was chartered: 550 l of a 5% aqueous solution of niclosamide was applied from a height of 3–10 m at 144 k.p.h. at the maximum discharge rate of 13.6 l/acre; this rate was calculated to produce an average concentration of one p.p.m. if the marsh was 75 mm deep in water in the designated area.

Heavy rain filled most of the marsh on 14 December and the chemical

Table 6.6. *Cul de Sac valley: summary of results of aerial spraying observed*
at three unobstructed and three obstructed sites

	Unobstructed sites	Obstructed sites
No. of droplets	36/cm²	19/cm²
Molluscicide concentration	0.0025 mg	0.0009 mg
Molluscicide in ground water	0.105 mg/l	0.045 mg/l
Snail mortality[a]		
Caged snails	68.4%	5.3%
Natural populations	45.6%	0%

[a] Adjusted for control mortality.

Fig.6.8. Cul de Sac valley: sketch map of valley mouth showing marsh
area treated by aerial spray.

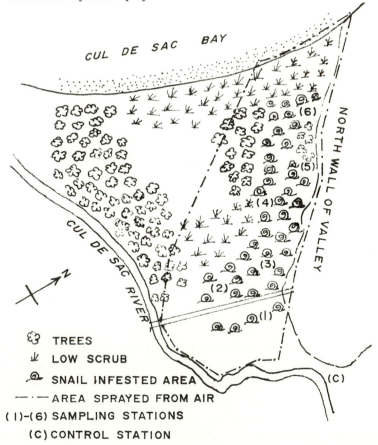

CUL DE SAC BAY

NORTH WALL OF VALLEY

CUL DE SAC RIVER

(1)–(6) sampling stations

(C)

£3 TREES

⅄ LOW SCRUB

@ SNAIL INFESTED AREA

— · —AREA SPRAYED FROM AIR

(I)-(6) SAMPLING STATIONS

(C) CONTROL STATION

was applied in the afternoon two days later, livestock having first been removed. The weather was sunny but a variable offshore wind made flying conditions a little difficult and caused some drift towards the sea within the treated area. The steep north wall of the valley and several clumps of trees further complicated the task of the pilot and resulted in some of the chemical falling on the marsh outside the designated area, but none landed on the banana fields. The whole operation, including loading the aircraft, flying to and from the marsh, spraying and cleaning the spraying system, took less than 2 hours. There was light rain about 2 hours after the application and heavier rain the following day.

The effectiveness of the treatment was assessed in four ways:

(a) With polythene sheeting to detect the dispersion of the droplets.
(b) Chemical analysis of ground water.
(c) Bio-assay with caged snails exposed for 24-hours starting just before treatment was applied.
(d) Quantitative quadrat samples of the natural snail population 24-hours before and 24 and 120-hours after the treatment.

All four methods were used at each of the six stations shown on the map of the area (Fig. 6.8). Stations 1, 2 and 3 in the open centre of the marsh were not obstructed by trees or the hillside as were stations 5 and 6. Station 4 was on a main drain and was partly obstructed by scrub. The results are summarised in Table 6.6.

Although these results are not impressive they demonstrate the feasibility of aerial spraying in unobstructed open areas and show that the chemical had penetrated the overlying vegetation and gradually built up a lethal concentration. A more suitable spraying system and more molluscicide would probably have produced better results.

The speed with which large areas can be treated is clearly advantageous. Minimal ground supervision is needed, and the only other labour required is the pilot and one man to clean the spraying system. The total cost per acre, excluding the cost of the chemical was estimated at less than US $0.50 per acre compared with $7.50–10.00 for hand spraying (Barnish & Sturrock, 1973; Sturrock & Barnish, 1973).

Death of other aquatic biota. Regrettably, many other aquatic animals were killed by mollusciciding, but populations recovered rapidly due to immigration from untreated areas of the valley. The environmental effect was therefore much less than many people feared and was much less than might have been the case had chemical control been applied to all water habitats in the valley. Specimens of shrimps and fish were sent for identification, while others were mounted for display and reference at the Research and Control Department (Appendix 6).

Allergic skin reaction to molluscicide. During the course of the mollusciciding programme one of the spraymen developed an itching papular reaction on the fingers of both hands soon after the programme started. The condition responded to hydrocortisone cream. Later, the man developed a pruritic vesicular cutaneous eruption on an indurated erythematous base where his molluscicide-drenched trousers touched his legs.

Patch testing with the emulsifiable concentrate of niclosamide at dilution of 1:1000 produced papules, at 1:100 and 1:10 dilution, vesicles, and undiluted, sloughing. No reaction occurred with patch testing with Bayer 73, the wettable powder formulation, nor with a saturated acetone extract of the active ingredient (saturated and diluted). It appears therefore that the reaction was due to one of the solvents or emulsifiers in the concentrate rather than the niclosamide itself (Cook, Sturrock & Barnish, 1972).

Site modifications. A few locations appeared suitable for site modification to render them less suitable for snails.

A spring was found to be the origin of a high level pond near Trois Piton on the northern side of the valley; it formed a pond and drained into a small marshy area supporting a large population of *B. glabrata*.

The seepage area was converted into a protected spring for use by the local inhabitants and although permission was refused to drain the marsh, it nevertheless did dry up with the subsequent elimination of the snail colony.

Two marshy sites at Ravine Poisson were drained into the nearby river and a third area of Soucis was canalised. Attempts to drain two other marshy areas were unsuccessful owing to their being below the level of the river. The total cost of these site modifications was $552 US.

Young seaside mahoe trees, *Thespesia populnea*, were planted in one marshy area in an endeavour to dry it out. These appeared to flourish temporarily, but long term effects were disappointing; despite fencing, they were damaged by cattle.

Snail findings in treated areas

Field B. glabrata. Between 1971 and 1975, snail colonies (defined as such when one or more snails were found) decreased considerably in number and size, and there was a significant reduction in the areas of the valley where snails were found (Table 6.7 and Fig. 6.9).

The general reduction in the number of sites yielding snails resulted in less molluscicide being necessary – in the last 12 months of the programme less than 200 l of niclosamide compared with 1260 l in the 1971–72 period.

As results of the annual parasitological surveys of children became available there were occasional indications that new infections occurred sporadically in areas where *B. glabrata* had not been found prior to the control and where mollusciciding was not being carried out. These areas were therefore subjected to intensive search for many months but no snails were found. The rest of the untreated areas were re-surveyed at 3–5 monthly intervals. A few colonies were found adjacent to known infested areas and brought into the surveillance treatment routine.

Table 6.7. *Cul de Sac valley: number of snail colonies found in different types of habitat during the mollusciciding campaign*

Year	Banana blocks	Marshes	Streams
1971–72	170	71	10
1972–73	150	60	0
1973–74	117	48	2
1974–75	71	30	2

Fig.6.9. Cul de Sac valley: areas infested with *B. glabrata* at start of control, 1970, and in 1975. (From Jordan, 1977.)

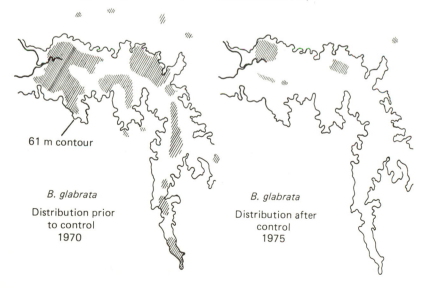

61 m contour

B. glabrata

Distribution prior to control 1970

B. glabrata

Distribution after control 1975

Initially, snails found were not systematically examined for infection, though some collections were screened in mass for cercarial shedding. From June 1972 all live snails were crushed and examined for sporocysts or cercariae (Table 6.8). Of the 11 infected snails, 9 were found between January and June (the dry season) and one each in July and September. All infected snails came from banana drains.

Examination of the pre-control index sites (comprising 4 pools, 5 marshes, 13 banana drains and 5 stream/river sites) continued until June 1973, when sampling stopped as the sites were included in areas receiving molluscicide and few *B. glabrata* were being recovered – a few in a static site two months after the initial blanket treatment, one hatchling snail in a stream site in June 1971 and a few young snails in a marsh site in January 1973.

In adjacent valleys surveys of index sites showed a build-up in snail populations in flowing sites in early 1971, with the seasonal burst of transmission associated with the dry season. Rainfall was below average in 1971 and 1972 so that colonies were not flushed out and infected snails were sporadically found throughout the year with a further increase in transmission in early 1972. In the early months of 1973 rainfall was well below average, sites dried up and the usual transmission burst did not occur. Stable colonies with sporadic infections were found in the static sites in the wetter months of the year.

Sentinel snail exposures. Two sites in each of the settlements of Ravine Poisson and Soucis were selected for exposing sentinel snails. Results are shown in Table 6.9.

The infection rate varied considerably from month to month but did not appear to be related to rainfall (Fig. 6.13), perhaps due to rain falling every month. The rates at Soucis are exceptional. One of the sites for exposure of snails was close to a bridge, frequently used as a latrine, on the main road through the valley. This could have been the site of a heavily infected

Table 6.8. *Cul de Sac valley: infection rates in field* B. glabrata

Year	Snails examined	Pre-patent		Patent		Total %
		No.	%	No.	%	
1972–73	6849	4	0.06	2	0.03	0.09
1973–74	5827	2	0.03	1	0.02	0.05
1974–75	4134	1	0.02	1	0.02	0.04

person regularly 'moving his bowels' and periodically giving high snail infection rates. If this were so, it appears he moved out of the area in early 1973.

Mouse exposures and cercariometry. Pre-control a low percentage of sentinel mice exposed in different habitats was found subsequently to have been infected.

Mouse exposures were continued for a year after the mollusciciding programme started (to December 1971) during which time 1451 mice were perfused (out of 1410 exposed). None was found infected and mouse exposures were discontinued.

Of 200 water samples examined from four streams none was found to contain detectable numbers of cercariae (Sandt, 1973*a,b*). In a neighbouring valley, 5 of 280 samples of water were positive with concentrations of 0.05–21.0 cercariae/litre.

Parasitological surveys
Pre-control investigations (1967–71)

The census and first stool survey was carried out between January and May 1967 when houses were numbered and details of households obtained. A second survey of children was made in 1969, and thereafter surveys were made annually to 1971 when the final pre-control survey of all age groups was made. (As noted above, mollusciciding started at the

Table 6.9. *Cul de Sac valley: results of yearly sentinel snail exposures, human infection data and crude index of potential contamination amongst 0–14-year-old children during different phases of control*

Year	Sentinel snails			Human infection[a]		
	No. exam.	No. infected	% infected	Prev. (%)	Intensity (GM)	Crude IPC (% × GM)
1971	1765	68	3.85	40	34	1360
1972	1823	82	4.49	60	22	1320
1973	1514	50	3.30	33	23	759
1974	1684	19	1.13	25	35	875
1975[b]	1709	7	0.41	16	20	320
1976[b]	1722	8	0.46	7	13	91
1977	1320	2	0.15	2	10	20
1978–81	3480	1	0.03	1	10	10

[a] Based on data from Ravine Poisson and Soucis.
[b] The population was offered treatment after surveys in 1975 and 1976.

Table 6.10. *Cul de Sac valley: overall prevalence by settlement at 1967 survey and subsequent incidence of new S. mansoni infections amongst children 0–7 years – in order of incidence between 1969 and 1970*

Settlement	Overall prevalence (%) 1967	1967–69[a]		1969–70		1970–71		Overall prevalence (%) 1971
		No. neg.[b]	% inc.[c]	No. neg.	% inc.	No. neg.	% inc.	
Ravine Poisson	57	30	10.0	63	30.2	77	31.1	47
Soucis	62	20	20.0	30	26.6	28	17.9	46
L'Abayee	65	17	11.7	52	23.0	67	17.9	50
Goodlands	34	28	3.6	49	22.4	23	8.7	23
Deglos	39	14	14.3	22	18.1	17	5.9	45
Bexon	55	30	10.0	65	16.9	65	10.8	41
Deglos Junction	50	5	0	24	12.5	23	4.3	31
Ti Colon	45	17	5.9	36	11.1	30	0	18
Welsan	31	20	0	46	6.5	49	2.0	18
Tourrat	25	8	0	17	5.8	12	0	14
Barre Denise	11	70	1.4	122	5.7	103	3.9	7
Ferrands	40	45	2.2	65	4.6	8	0	33
Trois Pitons	12	45	2.2	65	4.3	35	0	12
Marc	23	39	5.1	47	4.2	50	0	14
Marc Estate	9	19	5.3	9	0	46	0	4

[a] Approximately 21 months between surveys (% incidence *not* adjusted to 12-month rate).
[b] Number negative at first of two surveys.
[c] Percentage positive at second survey.

end of 1970; the time lag before the final survey allowed for maturation of infection accquired immediately prior to control.)

Between 1967 and 1969 (first and second surveys), transmission was at a very low level in all settlements, and in the 21 months between surveys there were only 19 new infections amongst 360 children aged 0–7 years who were negative in 1967. This low rate of transmission was associated with Hurricane Beulah in September 1967, and was confirmed by the biological findings of reduced snail populations and number of infected *B. glabrata* in the streams where most infection was believed to take place (Fig. 6.3). Between 1969 and 1970 transmission increased, but fell slightly in the next 12 months, but prevalence in 1971 was consistently lower than at the first survey. Rates varied considerably in different settlements, tending to be high in those on the valley floor and close to the river, and lower in those on the hillside (Table 6.10.)

The incidence of new infections varied between settlements and, for assessing results of control, these were categorised into high or low

Table 6.11. *Cul de Sac valley: Incidence of new* S. mansoni *infections by age amongst 0–7-year-old children in areas of high and low transmission prior to control*

Age in years[b]	1967–69[a]		1969–70		1970–71	
	No. neg.[c]	% inc.[d]	No. neg.	% inc.	No. neg.	% inc.
High transmission areas						
0 & 1	44	5.2	68	17.6	49	6.1
2 & 3	51	5.6	80	21.3	71	12.7
4 & 5	28	4.1	72	23.6	89	22.5
6 & 7	14	8.2	61	36.0	68	27.9
8 & 9					(46	39.1)
10 & 11					(35	40.0)
0–7	137	5.4	281	24.2	277	18.4
Low transmission areas						
0 & 1	51	0.0	78	1.3	61	0.0
2 & 3	73	0.8	86	4.7	97	1.0
4 & 5	65	0.9	102	5.9	116	6.9
6 & 7	34	6.7	113	10.6	91	3.3
8 & 9					(95	6.3)
10 & 11					(50	12.0)
0–7	223	1.5	379	5.5	365	3.3

[a] Incidence adjusted to 12 months from 21 months between surveys.
[b] Age at first of two surveys.
[c] Number negative at first of two surveys.
[d] Percentage positive at second survey.

transmission areas based on incidence amongst children aged 0–7 years being above or below 15% between 1969 and 1970. Six settlements, all close to the river, were included in the high transmission area – Ravine Poisson, L'Abayee, Bexon, Deglos, Goodlands and Soucis; in the pre-control investigations they showed incidence rates consistently higher than other settlements. In high and low transmission areas incidence increased with age (Table 6.11).

The final pre-control survey involved all age groups and was made in 1971 when 4852 persons were recorded, 2362 and 2490 being in the high

Fig.6.10. Cul de Sac valley: changes in *S. mansoni* prevalence between 1967 and 1971 (pre-control) among males and females in high (solid lines) and low (broken lines) transmission areas.

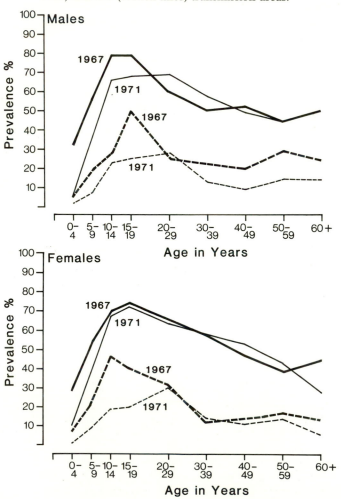

and low transmission settlements respectively. Of these, 75% provided stools for examination; the pattern of response was similar to that at the 1967 survey, with a higher response rate amongst females than males, but in both sexes a poor response amongst young adults. Although prevalence rates were lower in 1971 than in 1967, the pattern of change was not consistent – in high and low transmission areas prevalence was lower among age groups to 19 in both sexes; there was little change amongst the older age groups, but prevalence among males in the low transmission areas was significantly lower in 1971 ($Z = 3.29$, sig. at 0.1% level) (Fig. 6.10).

A cohort study of those examined at both surveys showed a C/R ratio of 1.17 amongst children (0–14) in the high transmission areas – much lower than usual for an uncontrolled area: the C/R ratio of 0.67 amongst the older age groups reflects the usual loss of infection in this segment of the population (Table 6.12).

The 1971 prevalence and intensity of infection were similar in the two sexes. In general, the age groups with high prevalence rates were associated with high levels of egg excretion, and by calculating the relative IPC, the 5–19-year-old age group were potentially responsible for 65% and 56% of contamination of the environment with *S. mansoni* ova in the high and low transmission areas respectively (Table 6.13).

The frequency distribution of egg output was typical of endemic areas, the majority of persons excreting few *S. mansoni* ova. In the high transmission areas 20% of egg counts were greater than 100 e.p.ml of faeces compared with only 7% in the low transmission areas.

Table 6.12. *Cul de Sac valley: results of a 1967–71 cohort study showing change in status of* S. mansoni *prior to control*

Age groups		High transmission		Low transmission	
		0–14	15 +	0–14	15 +
No. exam.		440	314	389	315
No. +ve (%)	1967	248 (56)	188 (60)	65 (17)	67 (21)
Conversions[a]		62	39*	16*	16**
Reversions[b]		53	61*	31*	36**
C/R ratio		1.17	0.64	0.51	0.44
No. +ve (%)	1971	257 (58)	166 (53)	50 (13)	47 (15)

[a] Conversions – negative 1967, positive 1981.
[b] Reversions – positive 1971, negative 1981.
* Difference between Conversions and Reversions significant at 5% level.
** Difference between Conversions and Reversions significant at 1% level.

Table 6.13. *Cul de Sac valley; prevalence and intensity of S. mansoni infection and corrected index of potential contamination (IPC) in 1971*

Age in years	Males			Females			Both sexes			Corrected IPC[b]	Relative IPC (%)[c]
	No. exam.	Prev. (%)	GM[a]	No. exam.	Prev. (%)	GM	% of pop. (1)	Prev. (%) (2)	GM (3)		
High transmission areas											
0–4	162	7	18	151	10	24	17.2	8	21	29	2
5–9	218	37	35	208	39	25	20.2	38	30	230	14
10–14	129	66	42	153	67	54	14.7	67	48	473	28
15–19	56	68	67	92	72	48	10.0	70	55	385	23
20–29	45	69	24	108	63	38	12.0	65	33	257	15
30–39	58	57	27	81	58	25	8.2	58	26	124	7
40–49	71	49	21	67	54	25	7.0	51	24	86	5
50–59	32	44	16	37	43	21	5.3	43	18	41	3
60+	42	50	30	52	30	25	5.4	27	28	41	3
0–14	509	35	37	512	39	37	(100)	37	37	(1666)	(100)
15+	304	57	30	437	55	32		56	31		
Low transmission areas											
0–4	187	2	15[d]	184	1	21[d]	17.2	1	18[d]	3	1
5–9	204	8	15[d]	228	9	21[d]	20.2	9	18[d]	33	10
10–14	149	23	24	129	19	32	14.7	21	27	83	27
15–19	56	25	29	71	20	20	10.0	26	24	62	19
20–29	60	28	24	129	30	24	12.0	30	24	86	27
30–39	56	13	17	101	14	27	8.2	13	24	26	8
40–49	64	9	19	74	11	11	7.0	10	14	10	2
50–59	52	14	20[d]	56	14	11[d]	5.3	14	15[d]	11	3
60+	29	14	20[d]	52	9	11[d]	5.4	9	15[d]	7	2
0–14	540	10	21	541	9	26	(100)	10	23	(321)	(100)
15+	317	17	23	483	18	20		17	21		

[a] Geometric mean of egg output of infected persons.
[b] Product of (1) × (2) × (3)/100 for each age group.
[c] Expressed as a percentage of the sum of the product of all age groups [b]
[d] Based on GM of 0–9 and 50+ age groups owing to a few infected persons.

During control

The incidence of new infections in the high transmission areas gradually declined from 23.2% in 1970–71 to 5.7% in 1974–75 (Table 6.14). Similar data from the comparison areas show no such decline (Table 4.9). In the low transmission areas the decline was from 4.7% to 2.3%.

The lower incidence inevitably led to a marked lowering of prevalence amongst children and, with a reduced risk of re-infection, prevalence and intensity of infection declined amongst the older age groups. males and females were similarly affected.

Overall prevalence was reduced from 45% to 24% and from 13% to 7% in the high and low transmission areas respectively; intensity of infection from 34 to 22 and 22 to 17 e.p.ml faeces (geometric mean), and the crude IPC by 63% and 53% in the two areas (Table 6.15).

In the comparison area between 1970 and 1975 prevalence increased slightly from 49% to 53% in the high transmission areas and decreased

Table 6.14. *Cul de Sac valley: annual incidence of new infections by age during area-wide mollusciciding compared with last pre-control data of 1970–71*

Age in years[a]	1970–71		1971–72		1972–73		1973–74		1974–75	
	No. neg.[b]	% inc.[c]	No. neg.	% inc.	No. neg.	% inc.	No. neg.	% inc.	No. neg.	% inc.
High transmission areas										
0 & 1	49	6.1	49	8.2	59	5.1	56	3.6	55	5.5
2 & 3	71	12.7	69	8.7	60	1.7	100	1.0	90	2.2
4 & 5	89	22.5	81	9.9	92	3.3	100	5.0	90	3.3
6 & 7	68	27.9	77	18.2	94	11.7	117	12.0	115	1.7
8 & 9	46	39.1	56	29.0	65	20.0	87	5.7	116	6.9
10 & 11	35	40.0	31	29.0	38	15.8	65	7.4	80	16.3
0–11	358	23.2	363	16.5	408	9.1	525	7.4	546	5.7
Low transmission areas										
0 & 1	61	0	89	1.1	84	0	95	0	74	1.4
2 & 3	97	1.0	88	3.4	108	0.9	133	0	119	0
4 & 5	116	6.9	109	1.8	120	4.2	122	1.6	136	2.2
6 & 7	91	3.3	112	3.6	124	1.6	151	0	146	2.1
8 & 9	95	6.3	102	9.8	113	5.3	128	4.7	143	2.8
10 & 11	50	12.0	67	14.9	88	3.4	105	6.7	124	4.8
0–11	510	4.7	567	5.3	637	2.3	734	1.9	742	2.3

[a] Age at first of two surveys.
[b] Number negative at first of two surveys.
[c] Percentage positive at second survey.

Table 6.15. *Cul de Sac valley: prevalence, intensity of infection and crude IPC in high and low transmission areas in 1971 and at end of different phases of control project*

Age group	1971 No. exam.	% +ve	GM[a]	1975 No. exam.	% +ve	GM	1977 No. exam.	% +ve	GM	1981 No. exam.	% +ve	GM
High transmission areas												
0–4	313	8	21	334	2	15[c]	259	<1		174	0	
5–9	426	38	30	447	6	15[c]	409	2		287	1	
10–14	282	67	48	430	28	24	391	5		268	1	
15–19	148	70	55	236	45	28	216	10	Mean	173	9	Mean
20–29	153	65	33	210	51	25	212	13	for	141	15	for
30–39	139	58	26	164	37	19	149	9	all	113	10	all
40–49	138	51	24	142	31	16	135	9	ages	98	7	ages
50–59	69	43	18	132	22	23	127	10	13	95	6	20
60+	94	37	28	117	33	16	118	7		94	7	
0–14	1021	37	37	1211	13	21	1059	3		729	0	
15+	741	57	31	1001	39	22	957	10		714	10	
Crude IPC[b]	15061			5560			858			1140		
Reduction by phase				63%			85%			Increase		
Cumulative reduction				63%			94%			92%		

Low transmission areas

	GM[a]		[c]	GM[a]		[c]	GM[a]			GM[a]	
0–4	371	1	18[c]	417	<1	17[c]	274	<1		138	<1
5–9	432	9	18[c]	525	3	17[c]	502	<1		280	<1
10–14	278	21	27	445	6	12	414	3	Mean for all ages 13	248	<1	Mean for all ages 14
15–19	127	26	24	213	17	20	208	7		121	5
20–29	189	30	24	257	21	16	218	10		91	11
30–39	157	13	24	172	17	21	151	8		87	12
40–49	138	10	14	185	9	14	150	1		87	10
50–59	108	14	15[c]	104	6	19[c]	98	5		75	3
60+	81	9	15[c]	86	8	19[c]	89	0		60	3
0–14	1081	9	23	1389	4	14	1190	1		666	<1
15+	800	18	21	1017	13	18	914	6		521	8
Crude IPC	2888			1365			468			662	
Reduction by phase				53%			66%			Increase	
Cumulative reduction				54%			84%			77%	

[a] Geometric mean of e.p.ml faeces.

[b] Sum of product of prevalence and GM of each age group.

[c] Based on GM of 0–9 and 50+ age groups owing to few infected persons.

from 29% to 22% in the low transmission areas. Crude IPC declined by 28% and 56% respectively (Table 4.11).

In a cohort study of children in the high transmission areas, lost infections (98) exceeded new infections (33) (C/R ratio 0.34), so that, in the age groups in which prevalence is normally increasing, there was a reduction in prevalence from 34.1% to 23.8%, although the children were 4 years older. In a similar study in the high transmission comparison area, prevalence increased from 35.2% to 62.5% as new infections (222) outnumbered those lost (56), C/R ratio 3.96 (Fig. 6.11). In the low transmission areas a similar pattern was found (Table 6.16) but changes were less pronounced.

(ii)   A focal surveillance programme supplemented by chemotherapy (1975–77).

Focal surveillance mollusciciding

While the area-wide snail control demonstrated that mollusciciding had reduced transmission to a very low level, such a regime was not considered satisfactory for the Government Public Health Department to run on a routine basis: a cheaper and simpler regime was necessary, particularly when prevalence was at a low level (Barnish, Christie & Prentice, 1980).

Fig.6.11. Cul de Sac valley: *S. mansoni* prevalence in 1971–75 cohort study of 1–14-year-old children and similar data from high transmission comparison area. (1975 T – theoretical finding if transmission ceased for 4 years; it does not allow for worm deaths.)

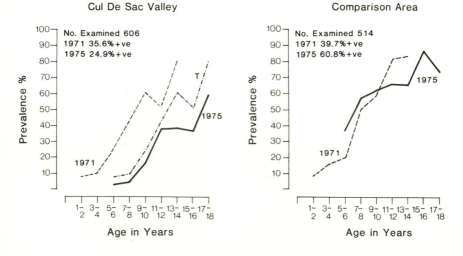

Accordingly, a system of focal surveillance mollusciciding was devised with only those flowing water habitats believed to be potentially important in transmission being checked for *B. glabrata*. Thus 145 streams, main drains and drains alongside footpaths were searched once every two weeks. The labour force and vehicles required were about half those necessary for the area-wide control; molluscicide and related stores were similarly much reduced in quantity.

When snails were found, as many as possible were collected prior to mollusciciding. They were examined for sporocysts after crushing. Between 1975 and 1977 from the 60 ravines regularly checked only 2 of 942 snails (0.21%) were infected, and from the 90 banana drains there were only 6 of 13 543 (0.04%).

With the change in control strategy, the 28 original index sites (the majority of which were subject to mollusciciding in the area-wide campaign and in which observations had ceased at the end of 1973) were again

Table 6.16. *Cul de Sac valley: results of a 1971–75 cohort study showing the change in status of* S. mansoni *during the consolidation phase of routine focal mollusciciding and data from the comparison area for 1970–75 (See also pre-control data (Table 6.12)*

Age group		High transmission		Low transmission	
		0–14	15+	0–14	15+
Cul de Sac					
No. examined		632	361	665	319
No. +ve (%)	1971	216 (34)	197 (55)	48 (7)	66 (21)
Conversions[a]		33**	30**	22*	10**
Reversions[b]		98**	96**	32*	42**
C/R ratio		0.34	0.31	0.71	0.24
No. +ve (%)	1975	151 (24)	131 (36)	38 (6)	34 (11)
Richefond (comparison)					
No. examined		601	345	275	180
No. +ve (%)	1970	212 (35)	248 (72)	37 (13)	100 (56)
Conversions		222**	31**	54**	15**
Reversions		56**	90**	16**	43**
C/R ratio		3.96	0.34	3.38	0.35
No. +ve (%)	1975	378 (63)	189 (55)	75 (27)	72 (40)

[a] Conversions – negative 1977, positive 1981.
[b] Reversions – positive 1977, negative 1981.
* Difference between Conversions and Reversions not significant.
** Difference between Conversions and Reversions significant at 1% level.
From Jordan *et al.*, 1978.

brought under surveillance, but in only one site were snails found. In the 2 years of over 3400 sentinel snails examined only 15 (0.44%) were infected due to the much reduced IPC (Table 6.9).

Chemotherapy campaigns (1975 and 1976)

The four years of mollusciciding reduced transmission significantly. However, the many persons infected prior to control, and whose infections had not spontaneously died out, remained a reservoir of infection capable of leading to a resurgence of transmission if snail control was relaxed.

In order to reduce the magnitude of this reservoir, 702 persons found infected at the 1975 survey were offered treatment. Hycanthone at a dose of 2 mg/kg body weight was given to 640 persons; 9 others received 'Ambilhar' or lucanthone. Forty-two patients failed to attend for treatment and 18 who were pregnant were not treated until after childbirth.

The day after hycanthone treatments, patients were visited at home to check on side effects. These were found to be of short duration and invariably ended within 24 h. Amongst the 62% with complaints, 12% vomited and in one person it was reported to be severe. The patient, a 22–year-old male, vomited only once after being admitted to the research ward for observation, but he remained anorectic for 2 weeks and lost 2 kg in weight. Hepatocellular enzymes were only slightly elevated, and he had no jaundice though his liver was moderately enlarged and tender.

Although hycanthone had been accepted by the population, there was still concern regarding its toxicity and mutagenicity (Hartman *et al.*, 1971). Thus with oral oxamniquine being available this drug at a dose of 15 mg/kg body weight was offered to 310 infected persons in 1976; 264 accepted including 58 persons from a village in the neighbouring valley of Roseau but whose inhabitants had close contact with Cul de Sac. Side effects, again assessed by a home visit, were experienced by only 14%, mild dizziness being the most common complaint (7.7%).

With further experience in the use of oxamniquine, it was considered unnecessary to continue to check on side effects and these were subseqently stopped. In the two campaigns, the cost of checking on side effects had amounted to 12.6% and 5.1% respectively of total costs, which are shown in Table 6.17. The higher cost per person protected with oxamniquine ($1.31) compared to the hycanthone ($1.04) was due to (i) the higher cost of oxamniquine: $5.65 per patient compared with $1.1 for those given hycanthone, (ii) salaries had been increased by approximately 20%, and (iii) a special Health Education effort made in 1976 in order to get as many persons treated as possible.

Table 6.17. *Cul de Sac valley: cost analysis of chemotherapy in 1975 (hycanthone) and 1976 (oxamniquine), and proportionate distribution of costs*

	1975			1976		
	Comment	Cost (US$)	% of total	Comment	Cost (US$)	% of total
Case detection						
Stool Collection:						
Number of specimens	4618			4437		
Survey team (man hours)	992	1096		1054	1529	
Transportation (miles)	965	206		1282	329	
Stool containers	5850	614		5676	524	
Stool examination (man hours)	1385	1337	62.5	1479	1834	64.3
Health education:						
Publicity (man hours)				115	235	
Transportation (miles)				224	48	4.3
Therapy	(649 treated)			(264 treated)		
Tracing patients (man hours)				8	20	
Transportation (miles)				33	6	
Nursing team (man hours)	249	245		82	115	
Transportation (miles)	406	97	6.6	144	34	2.7
Drugs and materials:						
Hycanthone/Oxamniquine	319 vials @ $2.25	718	13.8	1092–250 mg capsules @ $1.366	1492	22.8
Pregnancy tests		133			37	
Syringes, cards, etc.		102	4.5		16	0.8
Therapy follow-up etc.:						
Field team (man hours)	370	367		177	220	
Transportation (miles)	1314	288	12.6	597	114	5.1
Total		5203			6553	
Cost per: Stool examined		0.70			1.01	
Case detected		4.51			14.51	
Person treated		8.02			24.82	
Person protected		1.04			1.31	

From Jordan *et al.* 1980*b*.

It was calculated that if hycanthone instead of oxamniquine had been used in the 1976 campaign, the cost per head of population protected would have been reduced from $1.31 to $1.08, a cost comparable to the $1.04 *per caput* of the first campaign.

Parasitological results

At a survey in 1977, after two years of the focal surveillance mollusciciding and two chemotherapy campaigns, a further decline in all indices of *S. mansoni* was recorded (Table 6.15: Fig. 6.12).

Although prevalence appeared to be at a very low level, it was calculated that, owing to infections being missed on stool examination and the number of uncooperative persons increasing with each additional survey, the prevalence was more likely to be about 23% and 17% in the high and low transmission areas respectively (Table 6.18) (Jordan *et al.*, 1980*b*).

In the absence of further snail control, transmission was likely to recur, but the focal surveillance mollusciciding programme was considered too dependent on supervision, relatively insensitive snail search techniques, and the cost still too high for public health control when the risk of schistosomal disease was minimal.

Accordingly, the snail control programme was revised and a routine focal mollusciciding scheme was introduced in April 1977 and evaluated over a 4-year period as a consolidation phase strategy.

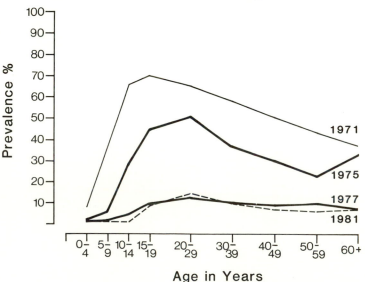

Fig.6.12. Cul de Sac valley: *S. mansoni* prevalence in 1971, prior to control, and after different control strategies.

Table 6.18 *Cul de Sac valley: calculations for assessing number of infected persons in population in 1977 but who were not detected on survey*

	High transmission		Low transmission	
Stools examined	2016		2104	
No. S. mansoni positive (%)		123 (6.1%)		70 (3.3%)
Calculated missed		184		153
Stools not examined	850		879	
1 Previously +ve	490		448	
(a) Treated (est. 10% +ve)	62	6	8	1
(b) Untreated (est. 50% +ve)	428	214	440	220
2 Previously −ve	235		273	
(a) Children (est. 5% +ve)	48	2	62	3
(b) Adults (est. 15% +ve)	187	28	211	32
Never examined				
(a) Children (est. 10% +ve)	20	2	53	5
(b) Adults (est. 25% +ve)	103	26	100	25
Total stools examined and not examined	2866		2983	
Total found and calculated +ve (%)		585 (22.8%)		509 (17.1%)

From Jordan et al., 1980b.

(iii)   **Consolidation phase – routine focal mollusciciding (1977–81)**

Biological studies.

Because of limited human contact with some of the sites treated in the focal surveillance programme, many were excluded for the consolidation phase and only 12 streams and 26 main drains were retained (Barnish, Jordan, Bartholomew & Grist, 1982). Routine application of molluscicide was made on a 4-weekly cycle: the work was completed by two men in five days. A major advantage of the system was that small numbers of snails that may have been undetected by normal searching techniques were subject to control at an early stage, preventing development of large colonies.

Initially, molluscicide was applied by drip-feed at a fixed dose depending on the average flow of each stream, but during the dry season of 1978 it was apparent this would lead to excessive use of molluscicide as habitats dried. A modification was introduced with the molluscicide dose being read directly from a V-notch weir.

Index sites

Observations at the original index sites had been terminated during the area-wide snail control strategy as they were subject to mollusciciding but, with a change to routine application of chemical, sampling was re-introduced in 25 of them (three sites had been destroyed in the development of the oil storage facility). Only one site was found to harbour snails, but none was infected. Forty additional index sites were introduced – 24 main drains, 12 primary drains and 4 marsh locations. They were searched every four weeks for 15 minutes. All types of habitat harboured snails at some time of the year, but no patent infections were found (by cercarial shedding) amongst over 4347 snails examined. Nearly 1000 additional snails from stream sites were examined, but again none was infected.

Sentinel snail exposures

Routine sentinel snail exposures were continued: in the four years of the project 3 of 4800 snails were infected (0.06%) (Table 6.9). A summary of the sentinel and field snail infection rates since control started in 1970 is shown in Fig. 6.13.

Lack of resistance to molluscicide

After nine years of applying niclosamide in Cul de Sac valley, the susceptibility of *B. glabrata* was compared with that of snails from two areas

Fig.6.13. Cul de Sac valley: *S. mansoni* prevalence among 0–14-year age group; rainfall, sentinel and field snail data from commencement of control in 1970 to 1981.

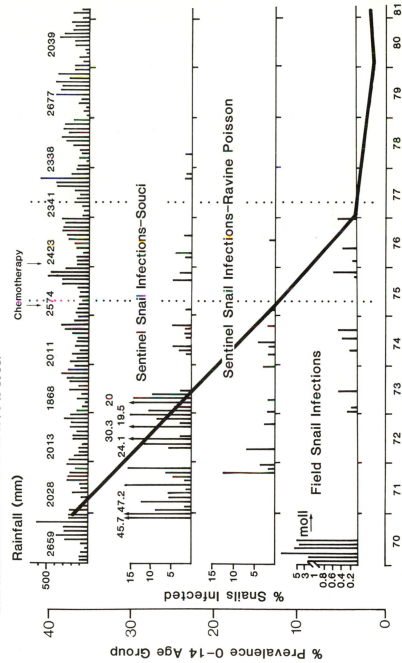

of St Lucia where molluscicide had never been used. Trials were made using methods recommended by WHO for standardised molluscicide trials.

There was no difference in susceptibility of snails from the three areas, nor was there a difference between the 1970 molluscicide trials with snails from Cul de Sac valley. It was concluded that after nine years of exposure to niclosamide there was no evidence of resistance developing (Barnish & Prentice, 1981).

Although it had been reported that Iranian *Bulinus truncatus* showed evidence of resistance to niclosamide after 10 years (Jelnes, 1977), it seems possible that the use of a 10-year-old laboratory strain of *B. truncatus* as a control may have resulted in this finding.

Parasitological results

The final parasitological survey was made at the beginning of 1981.

Incidence of new infections fell to zero between 1979 and 1980 but showed a slight rise the next year (Table 6.19), although only one of the four apparent infections was ELISA positive and known to have been infected from previous surveys.

Table 6.19. *Cul de Sac valley: annual incidence of new infections during consolidation phase of routine focal snail control (1977–81)*

Age in years	1977–78		1978–79		1979–80		1980–81	
	No. neg.	% +ve	No. neg.	% +ve	No. neg.	% +ve	No. neg.	% +ve
High transmission areas								
0 & 1	32	0	23	0	28	0	28	0
2 & 3	70	0	44	0	54	0	46	0
4 & 5	76	0	71	0	61	0	61	1.6
6 & 7	98	0	87	1.1	82	0	80	2.5
8 & 9	99	1.0	75	0	92	0	92	0
10 & 11	107	0.9	89	1.1	64	0	63	1.6
0–11	482	0.4	389	0.5	381	0	370	1.1
Low transmission areas								
0 & 1	35	0	32	0	29	0	22	0
2 & 3	63	0	57	0	42	0	52	0
4 & 5	126	0	80	0	64	0	54	0
6 & 7	138	0.7	107	0	95	0	89	0
8 & 9	121	0.8	106	0	93	0	80	0
10 & 11	108	0	88	0	74	0	84	0
0–11	591	0.3	470	0	397	0	381	0

Results of a 4-year cohort study (Table 6.20) indicate little change in status of infection. Although the C/R ratio greater than one implied that transmission was occurring, the differences between conversions and reversions were not significant.

There was thus little change over the 4-year period, suggesting the routine focal snail control consolidation phase strategy was successful in preventing a resurgence of transmission in spite of a reservoir of *S. mansoni* and colonies of *B. glabrata*.

Data on prevalence, intensity of infection and the index of potential contamination at different phases of the 10-year project are shown in Table 6.15. The changes in prevalence are shown in Fig. 6.12 and, in relation to biological findings, in Fig. 6.13. The changing pattern of the freqency distribution of intensity of infection as control progressed is shown in Table 6.21.

At the final stool survey, 118 people were found apparently infected; their past records were analysed (Table 6.22).

Table 6.20. *Cul de Sac valley: results of a 1977–81 cohort study showing change in status of* S. mansoni *over the period of routine focal mollusciciding*

Age group		High transmission			Low transmission	
		0–14	15+		0–14	15+
No. examined		490	417		485	294
No. +ve. (%)	1977	7 (1.4)	41 (9.8)	1977	2 (0.3)	9 (6.4)
Conversions[a]		10	24		4	12
Reversions[b]		6	26		(1.0)	14
C/R ratio		1.7	0.9		4.0	1.1
No. +ve (%)	1981	11 (2.2)	39 (9.4)	1981	5 (1.0)	21 (7.1)

[a] Conversions: negative in 1977, positive 1981.
[b] Reversions: positive in 1981, negative 1977.

Table 6.21. *Cul de Sac valley – high transmission areas: changing pattern of frequency distribution (%) of intensity of infection as control progressed*

Year	No. exam.	Egg load (eggs/ml faeces)					
		0	< 50	51–100	101–200	201–400	400+
1971	1762	54.9	30.1	6.4	5.1	2.1	1.4
1975	2212	75.5	19.6	2.8	1.6	0.5	—
1977	2016	93.9	5.8	0.2	0.1	—	—
1981	1368	94.5	5.1	0.2	0.1	—	—

Only 6 (all adults) had been treated, 7 had not previously been examined, 14 were immigrants since 1977, 24 had previously been examined but found to be uninfected, while 67 (57% of the total) had been known previously to be infected but had not been treated. Blood was taken from the 7 children with apparent new infections and the ELISA reaction was negative in all of them. The probability that these were 'mixed specimens' must therefore be considered. All other persons were treated with oxamniquine at a total cost of $9.73 *per caput.*

Survey of public sanitary facilities

Although Cul de Sac valley is the nearest rural community to the St Lucian capital, it has probably the poorest rural water supply in the island. The community water supply is not evenly distributed, and although 73% and 45% of households in high and low transmission areas

Table 6.22. *Cul de Sac valley: analysis of past records of 118 persons positive* for S. mansoni *in 1981*

Age	Previously +ve Not treated	Treated	Previously +ve	Not previously examined	Immigrants (since 1977)
0–4	—	—	1 (1)[a]	1	—
5–9	—	—	4 (4,6,7,8)	—	2
10–14	1	—	2 (9,11)	—	1
15–19	17	1	2 (7,10)	—	1
20–29	20	2	2 (4,5)	3	5
30–39	12	—	6 (1,1,1,2,3,4)	1	3
40–49	5	1	4 (1,2,3,3)	2	1
50–59	6	1	1 (2)	—	—
60+	6	1	2 (1,5)	—	1
Total	67 (57%)	6 (5%)	24 (20%)	7 (6%)	14 (12%)

[a] Number of previous negative stools from each individual.
From Barnish *et al.*, 1982.

Table 6.23. *Cul de Sac valley: the number and state of public facilities in Cul de Sac, May 1981*

Facility	Working	Not working	People/working unit
Tap	26	6	192
Laundry tub	26	12	192
Shower	14	6	357
Toilet	6	4	833

used a public standpipe as their main supply, 58% and 80% had to supplement this with river or stream water. Data in Table 6.23 stress the all too frequent finding in developing countries – the poor maintenance of expensive water supplies and latrine facilities. Although prevalence and intensity of infection were reduced to low levels, a reservoir of infection remained which could lead to a resurgence of transmission in the absence of adequate water supplies or some other form of control.

Cost of the three phases

The costs of the three phases of snail control are shown in Table 6.24: proportional costs of different aspects of the schemes are also shown.

Accurate comparison over the 10-year period is complicated due to the local currency (ECC) being tied to sterling until 1976 (£1 = ECC $4.80: US $1.00 = ECC $2.00) when it was tied to the US dollar at the rate of $2.70 ECC; however, for the purpose of this comparison the old rate of exchange is retained (see Chapter 3). A further complication was the world-wide inflation in recent years. This has been taken into account by using the mean Cost of Living Index (COLI) (published regularly in the St Lucia Gazette) (Fig. 3.8) for each of the three projects and relating it to the 1977–81 index, taken as zero (Table 6.24).

The area-wide mollusciciding project was labour intensive (65%) with minimal expenditure on imported (and costly) molluscicide (12%): in the routine focal mollusciciding programme the distribution of costs was reversed with chemicals accounting for 55% of costs and labour 27%. Such a scheme may be unacceptable to governments which may prefer a labour-intensive programme with minimal outlay of foreign currency for the importation of chemical. For this reason, the labour-intensive (68%) surveillance–mollusciciding programme, although more costly ($2.79 per head), may be more acceptable.

Parasitological results justify the use of the less costly routine focal mollusciciding programme which prevented a resurgence of transmission, but with prevalence at a level unlikely to be associated with *disease* it must surely be a difficult decision whether to continue expenditure on control (when the infection is a low health priority) or discontinue and risk a resurgence of transmission.

In view of findings in other parts of St Lucia the expenditure of US $13 000 between 1977 and 1981 on the routine focal snail control might have been better utilised in improving and efficiently maintaining water supplies and laundry/shower facilities, which may be as effective in a

Table 6.24. *Cul de Sac valley: comparison of actual and amended (to 1977–81 prices) costs of the three snail control programmes*

(*In US $*)

	Type of control		
	Area-wide 1971–75[a]	Surveillance– mollusciciding 1975–77	Routine focal 1977–81
Labour	50753 (65%)	13861 (68%)	3501 (27%)
Equipment	4095 (5%)	821 (4%)	588 (5%)
Molluscicide	9738 (12%)	703 (3.5%)	7066 (55%)
Transport	13847 (18%)	4977 (24.5%)	1754 (14%)
Total	78433 (55 months)	20362 (24 months)	12909 (48 months)
Cost/person/year[b]	3.42	2.04	0.65
COLI factor	2.27	1.31	0
Amended cost/person/year	7.76	2.79	0.65

[a] Calculations based on US $1 = $2 Eastern Caribbean for comparison with other programmes.
[b] Based on 5000 population.

consolidation phase strategy and provide additional social and medical benefits.

The cost of the chemotherapy campaigns of 1975 and 1976 (Table 6.17), $11 756, is not included in Table 6.24 and it may be questioned whether routine focal control would have been effective without the earlier chemotherapy and the surveillance–mollusciciding programmes. Likewise, would the latter programme have been effective without the area-wide treatment? Results from Fond St Jacques (see Part 2 below) suggest that routine focal control can be as effective as area-wide control; those from the Marquis valley (Chapter 5) indicate that chemotherapy alone can reduce prevalence dramatically, but that a consolidation phase control strategy is required to prevent renewed transmission. Thus it is calculated that if chemotherapy had been given on the results of a 1971 stool survey using the Kato technique approximately 1700 persons would have been found *S. mansoni* positive. Oxamniquine was not available in 1971, but using the 1975 cost of treating people with hycanthone (US$8.02) a treatment campaign would have cost about $13 600. If routine focal snail control had been used from the start and continued for 10 years, the cost, allowing for COLI factor, would have been US $23 523. With the estimated chemotherapy costs ($13 600) the 10-year programme would have cost US $0.74 per head of population compared with the actual cost of the three phases of snail control plus chemotherapy (US $11 756) or $2.47 per head of population. It must be remembered however, that although the area-wide scheme was a research project the cost of preliminary studies, on which the control strategy was based, has not been included, nor have lesser costs that would have been incurred in determining sites for routine focal control.

Summary and recommendations

In the area-wide snail control scheme from 1970–75, an initial blanket mollusciciding programme ensured the treatment of all known snail habitats in six weeks. This was followed by a 4–5-month re-treatment surveillance project, when all the previously treated areas were checked for live snails, and if found they were molluscicided. This procedure led to a routine surveillance treatment technique which lasted for five years – all the original snail infested areas were searched on a two-weekly basis and where snails were found mollusciciding was carried out. Overall prevalence was reduced from 45% to 24%.

A less costly focal surveillance–mollusciciding control programme plus two intensive chemotherapy campaigns were then implemented. The scheme lasted for two years (1975–1977) and almost 1000 people were treated, using either hycanthone or oxamniquine. A total of 145 potential transmission sites (56 streams, 2 rivers and 87 main drains) were checked on a routine fortnightly basis and were treated with molluscicide only if snails were found. This programme reduced prevalence from 24% to 6%.

A more efficient and cheaper system was required, and in April 1977 a routine focal mollusciciding programme was introduced. From the 145 sites which were checked in the previous scheme, 12 streams and 26 main drains were chosen for routine, four-weekly applications of molluscicide regardless of whether they had snails or not. This programme operated for four years. There was no resurgence of transmission, suggesting that in this area routine focal snail mollusciciding is an effective method of control in the follow-up phase after prevalence has been reduced to a low level.

Continuation of the programme is recommended in view of the reservoir of potential contamination remaining although this has been reduced by 92% in the high transmission areas. The reduction was less (77%) in the low transmission settlements, but generally these are on the hillsides, away from snail infested areas, and are probably of little importance in transmission. Government should expedite improved water supplies and provide, and maintain, additional standpipes and laundry shower units, particularly in those villages near the river: a minimum of one tub and one shower to every 10 households is suggested. Settlements which should be given priority were considered to be Ravine Poisson, L'Abayee, Bexon, Crown Lands, Soucis and Ti Colon.

PART 2 FOND ST JACQUES

Routine focal snail control

By 1974 results from Cul de Sac Valley indicated that area-wide snail control was having a marked effect on transmission of *S. mansoni*, but the cost was high. In view of the focality of transmission the effect of limiting the application of molluscicide only to transmission sites was investigated. Less chemical would be needed to kill potentially infected snails: a more cost-effective strategy should therefore result. This was investigated at Fond St Jacques, where a two-year period of pre-control studies (1974–76) was followed by a four-year period of routine focal snail control (Prentice, Jordan, Bartholomew & Grist, 1981).

The study area

As a result of surveys at schools in Soufriere and Fond St Jacques, a small comparatively isolated focus of transmission was found in the south-west of the island inland of the coastal town of Soufriere and close to Mount Gimie, the island's highest peak. Five communities occupy what little level ground there is in a narrow valley surrounded by hills. To the north the valley wall is precipitous, and as rainfall is very high (over 2550 mm) the streams are often torrential with no suitable snail habitats. The southern wall is less steep with numerous small dasheen (*Colocasia esculenta*) and water cress marshes on the lower slopes which are invariably infested with *B. glabrata*. (In Asia, dasheen is known as taro and in West Africa as coco-yam.) As flat land for agricultural purposes is scarce the hillsides have been cleared of vegetation for cultivation but, without terracing, the 'gardens' are quickly eroded and landslides are common.

The main stream in the area, Ravine Migny, arises from a grassy seepage at an altitude of about 533 m. It falls steeply and is joined, near the valley floor, by other streams from adjacent snail-infested marshes. At an altitude of about 250 m the gradient is less steep and the valley floor widens enough to allow human settlement in the villages of Migny, Ti Bourg (known collectively as Fond St Jacques) and, further downstream, St Phillip, Esperance and Ravine Claire. (Fig. 6.15) Owing to the shortage of flat ground, houses are close to each other and to the river. The settlements house a population of about 1250 persons. In 1971 a gravity-distributed piped water supply from a high altitude stream was provided by Government to the five communities. By 1980 approximately 50% of houses had an individual yard water supply, 7% depended on the rivers or streams and the rest used six public stand pipes. A laundry shower unit with six tubs, two showers and two latrines was constructed in Ti Bourg during 1978. Pit latrines were present in 82% of houses, septic tanks in 7%, while the remaining 11% had no waste disposal facilities. The communities are served by a church, a school and a health centre. A road connects the settlements to the coastal town of Soufriere at which point the Migny stream joins the Caribbean Sea.

In preliminary studies, although *B. glabrata* were frequently found in the marshes, very few were infected even in areas where adjacent stream populations were heavily infected. Infected snails were however commonly found in stream sites where direct defaecation during periods of gentle flow was likely to be the most important source of contamination.

Biological studies
Pre-control (1974–76)

The main objective was to investigate the dynamics of transmission and to develop a suitable focal control strategy. All streams and marshes were examined qualitatively for infected *B. glabrata*: based on these findings index sites in both types of habitat were selected. Snails were screened for infection in the field, and uninfected snails were returned to

Table 6.25. *Fond St Jacques: distribution of* B. glabrata *in stream and marsh index sites pre- and post-control*

	Pre-control (2 years' data)			Post-control (4 years' data)		
	No. exam.	No. +ve	% +ve	No. exam.	No. +ve	% +ve
Stream sites						
Ravine Claire (I1)[a]	1983	55	2.8	113	0	—
St Phillip (I2)	2918	187	6.4	7	0	—
Ti Bourg (I3)	3024	280	9.3	236	5	2.1
Belvedere (I4)	2979	7	0.2	1	0	—
Total	10904	529	4.9	357	5	1.4
Marsh sites						
Jeremie (I5)	1601	0	—	1409	0	—
Etang (I6) (Stream irrigated watercress)	1837	41	2.2[b]	—	—	—
Ti Bourg (I7) (Watercress)	2038	3	0.1	3114	0	—
Ti Bourg (I8) (Dasheen)	1661	27	1.6	4616	0	—
Ravine Claire (I9) (Dasheen)		—		7563	1	0.01
Belvedere (I10) (Dasheen)		—		7646	1	0.01
Total	5300	30	0.6	24349	2	0.008

[a] See Fig. 6.15.
[b] This site is excluded from the pre-control marsh total because it was irrigated by stream water.
Adapted from Prentice *et al,* 1981.

Fig.6.14. Fond St Jacques: pre-control snail data from Ti Bourg index sites showing effect of tropical storms on snail populations. (From Prentice *et al.,* 1981.)

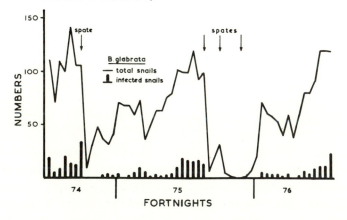

their original site: for ethical reasons infected snails were not. Sentinel snails were used to monitor miracidial densities at six sites.

The effect on snail populations of tropical storms was soon apparent; colonies in the streams were almost completely destroyed but were replenished with snails from the marshes. As these snails were uninfected there were periods of six weeks – or longer, when tropical storms were frequent – when no infected snails were present (Fig. 6.14).

Over the two-year period over 5000 field snails from six marsh index sites were examined and only 0.6% were infected compared with 4.9% of nearly 11 000 collected from four stream sites (Table 6.25).

The low infection rate in snails from the marshes confirmed that they played little part in transmission which was predominantly dependent on the stream colonies. Thus, if these could be reduced by mollusciciding at sites of human water contact, there would be considerable saving in the quantity of chemical required, particularly as control of snails in marshes had proved difficult elsewhere.

In view of the 4.9% cercarial infection rate amongst snails from stream index sites the low rate amongst sentinel snails, 0.29% (8 of 2747) in 1974 and 1975 (Table 6.26) was disappointing and could have been the result of a change in the susceptibility to infection of the laboratory bred snails. However, when snails were individually exposed to miracidia, infection rates similar to those obtained in previous years were obtained and in 1976 a much higher infection rate of 0.72% (17 of 2373) was obtained (Table 6.26).

Table 6.26. *Fond St Jacques:* S. mansoni *infection rates in sentinel* B. glabrata

	Ti Bourg			All sites		
	No. snails examined	No. infected	% infected	No. snails examined	No. infected	% infected
1974 (6 months)	101	2	1.98	746	4	0.54
1975	588	1	0.17	2001	4	0.20
1976	957	16	1.67	2373	17	0.72
1977	824	2	0.24	2056	2	0.97
1978	641	9	1.40	1591	17	1.07
1979	527	6	1.14	1304	20	1.53
1980	922	19	2.06	2279	55	2.41
1981[a] (6 months)	454	3	0.66	1134	8	0.71

[a] The lower rates in the first six months of 1981 were probably the result of chemotherapy offered after the last survey at the end of 1980.

Control strategy

Based on the above findings a strategy was devised whereby stretches of stream in which infected *B. glabrata* had been found, and which were human contact points, would be treated with niclosamide routinely at six-weekly intervals without prior surveillance.

Molluscicide carriage in streams was investigated by immersing caged snails at varying distances from a drip feed in the Migny stream. Although satisfactory kills were obtained within the required area of the molluscicide was ineffective beyond 2 km from the application point. This was a surprisingly poor carry in a fast flowing stream with a discharge of approximately 3 cusecs, and although the matter was taken up with the manufacturers no satisfactory explanation was forthcoming.

Parshall flow-rate measuring flumes were permanently built into the streams at appropriate points. A single flume served to measure the flow of several tributaries since frequent measurements had shown that the ratio of their individual discharges was reasonably constant. Tables were prepared which directly related the gauge reading to the required quantity of chemical. The lower limit of 0.5 l of concentrate ensured that very small streams were all over-dosed. This helped to compensate for molluscicide losses in these situations caused by their high perimeter to volume ratio. An upper limit of stream flow was also designated above which mollusciciding was unnecessary as snails would be flushed out. Niclosamide was applied at twelve dosing points from constant-flow drip cans (Prentice, 1971) at a target dose of 8 mg/l. If streams pooled out in the dry season their course was sprayed with a standard concentration of niclosamide.

Control: 1976–80

Mollusciciding started in October 1976 (during the rainy season) and was continued at monthly intervals. Molluscicide dispensing points are shown in Fig. 6.15.

Good control of stream snail populations was achieved from the outset. However, as stream flows decreased in the particularly dry season in 1977, relict pools formed at the stream edge and some contained snail populations. These were left to test the efficacy of the routine treatment, and in June and July four infected snails were found in a pool in Ravine Migny.

The last infected snail to be detected was found in the same pool in September; the colony was flushed free of snails the following month, and in the dry seasons of 1978 and 1979 fewer pools formed. In only one of these, alongside the St Phillip stream, were snails found in 1978. A few were found in 1979 but none was infected. Results of snail findings in index sites are shown in Table 6.25.

During the course of the programme two additional marsh sites were placed under surveillance as two of the original index sites were partially destroyed when they were cultivated. Apart from this, snail populations thrived, but only two snails (from the new sites) were infected in March 1979 (Fig. 6.16). Although heavy storms reduced snail populations slightly the effect was very temporary but numbers were drastically reduced in early 1981 after the final evaluation.

The quantity of molluscicide used varied from month to month in relation to flow rates. During the drier months of the year (January to June) the mean quantity of niclosamide was 13.4 l of 25% emulsifiable concentrate (range 11.3–16.0 l) compared with 17.6 l (range 14.7–20.5 l) in the rainy season. No treatment was given in August 1980 in the aftermath of Hurricane Allan.

Throughout the mollusciciding programme sentinel snail exposures continued. In general, and particularly in Ti Bourg, more infections were found from 1977 onwards (Table 6.26) which was consistent with an observed apparent increase in faecal contamination of the rocks in and on

Fig.6.15. Fond St Jacques: study area and location of index and sentinel snail sites, measuring flumes and treatment points. (Adapted from Prentice *et al.*, 1981.)

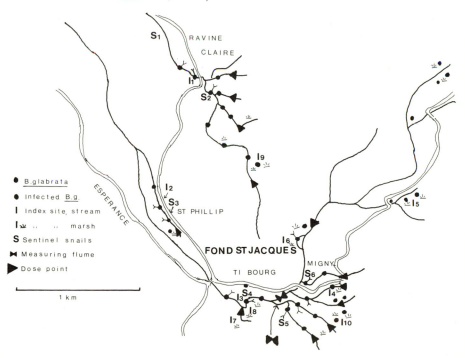

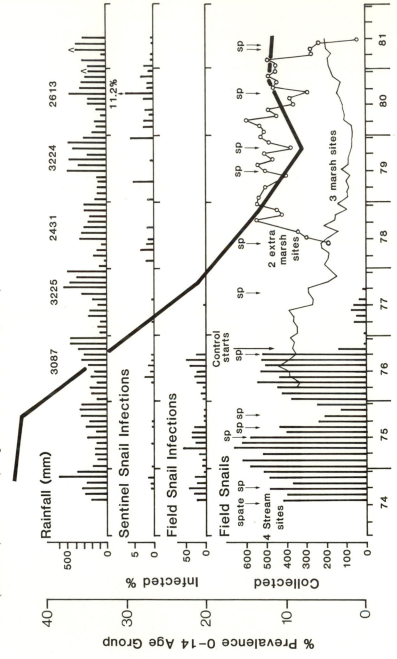

Fig. 6.16. Fond St Jacques: *S. mansoni* prevalence, sentinel and field snail data from stream (treated) and marsh (untreated) index sites. (Adapted from Prentice *et al.*, 1981.)

the edge of the streams. This may be because people were even less inhibited about disposal of faeces in the streams once control measures were operating. This attitude may have been reinforced with the construction of the laundry/shower unit in 1978, since elsewhere in St Lucia it was observed that the contamination level increased when streams were no longer essential for domestic purposes. (See p. 251.)

During the course of the mollusciciding the team was once attacked by a rock-throwing Rastafarian who objected strongly to the molluscicide passing through his dasheen garden. Further incidents and threats necessitated police intervention, following which there was no further trouble.

The main measuring flume was washed out in a tropical storm; since the flume was 'permanently' set in concrete the occurrence emphasises the violence of river flow which can follow such a deluge. The flume was replaced more securely in a more suitable place. In the absence of the flume, stream flow was measured by a flow meter.

Parasitological surveys

Pre-control

The first household census and stool survey of all age groups was made in 1974. A population of 625 males and 629 females was recorded. A survey was made of children in the following year and the final pre-control survey of all groups in 1976.

Prevalence varied in different settlements which were categorised into high and low transmission areas based on incidence of new *S. mansoni* infections being above or below 15% amongst 0–11-year-old children between 1974 and 1975 (Table 6.27).

Although incidence was lower between 1975 and 1976 than in the previous year, the difference was not significant (Table 6.30).

Table 6.27. *Fond St Jacques: overall prevalence by settlement in 1974 and 1976 with intervening incidence of new infections among 0–11-year-old children*

| Settlement | Overall prevalence (%) 1974 | 1974–75 | | 1975–76 | | Overall prevalence (%) 1976 |
		No. neg.	% inc.	No. neg.	% inc.	
Ti Bourg	54	31	29.0	25	20.0	38
Esperance	52	33	21.2	29	13.8	31
St Phillip	51	16	18.8	19	10.2	36
Ravine Claire	15	48	8.3	47	2.1	10
Migny	11	98	4.1	74	8.1	9

Changes in prevalence between 1974 and 1976 in the two sexes in the high and low transmission areas are shown in Fig. 6.17. Although overall prevalence was lower in 1976, the changes were not consistent. Amongst males, in the high transmission areas prevalence in 1976 in age groups to 50 years was significantly lower (at 5% level Z = 2.06), as it was among all age groups in the low transmission areas (Z = 2.29). Only among

Fig.6.17. Fond St Jacques: changes in *S. mansoni* prevalence between 1974 and 1976 (pre-control) among males and females in high and low transmission areas (solid and broken lines resp.).

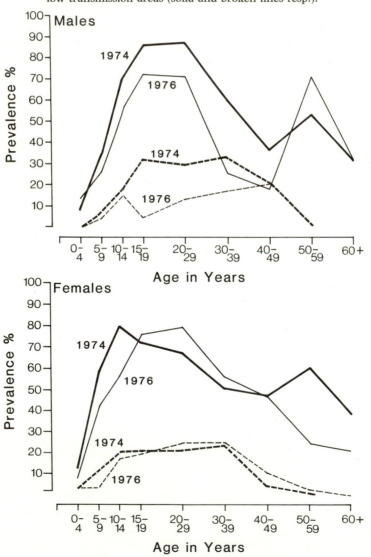

females to the age of 15 years in the high transmission areas was there a significant lowering of prevalence in 1976 compared with the 1974 rate ($Z = 2.57$, significant at the 1% level).

A pre-control cohort study showed the typical pattern of an endemic area with the C/R ratio among children being greater than 1, while amongst adults it was less than 1 with a corresponding decline in prevalence (Table 6.28).

The prevalence, intensity of infection and index of potential contamination at the start of control are shown in Table 6.29.

Effects of control

The effect on *S. mansoni* transmission of the focal snail control was monitored by annual stool examination of children to assess the incidence of new infections and by a final survey of all age groups in 1980. However, over the years the area had become one of the main centres of the Rastafarian movement in St Lucia and the response of the population to requests for stools at the 1976 and 1980 surveys left much to be desired, with even the children being less co-operative than usual; at the final survey only 52% of males and 66% of females submitted stool specimens for examination compared with 61% and 79% in 1976 and 82% and 85% in 1974.

Incidence of new infections in the high transmission settlements dropped from 15.1% to 5.6% in the first year of control, but showed no further decline thereafter. However, the 7.6% level in the last year of the study was significantly lower (at 0.5% level) than the pre-control 15.1% ($Z = 2.30$) (Table 6.30). In the low transmission settlements incidence was gradually reduced from 5.7% to 1.2% in the last year of control.

Table 6.28. *Fond St Jacques: summary of pre-control cohort study (1974–76)*

Age group		High transmission		Low transmission	
		0–14	15+	0–14	15+
No. examined		183	127	189	136
No. +ve (%)	1974	74 (40)	73 (58)	14 (7)	18 (13)
Conversions[a]		26	17	15	4
Reversions[b]		20	22	7	10
C/R ratio		1.30	0.77	2.14	0.40
No. +ve (%)	1976	80 (44)	68 (54)	22 (12)	12 (9)

[a] Conversions – negative in 1976, positive at 1980 survey.
[b] Reversions – positive in 1976, negative at 1980 survey.

Table 6.29. *Fond St Jacques: prevalence and intensity of S. mansoni infection and corrected index of potential contamination (IPC) in 1976*

	Males			Females			Both sexes				
Age in years	No. exam.	Prev. (%)	GM[a]	No. exam.	Prev. (%)	GM	% of pop. (1)	Prev. (%) (2)	GM (3)	Corrected IPC[b]	Relative IPC (%)[c]
High transmission											
0–4	35	14	13	37	8	17	17.2	11	15	28	3
5–9	50	26	29	43	42	14	20.2	28	19	107	11
10–14	35	57	26	36	56	21	14.7	56	24	198	21
15–19	29	72	38	25	76	25	10.0	74	31	229	24
20–29	17	71	30	24	79	17	12.0	76	22	200	21
30–39	12	25	25[d]	25	56	17[d]	8.2	46	23	87	9
40–49	11	18	25[d]	19	47	17[d]	7.0	37	16	41	4
50–59	14	71	25[d]	17	24	17[d]	5.3	45	19	45	5
60+	13	4	25[d]	14	21	17[d]	5.4	26	10	13	2
0–14	120	32	25	116	35	17	(100)	31	21	(948)	(100)
15+	96	54	31	124	55	18		55	23		

GM: Males — Mean for all groups 14; Females — Mean for all groups 16; Both sexes — Mean for all groups 15.

	Males			Females			Both sexes				
Age in years	No. exam.	Prev. (%)	GM[a]	No. exam.	Prev. (%)	GM	% of pop. (1)	Prev. (%) (2)	GM (3)	Corrected IPC[b]	Relative IPC (%)[c]
Low transmission											
0–4	39	0		31	0		17.2	0		0	0
5–9	54	4		56	11		20.2	7		1	8
10–14	48	15		41	20		14.7	17		3	23
15–19	23	4		36	19		10.0	14		2	15
20–29	8	13		28	21		12.0	19		3	23
30–39	6	17		17	24		8.2	22		3	23
40–49	10	20		25	4		7.0	9		1	8
50–59	11	0		20	0		5.3	0		0	0
60+	11	0		15	0		5.4	0		0	0
0–14	141	6	14	128	11	16	(100)	8	15	(13)	(100)
15+	69	7	14	141	13	16		11	15		

GM: Males — Mean for all groups 14; Females — Mean for all groups 16; Both sexes — Mean for all groups 15.

[a] Geometric mean of e.p.ml faeces of infected persons.
[b] Product of (1) × (2) × (3)/100 for each age group.
[c] Expressed as a percentage of the sum of the product of all age groups ([b]).
[d] GM of age groups owing to few infected persons.

Table 6.30. *Fond St Jacques: changes in incidence of new S. mansoni infections among children to 11 years of age: 1974–76 pre-control, 1976–80 during routine focal control*

Age[a] in years	1974–75 No. neg.[b]	1974–75 % +ve[c]	1975–76 No. neg.	1975–76 % +ve	1976–77 No. neg.	1976–77 % +ve	1977–78 No. neg.	1977–78 % +ve	1978–79 No. neg.	1978–79 % +ve	1979–80 No. neg.	1979–80 % +ve
High transmission areas												
0 & 1	14	0.0	13	0.0	11	0.0	2	0.0	1	0.0	4	0.0
2 & 3	21	29.0	15	26.7	20	5.0	21	0.0	18	0.0	12	0.0
4 & 5	16	25.0	19	10.5	17	0.0	20	0.0	23	0.0	18	0.0
6 & 7	13	23.1	13	15.4	17	0.0	20	15.0	19	5.3	20	5.0
8 & 9	11	45.5	8	25.0	16	13.3	21	19.0	14	14.3	15	13.3
10 & 11	9	33.3	5	20.0	8	25.0	13	15.3	18	16.7	10	30.0
0–11	84	22.6[d]	73	15.1[d,e]	89	5.6	97	9.3	93	6.5	79	7.6[e]
Low transmission areas												
0 & 1	15	0.0	15	0.0	10	10.0	12	0.0	8	0.0	7	0.0
2 & 3	17	0.0	16	0.0	25	0.0	23	0.0	21	0.0	19	0.0
4 & 5	20	5.0	18	11.1	28	7.1	25	4.0	13	0.0	17	0.0
6 & 7	33	3.3	31	3.2	22	4.5	24	0.0	13	0.0	18	0.0
8 & 9	27	18.5	21	9.5	28	0.0	25	4.0	13	0.0	16	0.0
10 & 11	21	0.0	20	10.0	23	17.4	21	4.7	7	14.3	8	12.5
0–11	133	5.3	121	5.7	136	5.9	130	2.3	75	1.3	85	1.2

[a] Age at first of two surveys.

[b] Number negative at first of two surveys.

[c] Per cent positive at second survey.

[d] Difference between incidence rates not significant at 5% level (Z = 1.42).

[e] Difference between incidence rates significant at 0.5% level (Z = 2.30).

Table 6.31. *Fond St Jacques: summary of changes in prevalence of*
S. mansoni *infection among males and females following routine focal snail*
control

Age group	Males				Females			
	1976		1980		1976		1980	
	No. exam.	% +ve	No. exam.	% +ve	No. exam.	% +ve	No. exam.	% +ve
High transmission areas								
0–14	120	32	91	4	116	35	79	20
15+	96	54	55	29	124	55	92	37
Total	216	42	146	14	240	45	171	29
Low transmission areas								
0–14	141	6	108	4	128	11	84	2
15+	69	7	47	9	141	13	105	7
Total	210	7	155	5	269	12	189	5

Fig.6.18. Fond St Jacques: changes in *S. mansoni* prevalence between
1976 and 1980 in high and low transmission areas after a four year
routine focal mollusciciding programme.

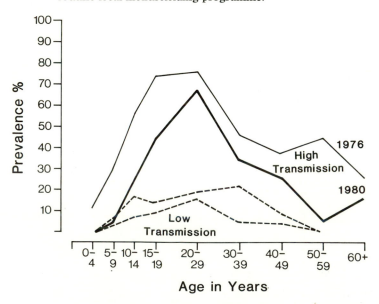

Reduced transmission led to a decline in prevalence from 44% to 22% and from 9% to 5% in the high and low transmission areas respectively (Fig. 6.18). In high transmission areas the decline tended to be greater amongst males than females; at the 1976 survey prevalence rates in children and adults were similar in the two sexes, but at the 1980 survey they were significantly lower amongst males ($Z = 4.94$, significant at

Table 6.32. *Fond St Jacques: prevalence, intensity of infection and crude IPC in high and low transmission areas in 1976 and after four years of routine focal mollusciciding*

Age group	1976 No. exam.	% +ve	GM[a]	1980 No. exam.	% +ve	GM
High transmission areas						
0–4	72	11	15	31	0	
5–9	93	33	19	77	5	
10–14	71	56	24	62	26	Mean
15–19	54	74	31	18	44	for
20–29	41	76	22	33	67	all
30–39	37	46	23	26	35	ages
40–49	30	37	16	19	26	21
50–59	31	45	19	19	5	
60+	27	26	10	32	16	
0–14	236	33	20	170	12	21
15+	220	55	23	147	34	21
Crude IPC[b]		8867			4703	
Reduction				47%		
Low transmission areas						
0–4	70	0		53	0	
5–9	110	6		79	3	
10–14	89	17	Mean	60	7	Mean
15–19	59	14	for	35	9	for
20–29	36	19	all	38	16	all
30–39	23	22	ages	19	5	ages
40–49	35	9	14	25	4	11
50–59	31	0		18	0	
60+	26	0		27	0	
0–14	269	8	14	192	3	11
15+	210	11	14	162	7	11
Crude IPC		1218			484	
Reduction				60%		

[a] Geometric mean of e.p.ml faeces.
[b] Sum of product of prevalence and GM for each age group.

0.01% level) (Table 6.31). In low transmission areas the reduction in prevalence was greater in females than in males. Intensity of infection was little affected and the IPC in the high and low transmission areas was reduced by only 47% and 60% (Table 6.32).

In spite of the poor response at the final survey, cohort studies confirmed that transmission had been reduced (Table 6.33).

Chemotherapy and further control

At the conclusion of the programme treatment was offered to all known to have been infected. A total of 254 (74%) received oxamniquine, but 90 persons did not accept treatment. In addition, *T. granifera* were introduced into the stream system (see Chapter 12).

Mollusciciding costs

A breakdown of costs of the four year project is shown in Table 6.34.

The programme was carried out by two semi-skilled workers who completed the treatment at 12 application points in two days.

Equipment costs included the measuring flumes and their installation in addition to drip feed equipment.

The mean annual cost per person protected($3.52) is relatively high owing to two factors: (i) the high transport expenditure due to the distance from Research and Control Department to the operational area, and (ii) the steep terrain which limits the number of persons living in the area. This

Table 6.33. *Fond St Jacques: summary of post-control cohort study (1976–80), cf. Table 6.28*

Age group		High transmission		Low transmission	
		0–14	15+	0–14	15+
No. examined		112	91	125	92
No. +ve (%)	1976	32 (29)	43 (47)	9 (7)	10 (11)
Conversions[a]		9	10	6	2
Reversions[b]		19	22	6	5
C/R ratio		0.47	0.45	1.0	0.40
No. +ve (%)	1980	22 (20)	31 (34)	9 (7)	7 (8)

[a] Conversions – negative in 1976, positive at 1980 survey.
[b] Reversions – positive in 1976, negative at 1980 survey.

is small in relation to the number and size of streams needing mollusciciding: the cost per person protected is, therefore, disproportionately high, but parasitological results show routine focal mollusciciding as effective as area-wide control in St Lucia (Chapter 9).

Summary and recommendations

The Fond St Jacques area was used to test the efficacy of routine focal snail control.

Pre-control studies began in 1974 and continued for two years. Transmission was shown to be associated with localised snail colonies near washing sites in several streams. Although *B. glabrata* was widespread and locally abundant in seepage marshes, these rarely contained infected snails and were important mainly as reservoirs of snails.

Following tropical storms snails re-populated stream index sites within two or three weeks, but infected snails were absent for six weeks or longer. This suggested that a control programme based on routine application of molluscicides at four week intervals to remove snails from limited stretches of the stream would be effective.

Twelve dosing points were selected. Stream flow was measured by reference to gauges on three Parshall Flumes set at strategic points and the quantity of molluscicide needed was read off from a table. Niclosamide was dripped into the streams from constant flow devices for one hour every month. Two semi-skilled workers were able to complete treatment in two days.

Control of the stream snail population began in October 1976 and was effective at once; a few snails persisted in relict pools towards the end of the 1977 dry season, but since then no *B. glabrata* were collected from

Table 6.34. *Fond St Jacques: breakdown in costs of four years of routine focal molluscicide control, 1976–80*

	Cost (US $)[a]	% of total
Labour	2129	12
Equipment and supplies	2642	15
Molluscicide	10204	58
Transport	2605	15
Total	17580 (48 months)	
Cost per person per year	3.52	

[a] Calculations based on US $1 = EC $2.

streams within the control area. From January 1981 the treatment interval was extended to six weeks within a 50% saving in costs.

The cost was US $3.52 per person protected. This figure is atypically high because the topography of the area severely limited population size.

Recommendations were made to Government to continue the routine focal mollusciciding and to supplement the standpipe water system (which has a good water supply) with more laundry/shower units.

7

Environmental control of transmission

Greany (1952), working in the Sudan, appears to have been the first worker reporting lower schistosomiasis prevalence rates amongst communities having access to well-water; later, in Egypt, it was reported that even the partial use of protected water markedly reduced prevalence rates (Farooq *et al.*, 1966*b*). However, the first deliberate attempts to control transmission by the installation of communal water supplies were made by Pitchford in South Africa and Barbosa in Brazil. In South Africa, in addition to providing water, simple swimming pools were built, and contact with infected water sources was prevented by the erection of wire fences (Pitchford. 1970); in Brazil latrines were provided (Barbosa *et al.*, 1971). In Venezuela communal water supplies were an integral part of the Public Health campaign to combat transmission (Jove & Marszewski, 1961).

Macdonald (1965) postulated that reduction of exposure to cercarial infested water by the provision of 'safe' water would also lead to lower snail infection rates as the risk of contamination of surface waters would be reduced if the population went to the river or pond less frequently for their domestic water requirements.

Since the development of water supplies in rural areas is of prime concern in many of the Third World countries, it was important to assess in depth their effect on transmission of schistosomiasis, as well as their other medical and social benefits. Water supplies in developing countries can, however, mean virtually anything – they may consist of simple protected springs or shallow wells, often barely capable of producing more than a few hundred litres of water a day, or, if piped water is provided, the supply is often unreliable and distributed through inadequate, poorly maintained communal standpipes. It has been shown that health benefits are greatest when water outlets are provided in the house or in the yard (Hollister, Beck, Gittelsohn & Hemphill, 1955).

In this chapter the effect on transmission of schistosomiasis of different water delivery systems is investigated: an individual household water supply was compared with a communal standpipe system in the comparison area. This system was later upgraded and the effect on transmission of additional laundry and shower units was studied. After chemotherapy the value of the household and standpipe water supplies in the consolidation or maintenance phase of control were investigated. The effect of an individual household supply was further investigated in two areas where populations were also offered selective population chemotherapy or latrines.

Part 1. RICHEFOND VALLEY

(i)   Individual household water supplies

If the provision of water was to be effective in reducing exposure to infested rivers, it was thought necessary to provide for *all* the domestic water requirements of the population at sites more convenient than the nearest potentially infected alternative water supply. It seemed essential also that *adequate* water be provided and that the system be *well maintained*.

Individual household supplies were planned for five settlements in the south-west of the Richefond (Mabouya) valley where *S. mansoni* was common. The effect of these water supplies was assessed and compared with the effect of a Government communal standpipe water system in settlements on the other side of the valley.

Water was obtained from three different sources. Thus, in the village of Grande Ravine water was provided from an infiltration gallery close to a stream which dried completely during periods of low rainfall between 1971 and 1974. The largest system, serving Thomazo, Grande Riviere and Morne Panache I, was supplied from surface water from a stream with a good flow, while in the smallest, supplying Debonnaire, surface water was collected from two streams with very limited flow and led to a storage tank to collect water at night to provide sufficient for the following day.

The study and comparison areas

Richefond valley is Y-shaped with a wide valley floor to the west narrowing towards the east where the main river, the Mabouya, enters the Atlantic. The valley is relatively isolated: to the north and west hills rise to over 350 m and apart from footpaths there is little communication with the sparsely populated adjacent Louvet valley to the north. There is no direct way into the Marquis valley to the north-west. The western boundary is formed by the Barre de l'Isle – the island's central mountain ridge – and to the south uninhabited hills rise to over 250 m, over which a single road winds to the Errard valley where *S. mansoni* transmission does not occur (Fig. 7.1).

Hills to the north of the valley are drained by the Derniere Riviere and other streams which enter the Mabouya river. The Grande Ravine, a stream from the Barre de l'Isle, flows across the centre of the valley to join the Derniere Rivere. The main river, the Mabouya, rises in the centre of the island, flows in a north-easterly direction and drains a large area of the eastern side of the Barre de l'Isle. Other tributaries drain the southern hillsides of the valley. The village of Grande Ravine is close to the stream with the same name: it is on a small promontory towards the western end of the valley. This village and others in the south-western corner of the valley – Thomazo on the main road down the Barre de l'Isle, Grande Riviere where the road reaches the valley floor, and Morne Panache I and Debonnaire on the foothills of the southern side of the valley – were selected for assessing the impact of water supplies on *S. mansoni* transmission.

On the north side of the valley, settlements of Belmont, Morne Panache II, Derniere Riviere, La Ressource and La Pearl are situated close to the river. A sixth settlement, Richefond, lies towards the southern side of the valley. Incidence rates in these six villages were similar to those in the high transmission areas of Cul de Sac and were used as comparison areas there, and for the five villages in the south west of the valley provided with experimental water supplies (EWS). Three settlements, Au Leon, Despinose and Gadette, higher on the northern hillside, were comparison areas for the low transmission areas of Cul de Sac (Chapter 5).

Under a Government water supply programme introduced in this area in 1969 to counter endemic typhoid, 16 public standpipes were constructed

Fig.7.1. Richefond valley: map of the study area.

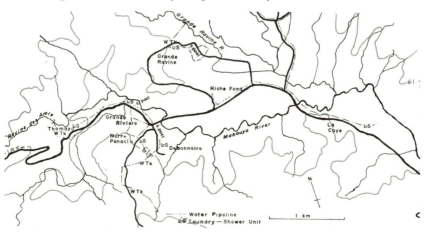

along the road at approximately 350 m intervals. Some householders paid for connections to be made to their homes.

The five settlements chosen for the experimental water supplies had a population of approximately 2000 persons living in the typical small wooden houses common throughout rural parts of St Lucia. Adequate sanitary facilities were generally lacking as in other areas, and water supplies consisted of one protected spring in Grande Riviere and an additional single pipe from a surface water stream (at one time heavily infected with schistosome cercariae) in Morne Panache I. Essentially the population was dependent on the main river or tributaries for domestic water which had to be carried a considerable distance up steep inclines to the houses (Table 7.1).

Investigations showed that on average 15 l per person per day were carried from the river over rough, steep paths to the houses (Unrau, 1975). For the 2000 population in the five villages to be provided with this water it was necessary to carry nearly 25 000 kg daily. Women and boys did most of this – the energy wasted by such an exercise was enormous (White, Bradley & White, 1972).

The floor of Richefond valley is used for banana cultivation; the root drainage system used in the sugar fields is still present. Recently there has been some diversification of crops and a considerable extension of the area under banana cultivation on the sides of the valley following illegal deforestation. This resulted in markedly reduced stream flows and the need to find a higher alternative source for the Government water supply.

Hydrological data: design of water systems

The rugged terrain, the hillside location of some of the houses, and, in spite of numerous small streams, the absence of a suitable river for a

Table 7.1. *Richefond valley south – experimental water supply (EWS) settlements: mean distance water was carried from source to house*

	Distance water carried (metres)	
	Range	Mean
Grande Ravine	137–480	342
Thomazo	37–549	217
Grande Riviere	14–549	226
Morne Panache I	4–494	304
Debonnaire	82–242	165

gravity fed distribution system, led to problems in finding water sources suitable for supplying *adequate* water. Estimated water requirements were based on a need to supply 114 l *per caput* per day and allowance was made for double the initial population. Consumption records of actual use proved this estimate to be high; thus designs based on 60 l/person/day would provide adequate capacity (Unrau, 1978). (After eight years of constant monitoring, consumption remained at *circa* 45 l/person.)

Flow rates of streams were determined at sites which might be suitable for intake points. In the Grande Ravine the flow rate of 1000 l/min was considered adequate for supplying the nearby village, but the use of surface water from this source was precluded since in some years it dried in the early months of the year and was subjected to a considerable amount of animal and human pollution. These problems could, however, be overcome by the use of an infiltration gallery (to filter the water) if a suitable location could be found. Five test wells were sunk close to the stream to determine the level of the water table, and the rate of water flow through the soil – found to be 57 l/min. From this, the effective trench area required for providing the necessary water was calculated. Although test wells were made during the rainy season, the infiltration gallery later provided adequate water in periods of low rainfall. The design of the infiltration gallery is shown in Fig. 7.2.

Water was pumped from the central well through a 5 cm diameter polyvinylchloride (PVC) line to an 83 m³ storage tank at an elevation 38 m above the well. The electric motor driving the pump was activated by a time clock to pump at appropriate times to ensure adequate stored water

Fig.7.2. Richefond valley – EWS settlements: design of infiltration gallery. (From Unrau, 1975.)

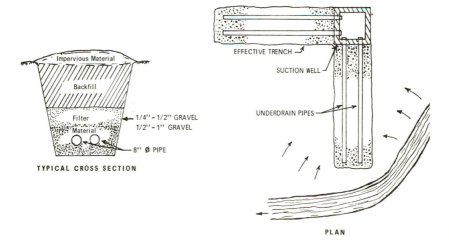

for peak usage times during the day. (Power lines were brought in specifically for the pump: this changed the settlement considerably as many houses paid for a connection for lighting (principally) and other uses. Laundry units were also initially provided with lights for night use, but vandals stole the light bulbs. A street light installed near the units was substituted for the unit lights.) A 5 cm main served a distribution loop of 2.5 cm pipe: household connections were made with 2 cm pipe.

The location of the storage tank was dependent on the ability of the pump to lift water a total dynamic head of 73 m (elevation plus friction losses). In order to provide for 10 houses above the tank a laundry and shower unit was provided. In addition, a simple cement-lined swimming pool for the children was constructed in the centre of the village.

The flow rate in the rock-strewn and fast flowing Ravine des Amis was 1700 l/min and adequate for supplying Thomazo, Grande Riviere and Morne Panache I. (Another village on the northern side of the valley has the same name: it is designated II.) An intake point, well away from human population, was found so that contamination was not a problem and surface water could be used safely.

A small dam was built across the stream; water was piped to a sedimentation chamber to remove sand etc. and then to a suction well from which it was pumped by means of a 15 kilowatt motor to a 159 m³ storage tank located at an elevation of 98 m on the top of Thomazo hill, requiring a dynamic head of 103 m. The galvanised steel tank was assembled from sections hauled up the very steep hillside on a skid with the help of shear legs at the top of the hill and a winch on the front of a truck at the bottom.

From the tank, distribution was by gravity through PVC mains to Thomazo and Grande Riviere, then by looped distribution lines. Owing to the varying elevations of houses to be supplied with water, low and high pressure distribution systems were required and pressure-reducing chambers and tanks were necessary in appropriate places. A few houses at Morne Panache I were above the point to which water would flow by gravity so that, as in Grande Ravine, a laundry and shower unit was built at the highest point water would reach.

Originally, Debonnaire, a village of 60 houses, was served by the most simple of systems – surface water from two small isolated streams with measured flows of only 475 l/m was collected by gravity, fed through a sedimentation tank and into an 83 m³ storage tank. A loop distribution system served the houses by gravity.

Later, however, owing to roadwork development near the original intake points, the sources of water became less satisfactory and an additional source higher on the hillside was found. A further 60 m³ storage tank was located at a higher elevation, enabling 10 additional houses to be served. As a safeguard against this small stream becoming dry, the system was connected to the Morne Panache supply.

Two swimming pools were built, one near a banana-packing shed at Grande Riviere, the other convenient for children of Debonnaire and Morne Panache I.

Water outlets to all houses were spring loaded Fordilla taps delivering about 7.5 l of water at each activation. (Fordilla taps are manufactured by Ford Meter Box Co., Wabash, Indiana, USA.) It was thought these taps could not be manipulated to provide a constant flow of water, but a St Lucian found a way! Appropriate modifications were subsequently made by the manufacturers (Fig. 7.3).

It had been hoped that the community could be motivated through health education to dig trenches for the main pipes, but while some progress was made it was too slow; subsequently household connections were made only when householders had dug the requisite trench to their home.

With an individual household water supply it was thought that washing of clothes in rivers would stop, and only two laundry and shower (L/S) units were planned at Grande Ravine and Morne Panache for the use of persons living in houses above an altitude to which water could be pumped economically.

Fig.7.3. Richefond valley – EWS settlements: householder shower arrangement with single Fordilla water tap. (From Unrau, 1975.)

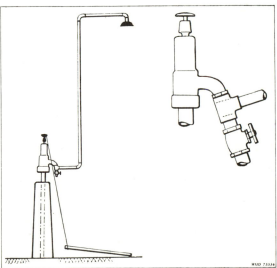

Fig. 7.4. Richefond valley – EWS settlements:: an operating laundry unit. (Note children who would normally be in the river while their mothers washed.) The shower unit is extreme left. (Photograph by G. O. Unrau.)

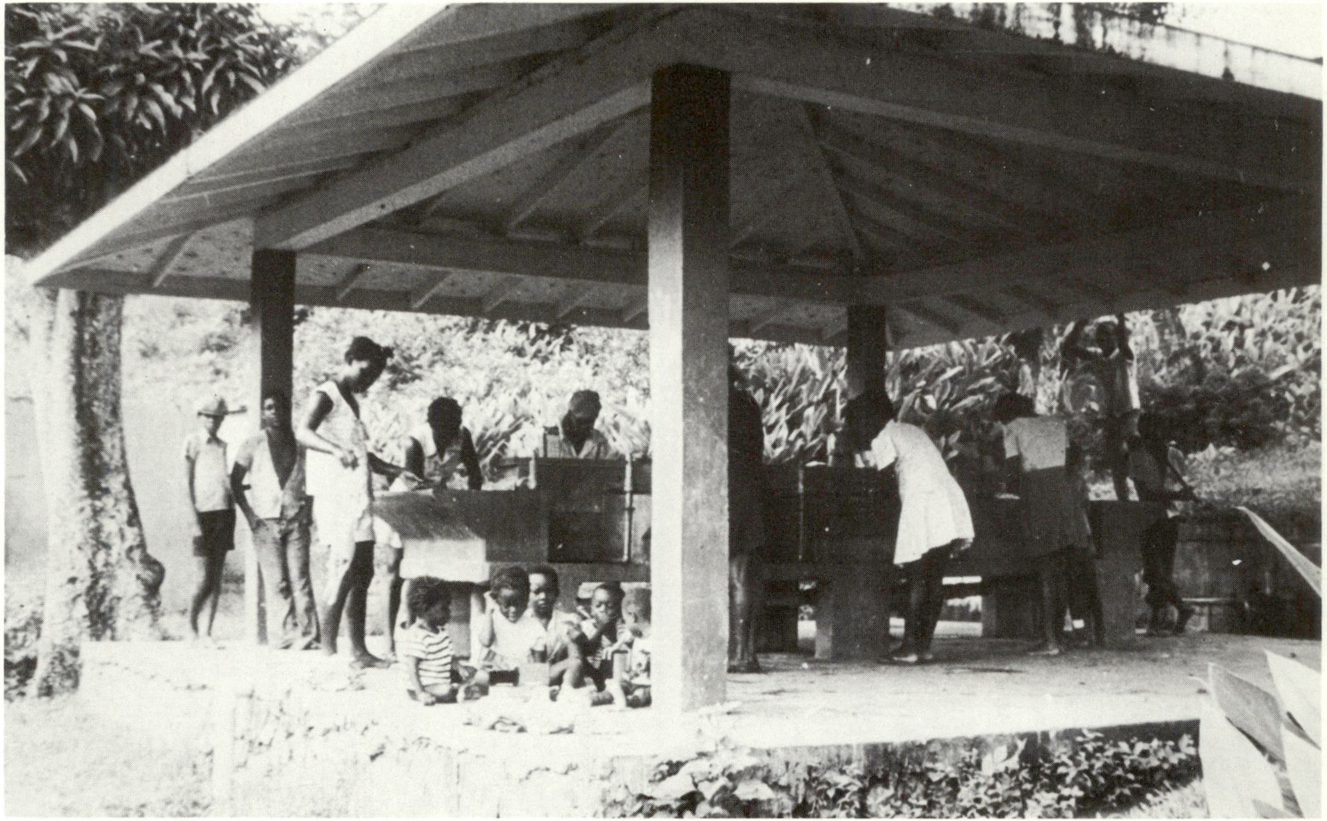

Although the household water supply was used for washing small quantities of clothes and by a few householders for the entire wash, the women at Grande Ravine and Morne Panache found their household taps inconvenient for large quantities of clothes and made use of the nearby laundry facilities. The stream previously used for washing at Grande Ravine was far from ideal, being slow flowing and tending to be muddy and, as at Morne Panache, at some distance from the village. It was soon apparent therefore that the laundry units, when conveniently located, were acceptable to the women and provided a meeting place for local gossip – said to make washing in rivers so popular (Figs. 7.4 and 7.5).

This was one of the reasons given by the women at the other settlements, Grande Riviere, Debonnaire and Thomazo, for continuing to wash in the river in spite of having a household water supply. A further reason was that they were used to a good flow of water for rinsing their clothes and there were good surfaces on sand, river banks, or rocks on which to spread their washing for bleaching by the sun.

There was some reduction in the numbers washing in the river after a health education campaign and the convenience of the L/S units was appreciated; the women agreed they would use laundries if provided at sites

Fig.7.5. Richefond valley – EWS settlements: laundry tubs are not only used for washing clothes. (Photograph by G. O. Unrau.)

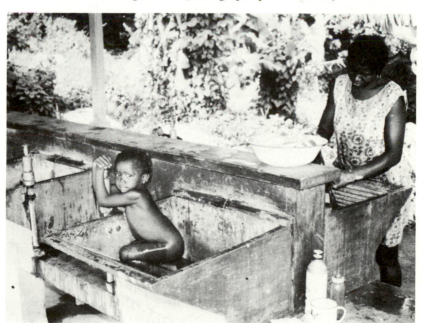

convenient to them. Additional units were therefore constructed at approved sites at Grande Riviere, Thomazo and Debonnaire.

Sites for laundry and shower units were either donated by land owners or compensation was paid, but it was apparent that if units were built on the land of unpopular families they would not be used by the rest of the community – the need for consultation with the women, particularly in respect of the siting of units, was therefore of paramount importance.

Experience showed that attention to a few simple aspects of construction of these units greatly facilitated their use and maintenance. Plumbing should be from one end of the unit, leaving the area beneath the tubs free of obstruction so as to make sweeping easier; the floor should be sloping to encourage drainage and there should be room on the bench adjacent to washing tubs for buckets or basins of clothes.

Water treatment in the different systems was simple, consisting only of plain sedimentation or the infiltration gallery, each combined with storage. Although chemicals were kept available no further treatment was required. Bacteriological analysis of water in the different systems was checked routinely and coliform counts were low except in one instance when they increased due to illegal pig farming on the bank of a tributary of Ravine des Amis. Once the offending animals had been removed the counts decreased.

The physical and chemical properties of the water supplied were within acceptable ranges. However, the iron and manganese content was near the upper limit in the Grande Ravine supply and mineral deposits in the pipe-lines reduced flow in the distribution system. Staining and discoloration, noticeable in the pool, were due to the chemical reaction with chlorination.

All the pools were chlorinated daily and cleaned as needed, but in general they were used less than expected; however, use varied with season and school sessions. Daily chlorination has little meaning to those unfamiliar with chemical treatment, and the local feeling that 'static' water is stale water may have been partly responsible for the limited use made of them. Clean water left in a bucket overnight is considered unfit for use and usually discarded.

Installation of water to the five settlements took $2\frac{1}{2}$ years. Grande Ravine, the first village supplied, received water in mid-1970; Grande Riviere, Thomazo and Morne Panache I in 1971 and Debonnaire in 1972.

Parasitological findings

Children were examined annually, 1968 to 1975, and adults in 1968, 1970, 1972 and 1975. Results thus show changes in the pre-control period (1968–70), during installation of water (1970–72), and when all villages had water (1972–75). Similar surveys were made in the comparison area.

Pre-control

Pre-control data from individual villages selected for the experimental water supply (EWS) are shown in Table 7.2.

Unlike other control valleys, villages with EWS have not been categorised into high and low transmission areas as Debonnaire was the only one with incidence less than 15% between 1969–70.

Except for Grande Ravine, settlements showed an increase in incidence in 1969–70 and overall prevalence in 1970 was higher than in 1968 in all five villages. The increase had not affected children to the age of 9 years, but among adults of both sexes the increase was significant at the 0.1% level ($Z = 4.06$ and 5.77 for males and females respectively) (Fig. 7.6 and cf. Fig. 4.4). At the 1970 survey, among adults, prevalence tended to be higher in females than males but intensities of infection were similar. The 5–19-year age group was potentially responsible for 67% of contamination (Table 7.3). Sixty-five and 68% of males and females respectively were examined.

During installation of water

Between 1970 and 1972, when water supplies were being installed, incidence of new infections was only a little lower than in the two previous years (Table 7.4) but, between 1971 and 1972 (when four

Table 7.2. *Richefond valley south – EWS settlements: overall prevalence by settlement at 1968 survey and subsequent incidence of new S. mansoni infections amongst children aged 0–9 years*

	Overall prevalence (%) 1968	1968–69[a]		1969–70		Overall prevalence (%) 1970
		No. neg.[b]	% inc.[c]	No. neg.	% inc.	
Grande Ravine	50	45	53.3	42	40.5	72
Thomazo	30	22	18.2	30	20.0	41
Grande Riviere	42	74	17.6	79	40.0	53
Morne Panache I	37	30	10.0	48	16.7	51
Debonnaire	34	34	8.8	28	10.7	49

[a] Approximately 18 months between surveys (% incidence *not* adjusted to 12 months rate).
[b] Number negative at first of two surveys.
[c] Percentage positive at second survey.

Fig.7.6. Richefond valley – EWS settlements: change in *S. mansoni* prevalence between 1968 and 1970 (pre-control) among males and females.

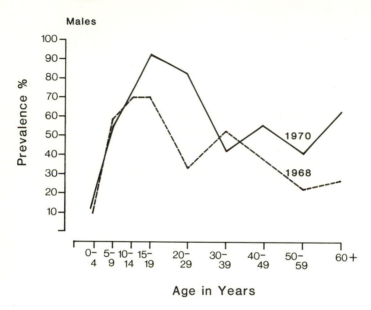

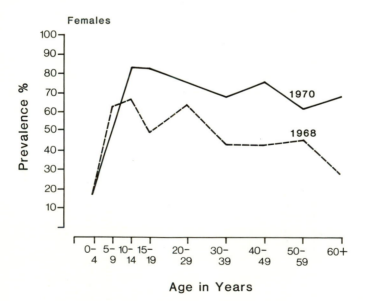

Table 7.3. *Richefond valley south – EWS settlements: prevalence, intensity of S. mansoni infection and index of potential contamination (1970)*

Age in years	Males			Females			Both sexes				
	No. exam.	Prev. (%)	GM[a]	No. exam.	Prev. (%)	GM	% pop.	Prev. (%)	GM	Corrected IPC	Relative IPC (%)
0–4	112	14	15	113	17	22	17.2	15	19	49	2
5–9	127	54	28	110	52	43	20.2	53	34	364	16
10–14	92	74	49	67	84	41	14.7	78	45	516	23
15–19	25	92	71	52	83	77	10.0	86	75	645	28
20–29	38	82	34	63	76	40	12.0	78	38	356	16
30–39	12	42	14	41	68	23	8.2	62	22	112	5
40–49	25	56	28	42	76	21	7.0	69	22	106	5
50–59	27	41	22	42	62	17	5.3	54	18	52	2
60+	19	63	19	25	68	18	5.4	66	18	64	3
0–14	331	46	33	290	46	38	(100)	46	36	(2264)	(100)
15+	146	66	34	265	73	31		71	32		

[a] Geometric mean of egg output.

of the five villages had water), it was significantly lower than in the comparison area where the incidence rose from 21% to 39.4% (Table 4.9).

After installation of water

Between 1972 and 1973, with water supplies in all villages, incidence dropped from 25.7% to 11.3% (Table 7.5), and was subsequently

Table 7.4. *Richefond valley south – EWS settlements: annual incidence of new S. mansoni infections amongst children (prior to control 1968–70) and during installation of water (1970–72)*

(cf. Table 4.9)

Age in years[a]	1968–69		1969–70		1970–71		1971–72[d]	
	No. neg.[b]	% inc.[c]	No. neg.	% inc.	No. neg.	% inc.	No. neg.	% inc.
0 & 1	42	9.5	48	16.6	35	8.6	50	6.0
2 & 3	67	14.9	63	12.7	52	17.3	70	20.0
4 & 5	42	16.6	55	29.1	47	23.4	70	24.3
6 & 7	30	46.6	32	43.8	35	31.4	46	28.3
8 & 9	24	50.0	35	34.3	20	40.0	30	46.7
10 & 11					(10	30.0)	(18	66.7)
0–9	205	25.9	233	27.9	189	22.2	226	22.9

[a] Age at first of two surveys.
[b] Number negative at first of two surveys.
[c] Number positive at second of two surveys.
[d] Debonnaire was the only village without water in this period.

Table 7.5. *Richefond valley south – EWS settlements: incidence of new S. mansoni infections after installation of water.*

(Note declining incidence in 0–5-year-olds)

Age in years	1971–72[a]		1972–73		1973–74		1974–75	
	No. neg.	% inc.	No. neg.	% inc.	No. neg.	% inc.	No. neg.	% inc.
0 & 1	50	6.0	40	5.0	29	3.4	21	0
2 & 3	70	20.0	55	10.9	49	8.2	59	5.1
4 & 5	70	24.3	56	14.3	43	9.3	54	5.6
6 & 7	46	28.3	50	14.0	58	19.0	63	19.0
8 & 9	30	46.7	24	12.5	47	17.0	50	20.0
10 & 11	18	66.7	6	0	25	24.0	39	28.2
0–11	284	25.7	231	11.3	251	13.5	286	13.6

[a] Debonnaire was the only village without water in this period.

Table 7.6. Richefond valley: summary of results of three cohort studies in the experimental water supply areas before, during and after installation of water and in comparison areas

	1968–1970 Before installation			1970–72 During installation			1972–1975 After installation		
		Age group (years)			Age group (years)			Age group (years)	
	Year	0–14	15+	Year	0–14	15+	Year	0–14	15+
Experimental water supply									
No. examined		341	195		455	217		507	257
No. +ve (%)	1968	145 (43)	88 (45)	1970	231 (51)	169 (78)	1972	257 (51)	183 (71)
Conversions		89**	70**		61*	23		38**	26**
Reversions		15**	8**		37*	28		105**	86**
C/R ratio		5.93	8.75		1.65	0.82		0.36	0.30
No. +ve (%)	1970	219 (64)	150 (77)	1972	255 (56)	164 (76)	1975	190 (37)	123 (48)
Comparison									
No. examined		390	332		614	349		635	342
No. +ve (%)	1968	164 (42)	165 (50)	1970	212 (34)	234 (67)	1972	343 (54)	266 (78)
Conversions		108**	89**		198**	52*		95	17**
Reversions		33**	21**		39**	29*		75	95**
C/R ratio		3.27	4.24		5.07	1.79		1.27	0.18
No. +ve (%)	1970	239 (61)	203 (61)	1972	371 (60)	257 (74)	1975	363 (57)	188 (55)

* Difference between conversions and reversions significant at 5% level
** Difference between conversions and reversions significant at 1% level.

always lower than in the comparison area. Although there was no consistent overall decline over the next few years, this was noted amongst those aged 0–5 years. The lack of decline among older children is probably due to their being exposed to infection in the comparison area, where many went to school, having to ford streams to get there.

The changes in transmission in the three phases of the project (pre-control, during installation and post-control), are apparent from cohort studies (Table 7.6). Amongst cohorts of children, between 1968 and 1970 in the EWS and comparison area conversions exceeded reversions, C/R ratio 5.93 and 3.27 respectively, and the prevalence of infection increased in both areas. Between 1970 and 1972 when EWS water was available in some villages, the C/R ratio fell to 1.65 and cohort prevalence increased only from 51 to 56%: at the same time in the comparison area the C/R ratio was a high 5.07 and cohort prevalence increased from 34 to 60%. Between 1972 and 1975, with water in all five settlements, the C/R ratio dropped to 0.36 with a consequent reduction in the prevalence rate among children from 51 to 37%. In the comparison area over the same three years conversions again exceeded reversions (C/R ratio 1.27) with an increase in cohort prevalence (54 to 57%).

Amongst adults, as the typical age prevalence curve shows declining rates in the older age groups, reversions would be expected to exceed conversions. In both study areas, therefore, the reverse finding between 1968 and 1970 was atypical and indicated unusually high transmission. Between

Fig. 7.7. Richefond valley – EWS settlements: change in *S. mansoni* prevalence among cohorts of 1–14-year-old males and females with individual household water supplies for four years (1971–75). (T – theoretical finding if transmission ceased for four years; it does not allow for worm deaths.)

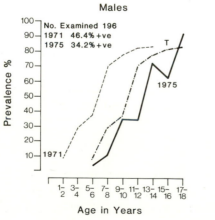
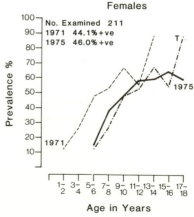

Males

Females

1970 and 1972 the same finding in the comparison area was associated with the very high incidence recorded for children between 1971 and 1972 (Table 4.9). In the EWS area reversions exceeded conversions, C/R ratio 0.82, compared with 8.75 in the previous two years, but in the following three-year period the decline continued with reversions greatly exceeding conversions (C/R ratio 0.30) and the prevalence in the adult cohort fell from 71% to 48%. In the comparison area at the same time a decline in cohort prevalence from 78 to 55% was noted, a usual finding when transmission is steady.

The lower incidence in the EWS settlements between 1970 and 1975 led to prevalence being reduced from 56% to 38% and intensity of infection from 34 to 17 eggs/ml, with a 68% reduction in the crude level of potential contamination compared with the 1970 data (Table 7.8). The decline in prevalence was greater in boys (C/R ratio 0.40) than girls (C/R ratio 1.16) (Fig. 7.7).

These findings indicate that in St Lucia the domestic water supplies reduced exposure to cercarial infested water and had a marked effect on transmission of *S. mansoni* over the period studied.

Chemotherapy supplement (1975–77)

By 1975 it was apparent that the individual household water supplies had reduced transmission markedly. A chemotherapy campaign was therefore planned. It was explained to the people that they were no longer getting infected and therefore treatment would be given to those infected as the risk of re-infection was slight. The news that new infections were not occurring was interpreted that the rivers were free of infection, there was a return to them for recreational purposes, and incidence increased to pre-control levels (Table 7.7). The very high incidence resulting from exposure for only a few months supports the views expressed elsewhere that rivers and streams are subjected to more pollution when they cease to be the source of a domestic water supply once piped water is available. After the 1975 survey 461 persons were treated with a further 290 after the 1976 survey. Oxamniquine was given in a single dose of 15 mg/kg body weight; in 1976 and 1977 this was increased to 20 mg/kg for children. In the year after the last treatment incidence was reduced to 6.4% (Table 7.7).

Maintenance phase (1977–81)

After the treatment in 1977 no further action was taken, but transmission was monitored until 1981 to assess the value of the water supplies in the maintenance phase of control (Table 7.7). Although there

Table 7.7. *Richefond valley south – EWS settlements: annual incidence of new S. mansoni infections following chemotherapy in 1975 and 1976 and in the maintenance phase 1977–81*

Age in years	1975-76		1976-77		1977-78		1978-79		1979-80		1980-81	
	No. neg.[a]	% inc.[b]	No. neg.	% inc.	No. neg.	% inc.	No. neg.	% inc.	No. neg.	% inc.	No. neg.	% inc.
0 & 1	40	5.0	23	0	11	0	15	0	13	0	14	0
2 & 3	55	14.5	53	3.8	47	2.1	35	2.9	20	5.0	21	0
4 & 5	77	20.8	58	12.1	41	4.9	53	3.8	32	6.3	22	0
6 & 7	60	48.3	50	16.0	51	5.9	45	1.0	31	12.9	36	5.6
8 & 9	72	31.9	61	16.4	58	3.4	48	8.3	37	8.1	35	2.9
10 & 11	52	42.2	57	21.1	59	15.3	49	4.1	27	0	35	2.9
0–11	356	28.7	302	12.9	267	6.4	245	10.4	160	6.3	163	1.0

[a] Number negative at first of two surveys.
[b] Percentage positive at second survey.

Table 7.8. *Richefond valley south – EWS settlements: prevalence, intensity of infection and level of potential contamination by phase of control programme*

Age in years	1970			1975			1977			1981		
	No. exam.	% +ve	GM[a]	No. exam.	% +ve	GM	No. exam.	% +ve	GM	No. exam.	% +ve	GM
0–4	225	15	19	208	7	13	140	2	18[b]	105	1	10[b]
5–9	237	52	34	278	23	17	230	11	18[b]	169	3	10[b]
10–14	159	78	45	232	50	17	227	19	12	176	11	16
15–19	77	86	75	144	60	19	98	20	22	81	20	16
20–29	101	78	38	144	60	23	117	17	29	80	15	25
30–39	53	62	22	91	56	15	88	16	17	74	12	26
40–49	67	69	22	94	40	14	73	11	13[b]	67	10	11[b]
50–59	69	54	18	74	41	14	59	10	13[b]	53	4	11[b]
60+	44	66	18	75	39	15	71	11	13[b]	46	2	11[b]
0–14	621	46	36	718	27	17	597	12	14	450	6	17
15+	411	71	32	622	51	17	506	15	19	401	12	17
Crude IPC[c]	20053			6411			2083			1399		
Reduction by phase	68%			68%			33%					
Cumulative reduction				68%			90%			93%		

[a] Geometric mean of egg output/ml faeces.
[b] Based on GM of 0–9 and 40+ age groups owing to few uninfected persons.
[c] Sum of product of prevalence and GM for each age group.

Fig.7.8. Richefond valley – EWS settlements: *S. mansoni* prevalence in 1970, prior to control; after provision of water, 1975; after chemotherapy, 1977; and at conclusion of programme.

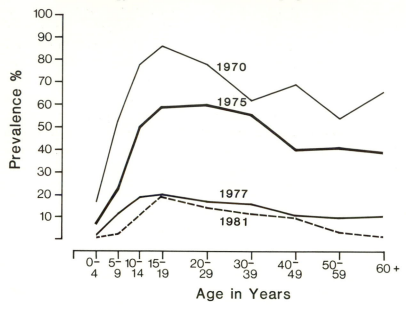

Fig.7.9. Richefond valley – EWS settlements: *S. mansoni* prevalence among children to 14 years of age, rainfall and sentinel and field snail data.

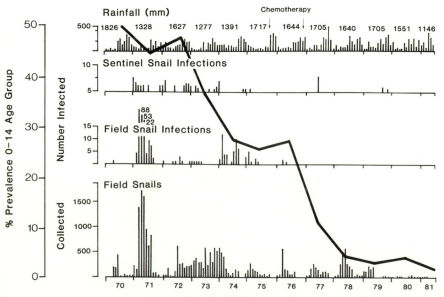

was evidence of a low level of transmission among children aged 6 to 11 years, no new cases were detected in chidren below this age between 1980 and 1981.

The final survey was made in 1981 when the prevalence was found to be 8.6% compared with 56% in 1970. Intensity of infection was reduced from 34 e.p.ml to 17 e.p.ml and the crude IPC by 93% (Table 7.8). Changes in prevalence in all age groups over the years are shown in Fig. 7.8 and in relation to biological findings in Fig. 7.9.

The past history of *S. mansoni* in the 73 infected persons is shown in Table 7.9. Of those 'previously negative', 11 were children who had been negative on numerous occasions, new infections being consistent with a continuing low level of transmission. However, the greatest reservoir of infection was amongst those known to have been positive from previous surveys but who had not had treatment (30%).

Table 7.9. *Richefond valley south – EWS settlements: past known history of* S. mansoni *infections in the 73 persons found infected at 1981*

| Age | Previously +ve | | Previously −ve | Not prev. examined | Immigrants |
	Not treated	Treated			
0–4	—	—	—	—	—
5–9	1	—	4 (2,3,4,5)[a]	—	—
10–14	3	4	7 (3,4,5,6,7,9,11)	7	2
15–19	5	4	1 (1)	1	1
20–29	6	—	1 (3)	4	3
30–39	4	2	1 (1)	2	—
40–49	2	2	2 (1,2)	—	1
50–59	—	1	—	1	—
60+	1	—	—	—	—
	22 (30%)	13 (18%)	16 (22%)	15 (21%)	7 (10%)

[a] Number of previous negative stools from each individual.

Table 7.10. *Richefond valley south – EWS settlements: changing pattern of frequency distribution (%) of intensity of infection as control progressed*

| Year | No. exam. | Egg load (eggs/ml faeces) | | | | | |
		0	<50	51–100	101–200	201–400	>400
1970	966	44.3	35.1	8.0	7.5	3.3	1.8
1975	1340	61.9	34.0	2.5	1.2	0.4	—
1977	1103	86.6	11.9	0.8	0.4	0.3	—
1981	851	91.5	7.2	1.2	0.1	—	—

As control of transmission progressed, the frequency distribution of intensity of infection changed so that the level of egg output in 1981 was such that schistosomal disease was unlikely to occur (Table 7.10).

Results of this programme indicate that in St Lucia individual household water supplies when properly maintained were effective in reducing *S. mansoni* transmission and that after chemotherapy they prevented a resurgence of transmission in the consolidation or maintenance phase of control. The changes in prevalence at different times during the programme are shown in Fig. 7.8.

Cost analysis

A breakdown of the total capital cost of the water installations is given in Table 7.11. The materials were imported into St Lucia free of duty and shipping costs and senior staff salaries are not included. The Grande Ravine laundry and shower unit was constructed in co-operation with the Government Public Health Engineering Unit; later units were built by local contractors. The systems were designed for more than double the present population – on the basis of the design capacity of 4500 the cost was US $16 *per caput*, but it is stressed that the scheme was basically to test the concept that in a highly endemic area transmission of *S. mansoni* could be reduced by water supplies which have additional social and medical benefits.

Capital costs of the simple system at Debonnaire might have been expected to be lower *per caput* than the other systems. However, labour costs of installation were high and amounted to 35% of total costs compared with only 12% at Grande Ravine and 19% in the Grande Riviere/Thomazo/Morne Panache I supply. This was due to there being no road to the Debonnaire intake and labour was required to carry tank sections, cement, sand, etc. a quarter mile to the site. Transport was, however, able to reach the intake site at Grande Ravine (hence low labour costs), but the other system required the storage tank and other materials to be hauled to the top of a hill for gravity distribution of water. Although installation costs at Debonnaire were therefore disproportionately high, the system demonstrated that small streams with minimal flow could provide water for small communities.

The maintenance costs from 1972–81 are shown in Table 7.12. The unit cost of electricity went up from US 6.7 cents in 1970 to 40.9 cents in 1981 (Table 3.7), and with power needed in two systems electricity costs amounted to nearly 50% of maintenance expenditure over the 10-year period. If maintenance costs of items other than electricity are apportioned to the schemes on the basis of population served, and all electricity costs

Table 7.11. *Richefond valley south – EWS settlements: breakdown of capital costs of individual household water supplies* ($ US)

	Equipment and materials	Labour	Trucking	Miscellaneous		Total
1. Grande Ravine (Design capacity 750)						
Intake, tank and distribution	7745	374	32	Site	30	8521
				Equip. rental	250	2387
				Tools etc.	90	820
Laundry and shower	903	1418	66			
Pool, sidewalk and fencing	642	173		Equip. rental	5	
Electricity				Power-line	4500	4500
Total:	9290	1965	98		4875	16228
2. Grande Riviere, Thomazo, M. Panache (Design capacity 2500)						
Intake, tanks (2) and distribution	19420	3735	82.	Site	56	23237
Laundry and showers (3)	2822	2172		Equip. rental	10	5050
Pools (2), sidewalks and fencing	1574	380		Power-lines	2793	1964
Electricity						2793
Total:	23816	6287	82		2859	33044
3. Debonnaire (Design capacity 750)						
Intake, tank and distribution	7180	4131	65			11376
Laundry and shower	1248	508				1756
Total:	8428	4639	65			13132
4. Other charges						
Bridges (2)	117	213				330
Transportation					1086	1086
Supervision					8890	8890
Total:	117	213			9976	10306
Grand total:	41319	12992	245		17710	72266

Table 7.12. *Richefond valley south – EWS settlements: breakdown of maintenance costs of individual household water supplies* ($ US) and % distribution

Year	Electricity $	%	Materials $	%	Labour $	%	Miscellaneous $	%	Total	Payments received	Cost/ person
1972–73	2008	40	394	8	2612	52	—	—	5104	111	2.51
1973–74	2934	52	354	6	2147	38	228	4	5663	80	2.83
1974–75	2965	36	1647	20	3469	42	171	2	8252	166	4.14
1975–76	3262	38	172	2	3847	45	1363	16	8644	303	4.32
1976–77	4366	44	328	3	4473	45	783	8	9950	336	4.97
1977–78	6504	50	1331	10	4582	35	704	5	13121	299	6.56
1978–79	6140	39	978	6	7904	50	848	5	15870	489	7.94
1979–80	10504	48	1206	6	9516	43	715	3	21941	583	10.97
1980–81	13284	57	1163	5	8625	37	110	1	23182	454	11.59
Total	51967	46	7573	7	47175	42	4922	5	111637	2821	6.20

debited to the systems using power, the mean maintenance cost *per caput* per year amounted to $6.92, compared with $3.32 for the gravity dependent scheme.

In 1978, with the development of a new water intake high on the northern side of the valley wall, the Grande Ravine water storage tank was filled by gravity, and, in the last two years of the programme, electricity charges for this system amounted to less than 1% of the total electricity charges as compared with 20% before. This new source of water also enabled the few houses above the Grande Ravine tank to be supplied: necessary extensions to the pipe-line were therefore made.

At the end of the project work was being carried out to pipe water from the new intake into the Thomazo tank by gravity. It was anticipated that electricity charges would thus be minimised for the Central Water Authority who took over the scheme when the Research and Control Department closed.

Maintenance included wages for 'caretakers' at each of the laundry and shower units, keeping the surrounds of pools clean, and cleaning, painting and chlorinating them, clearing overgrown drains etc. Fluctuations in the voltage of the electricity led to numerous electric motors being burnt out, necessitating costly repairs. The Fordilla taps gave little trouble though springs and washers had to be replaced occasionally. This applied also to the frequently used taps over the laundry tubs. Towards the end of the project mineral deposition in the Grande Ravine pipe-line required each pipe to be cleared, during which time public standpipes provided water.

Emergency work (included under miscellaneous charges) was sometimes needed: extensive damage was sustained at the Thomazo laundry unit when the nearby road was being widened, and the roof of the Grande Ravine unit was blown off during Hurricane Allan.

Over the years maintenance costs increased from US $2.51 per person in 1972 to US $11.59 in 1981. In the three years 1972–75, they averaged $3.16, a little less than control in Cul de Sac where the *per caput* cost of area-wide control was $3.42. However, even if the system had been completely gravity fed in the last four years of the project, and maintenance costs only 50% of those recorded (i.e. US $9264 per year), the cost per head, US $4.63, would have been greatly in excess of the $0.65, the cost of the maintenance phase routine focal snail control (Table 6.24).

Water contact studies
Pre-control observations

Since the object of providing domestic water supplies was to encourage people to avoid contact with infected surface water, an immediate indication of success in this respect would be obtained from quantitative water contact studies before and after water was provided. Such observations also provide information on the most important aspect of the epidemiology of the infection – why and when exposure to infection occurs. The method used for carrying out the studies has been described in Chapter 3. They were carried out over a period of 15 months at 15 popular sites (A–O) in rivers and streams. Observations showed fairly well-defined patterns of contact that varied by day, week and month and were influenced mainly by rainfall, season and agricultural activities (Appendix 2).

The daily cycle began between 5 and 6 a.m. when peasant farmers left home for work, often crossing streams on the way. Water carriers usually between the ages of 5 and 9 years, carried buckets or other containers to the rivers for domestic water supplies before going (often late), to school. Children frequently stepped into the river and usually got their arms wet while filling containers. Although this took only a short time, they would remain in the water for 3–4 minutes before returning home. Contact at this early hour was, however, limited, owing to the fear of 'chill' which has a strong cultural influence on life in St Lucia. In the home, water was mainly used for drinking, washing dishes and sponging the body. During the rest of the day, women occasionally carried water, but in the evening it was again the duty of the children.

Around 9 a.m. women arrived at the river with basins of clothes on their heads. They were often accompanied by pre-school-aged children when there was no-one at home to look after them. Girls began to wash clothes at an early age (5–9 years), but the children may spend many hours in and out of the water while mothers washed. In most cases the women squatted by the side of the river with only their feet and hands in contact with water: often the washing was done in a bucket and soap was commonly used. Less frequently, the women stripped to the waist and got into deeper water to do their laundry.

At a typical washing site, between 9 a.m. and 4 p.m. a small group of women engaged in the various phases of washing, rinsing and bleaching of clothes (by spreading them on rocks or bushes) could be seen. The washing sites offered an informal community centre, providing an opportunity for householders to break the monotony of housework and to meet their friends.

In general the degree of bodily exposure while washing was minimal but sometimes prolonged. The effect of soap on cercarial survival has been inadequately investigated but there is evidence that it is strongly cercaricidal (Jordan, 1960). After completing their clothes washing, the women

Table 7.13. *Richefond valley south – EWS settlements: number of water contacts categorised by age and sex in relation to various activities before installation of water*

| | Age group (years) | | | | | | | | |
	0–4	5–9	10–14	15–19	20–29	30–39	40–49	50+	Total
Males									
Water carrying	2	57	78	17	6	4	2	5	171
Washing	0	10	22	2	3	4	2	1	44
Bathing	107	109	56	19	19	5	6	15	336
Swimming	120	145	64	9	2	1	0	1	342
Fording	6	69	48	29	43	37	19	57	308
Other	1	3	16	1	0	1	0	1	23
Total	236	393	284	77	73	52	29	80	1224
% of total contacts	19.2	32.1	23.2	6.2	5.9	4.2	2.3	6.5	
Females									
Water carrying	10	47	97	88	85	47	22	31	427
Washing	4	47	116	145	160	131	58	57	718
Bathing	98	113	73	67	49	26	18	16	460
Swimming	80	128	59	5	4	1	2	0	270
Fording	22	33	82	88	40	34	40	31	370
Other	3	4	28	13	17	7	3	1	76
Total	217	372	455	406	355	246	143	136	2330
% of total contacts	9.3	15.9	19.5	17.4	15.2	10.5	6.1	5.8	

P. Dalton; personal communication.

frequently washed themselves, involving considerable exposure but of limited duration.

Fording the river was observed on many occasions. The main reasons were going to school, carrying fruit to the buying points on 'banana days', visiting other villages and for reaching 'gardens'; a large number of men wore Wellington boots for this work. Other reasons for observed contact were collecting river sand for building, washing cars, washing the possessions of the deceased, and cray-fishing.

An analysis of observed pre-water supply contacts on 105 observation days is shown in Table 7.13. As is common in all such studies, the number of observed contacts was much greater for females than for males.

Post-control studies

As Grande Ravine was the first community to receive household water supplies, their effect was assessed on eight observation days, August–December 1970, on the same days of the week that observations had been made the previous year (as part of the 15 months pre-control study). The number of contacts were found to have been reduced by 82%, and their duration by 96%. All activities were affected except fording, which was mainly by farm and agricultural workers and children on their way to and from school; a foot bridge was therefore built across the main stream (Table 7.14).

Table 7.14. *Richefond valley south: number and duration (in minutes) of water contact at two sites before and after water was supplied in Grande Ravine*

| | 1969 | | 1970 | |
| | No. of contacts | Total duration | No. of contacts | Total duration |
Age in years				
0–4	48	2320	3	1
5–9	104	3299	9	9
10–14	84	2767	23	31
15–19	71	1414	5	89
20–29	38	953	3	81
30–39	21	536	7	6
40–49	2	89	5	156
50+	7	185	11	70
Total	375	11563	66	443

From Dalton, 1976.

The source of water for Grande Ravine was a small, slow-flowing and often muddy stream some distance from the village. It was not surprising therefore that the piped water supply, laundry and shower units and the pool were immediately popular in this settlement.

Further extended water contact studies were carried out from January 1972 for 15 months at the same sites and using the same random block design as before. Observations from January to May showed a 55% reduction in water contacts, mainly in the number collecting and carrying water to the home (Fig. 7.10). Some women were found to be washing clothes at home but taking them to the river to rinse and bleach them. An intensive health education programme was therefore launched and in the next five months contacts fell by 72% of pre-control figures. In the succeeding five months, contacts declined further to give a 92% reduction of pre-control domestic related contacts: those associated with fording, fishing, sand collecting, washing possessions of the dead, etc. were not materially affected by the domestic water supplies. Over the whole 15 month observation period the total number of observed contacts were reduced by 68% (Table 7.15).

As a result of these changes, it was noticeable that sandbanks, previously used for spreading clothes for bleaching purposes, were overgrown with weeds and that soap marks on rocks near the river bank were no longer seen. It was also noted that the odour of faeces on the river bank was much greater than before; apparently with less need to use the rivers, people were less inhibited about using them as a latrine, an unfortunate change in

Fig.7.10. Richefond valley – EWS settlements: percentage reduction in observed water contacts during three 5-month post-control periods. ■ Jan.–May 1972; ▨ June–Oct. 1972; □ Nov.–Mar. 1973.

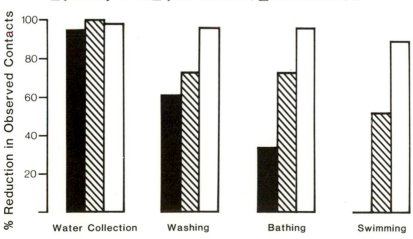

behaviour not foreseen by Macdonald who had anticipated less faecal pollution.

This finding increased the importance of maintaining water supplies, since, in the event of a breakdown, the community would be compelled to return to the river with a greater chance of becoming infected. For this reason temporary snail control should be considered in the event of a long interruption in water supplies, particularly during the dry (transmission) season. Although power-lines were down for six weeks after Hurricane Allan, with a consequent breakdown in water supplies and people having to use the river, mollusciciding was not carried out as snails would have been flushed out by the torrential rains. It was reassuring that no increase in incidence of new *S. mansoni* infections was detected at the next stool survey.

The Health Education programme

When it was apparent that some women continued to use the rivers and streams, a Health Education programme was instituted. From an initial survey it was apparent that a lack of knowledge of schistosomiasis and a failure to understand the role of the communities in the control scheme were, more than anything else, responsible for the limited response in reducing contact with rivers and streams.

The Health Education programme was designed therefore to increase the awareness of the community to the dangers of contact with water and the

Table 7.15. *Richefond valley south – EWS settlements: number of observed persons and contacts at 15 major water contact sites during 15 months of observations before and after installation of water supplies.*

Age in years	Pre-control		Post-control	
	No. persons observed	No. contacts observed	No. persons observed	No. contacts observed
0–4	215	453	39	96
5–9	322	765	91	265
10–14	233	739	72	236
15–19	149	483	49	152
20–29	141	428	49	128
30–39	115	298	45	103
40–49	84	172	15	51
50+	90	216	35	94
Total	1349	3554	395	1125

P. Dalton; personal communication.

need for disease control so that by their own actions or efforts they could help to solve the schistosomiasis problem.

Although some progress in community education had been made with the survey teams having to explain why stools were being collected, why rivers were being searched for snails and why piped water was being introduced, the population regarded the water supply as a social acquisition rather than a health promoting exercise. It had been hoped that involving the community in the digging of trenches for pipe-lines would heighten interest in the project, but this was not satisfactory as progress in trench digging was too slow. The 'self-help' approach was therefore restricted to houseowners having to dig a trench from the main distribution pipe to their own home in order to get water.

The Health Education programme to encourage greater use of the water supplies was aimed at developing good health practices and habits both in the young (forming a high proportion of the community), and amongst adults. Emphasis was on *changing* their attitudes towards health; it was not on 'don't do', but on change of habit since an alternative to going to rivers had been provided. It was considered that women in the community would not only be more receptive than men to the change (they were consistently more co-operative in giving stools for examination), but they might also be able to influence other members of the family.

Training of young people

In the six schools in Richefond Valley, children were in near homogeneous classes according to age and academic ability. Each class was supervised by a teacher who was responsible for instruction and direction for one year. A teacher was, therefore, very important in giving information on schistosomiasis and ensuring the practice of measures to control this and other diseases.

The Education Authorities gave permission for special training seminars for the teachers of three of the six schools. With the help of the WHO/PAHO Regional Advisor on Health Education, the teachers were instructed in methods of health education. Seminars took the form of talks on schistosomiasis, *Ascaris*, *Trichuris* and hookworms, and lectures, film shows and discussions. The School Health Education programme was then launched in three schools, with children being taught what schistosomiasis is, how it is transmitted, what it does to people, how it is treated, and how it can be prevented. After six months a survey was made to assess the children's knowledge of schistosomiasis; results were compared with those from a similar survey in three schools where health education had not been given.

In infant schools the pupils were aged 5–9 years; in primary schools they were 10–14 years; separate questionnaires were prepared for each asking for information on the infection and the parasite's life cycle. Teachers in infant schools were required to assist infants who were too young to read and interpret the questions correctly. As far as was practicable, older children were allowed to respond in their own way. Table 7.16 shows the survey results.

These indicated that the pupils who had health education were more knowledgeable than their counterparts in the schools without the Health Education programme and these children were then suitably instructed.

Further evaluation was through the water contact observations that revealed a dramatic reduction in the number of children in the streams (Fig. 7.10). As fording was only slightly affected, the possibility of making rubber boots available to the people at cost price was investigated but was not practicable.

Meanwhile, revision courses were given with films on schistosomiasis and other diseases being shown and discussed. Occasionally older pupils were given work assignments by the Health Educator. These took the form of essays on schistosomiasis, letters to relatives overseas about it, what was being done to control it and diagrammatic descriptions of the life cycle of the worm. In most cases the pupils' efforts were commendable. Two health education pamphlets were produced – 'You and bilharzia' and 'Compere Lapin tricks the king' based on a St Lucia folklore 'Tim-Tim' story; in

Table 7.16. *Richefond valley – average marks (%) given to questionnaire on schistosomiasis at infant and primary schools*

Age	Health education		No health education	
	La Resource	Richefond	Dennery	Derniere Riviere
Infant schools				
5–6	—	60	39	40
6–7	73	63	54	59
7–8	65	71	36	—
8–9	68	70	51	
Primary schools				
9–10	79		55	
10–11	82		50	
11–12	45		39	
12–13	53		29	
13–14	47		24	

addition, many school classes visited the Research and Control Department for further instruction.

Training of adults

Complementing the school programme, an adult health education programme was designed to obtain maximum use and benefit from the water provided by emphasising the importance of hand washing after defaecating and before preparing food, and the thorough washing of utensils and babies' bottles etc. The importance of parents supporting the efforts of teachers in the school programme was stressed.

The adult health education programme involved film shows on schisto-somiasis and later, on other diseases. These provided recreation (a rare commodity in rural areas) as well as instruction and relaxation. They were well attended, often with up to 350 persons, and the ensuing discussions were sometimes very lively. Whenever possible the people provided the accommodation, including electricity, as their contribution.

As follow-up to the film shows the Health Educator continued the discussion in the homes, at the laundry units and the now less popular river sites where a few people still did their laundry. These discussions were always with individuals or very small groups. The efforts were supported by the religious leaders in their pulpits, the public health nurse in her clinics, the public health inspector on his home visits and the teachers living in the communities. Emphasis was placed on meeting the people, but series of posters were prepared for display in Health Centres, rum shops and other centres where people gathered. A positive approach was adopted; showing people what they ought to do was considered more effective than showing what they should not do. Although posters were used, it was felt they made little impact on the community: their message may have been clear to the designer, but frequently it was not clear to the uneducated or semi-educated countryman. It is difficult for such people to understand the concept of enlarging things in drawings, such as a worm or a helminth ova, so that whenever possible, eggs under a microscope, or actual worms, were demonstrated.

With health education and the construction of the laundry and shower unit in Grande Riviere (completed in March 1973) there was a noted change in the attitude of the women, with those who previously insisted on washing in the river now using the laundry or their home water supply. Even when the laundry was filled women would await their turn, or fill a utensil with water and do their washing, gossiping as at the river sites. Children played near the laundry or in the nearby pool. A few recalcitrants returned to the river but community pressures were building up and very soon it was rare to see river washing. Discussions with residents indicated that they were fully aware of the hazards associated with rivers and streams and there was evidence that the communal laundries were preferred to the former river and stream sites.

Other effects of water supplies
Intestinal helminths
It had been hoped that the water supplies would have led to greater cleanliness and, with more frequent washing of hands and food, a reduction in the prevalence of *Ascaris* and *Trichuris*. Rates were lower in 1981 after household water had been available for 10 years, but they were similarly lower in the comparison area of the northern side of the valley. Prevalence of hookworm infections had also fallen in both areas, possibly due to a gradual improvement in the standard of living with greater numbers wearing shoes.

Morbidity surveys
Two questionnaire morbidity surveys were carried out in Grande Ravine, the first village to be supplied with water, in 1972 and 1981

Table 7.17. *Grande Ravine: frequency (%) of persons admitting to various symptoms in the course of two morbidity questionnaire surveys*

| | Under 20 years | | | | 20 years and above | | | |
| | Males | | Females | | Males | | Females | |
	1972	1981	1972	1981	1972	1981	1972	1981
No. interviewed	78	76	68	88	12	45	52	66
Abdominal pain	40	19	43	26	42	31	51	32
Diarrhoea	20	4	18	7	9	4	0	0
Blood in stool	13	4	16	3	9	6	11	17
Tenesmus	13	0	10	1	9	6	14	3
Vomiting	1	1	4	2	0	0	0	0
Abdominal cramps	5	0	9	0	17	2	30	18
Headache	24	11	25	18	25	26	65	55
Giddiness	1	4	6	3	0	4	6	11
Weakness	3	3	7	5	25	8	33	20
Body pains	4	1	6	6	33	22	39	27
Cold and fever	59	26	53	22	33	22	40	18
Skin complaints	4	5	0	0	0	0	0	0
Mean complaints/person	1.1	0.8	2.1	0.9	2.1	1.0	3.0	2.1

(Dalton, unpublished data). The questionnaire consisted of a check list of common complaints and persons were asked whether or not they had been suffering from them during the previous month. A St Lucian, well known in the area, conducted both surveys. Results are shown in Table 7.17.

While results of such questionnaires must be interpreted with caution, it is noteworthy that the mean number of complaints per person was reduced in all groups questioned. It cannot be assumed that the apparent improvement in 'well-being' was due to lighter *S. mansoni* infections (although there was a marked reduction in symptoms often associated with it, particularly in the younger age group), nor to the water supply directly, but this may be considered as leading the way to an improved standard of living which was noticeable in the village. Previously Grande Ravine was considered a back-water by most St Lucians, but with the water and electricity supplies, and a new road through the village, the population became more widely involved in the St Lucian community as a whole.

Biological studies

Only limited biological studies were made in Richefond valley but they confirmed the same general ecological conditions as in other valleys.

Index sites were selected for fortnightly sampling at Grande Ravine and Debonnaire; sites for sentinel snail exposures were also chosen. Results of field snail findings from 1971–79 are shown in Table 7.18.

The number of *B. glabrata* from index sites decreased markedly from 1971 as was noted on the northern side of the valley (Chapter 4), and from

Table 7.18. *Richefond valley south – EWS settlements: annual* S. mansoni *infection rates in field* B. glabrata

Year	No. examined	No. infected	% infected
1971	7462	207	2.70
1972	3691	27	0.73
1973	4494	3	0.06
1974	2129	47	2.21
1975[a]	1175	9	0.77
1976[a]	1232	3	0.25
1977[a]	461	0	0.00
1978	2321[b]	2	0.09
1979	988[b]	2	0.20

[a] Treatment was offered.
[b] Additional index sites examined.

1978 two additional sites were regularly searched. The reasons for the declining populations are obscure but the ecology of the area was changing. Initially Grande Ravine was at the end of a dirt track, but by 1976 it was a village on a surfaced loop road from the main valley road. This resulted in a nearby flowing water habitat being extensively dug out and widened, making it less suitable for *B. glabrata*. Agriculturally, major changes were noted – extensive areas of banana fields were taken over for growing okra, egg plants, tomatoes etc., and the root drainage system no longer existed. In addition, because of lower rainfall, overhead irrigation became necessary for the new crops as well as the remaining bananas.

The changing pattern of rainfall over the past 30 years is demonstrated in Fig. 1.4. The flow of water in streams and populations of *B. glabrata* they may have harboured were inevitably affected by these changes, but they could have been affected also by deforestation on the valley walls, uncontrolled until the effect on stream and river flows was manifest and necessitated the finding of a new source of water, as referred to above.

The proportion of infected snails declined from 1971 and 1973 (Fig. 7.9), but the marked increase in 1974 could have been the result of the increased faecal pollution of streams following the provision of piped water, referred to above, although sentinel snails did not show a similar increase of infections. It was, however, not until the introduction of the

Table 7.19. *Richefond valley south – EWS settlements: results of sentinel snail exposures (1971–81) with human infection data and crude IPC amongst 0–14-year-old children*

Year	Sentinel snails			Human infection		
	No. examined	No. infected	% infected	Prevalence (%)	Intensity GM	Crude IPC (% × GM)
1971	3098	18	0.58	45	33	1485
1972	3293	16	0.49	46	34	1564
1973	3172	9	0.28	39	28	1092
1974	2919	6	0.21	29	22	638
1975	2804	1	0.04	25	17	425
1976	2989	0	0.00	27	17	459
1977	2691	6	0.22	13	14	182
1978	2285	0	0.00	7	14	98
1979	2212	3	0.14	7	19	133
1980	2568	0	0.00	7	14	98
1981[a]	1304	0	0.00	6	14	84

[a] 1981 Observations from January to June (main transmission season).

chemotherapy that the proportion of infected snails was consistently low. From 1977 no infected snails were found.

The finding of a spontaneous reduction in the snail population emphasises the importance of biological investigations (and possibly anthropological) in research schemes, to monitor spontaneous changes that might affect transmission.

Results of sentinel snail infections and the changing level of potential contamination in the human population are shown in Table 7.19.

Sentinel snail infection rates declined slowly as water became available (1971–75) and sharply after the chemotherapy campaigns of 1975–77. Only sporadic infections occurred in the maintenance phase (1977–81) consistent with the lower level of potential contamination (Fig. 7.9).

Summary and recommendations

Results of the first four to five years of the scheme showed that by providing individual households with water and villages with communal laundry and shower units the population can be educated to use them rather than the rivers, thus reducing exposure to *S. mansoni* infection. In the first four years of evaluation prevalence dropped from 56% to 38%. The final four years of the scheme showed that after chemotherapy, water supplies prevented any resurgence of transmission: incidence varied between 4 and 6%, overall prevalence was reduced to 9%, intensity of infection from 34 to 17, e.p.ml faeces and the contamination potential was reduced by 93%.

Future indications are that as long as the water system is maintained there is little risk of any major breakdown in control, particularly as colonies of *B. glabrata* are now infrequently found. These may, however, give rise to infections, particularly among children.

(ii)   Community standpipe water supplies and laundry and shower units

The study area

A community standpipe water system is commonly used in villages in developing countries (an individual household system being considered too costly). A programme was designed, therefore, to investigate the effect on schistosomiasis transmission of a government water supply improved and supplemented by additional laundry and shower units. Three villages, Derniere Riviere, Belmont and Morne Panache II (Group I), where two government laundry and shower units had been built previously, were chosen for the investigation. They were adjacent and very close to each other, near the main river, and in the period from 1970 to 1975 incidence

Table 7.20. *Richefond valley north: annual incidence of new S. mansoni infections between 1968 and 1975 in two groups of high transmission settlements of comparison area*

Age in years	1968–69 No. neg.[a]	1968–69 % inc.[b]	1969–70 No. neg.	1969–70 % inc.	1970–71 No. neg.	1970–71 % inc.	1971–72 No. neg.	1971–72 % inc.	1972–73 No. neg.	1972–73 % inc.	1973–74 No. neg.	1973–74 % inc.	1974–75 No. neg.	1974–75 % inc.
Group I Derniere Riviere, Belmont, Morne Panache II														
0 & 1	29	10.3	53	5.7	33	9.1	25	24.0	20	15.0	35	17.1	24	8.3
2 & 3	60	13.3	73	16.4	45	15.6	42	35.7	23	26.1	33	36.4	35	22.9
4 & 5	58	17.2	72	22.2	59	15.3	63	41.9	22	31.8	33	27.3	24	25.0
6 & 7	34	11.8	56	32.1	64	35.9	63	55.6	20	40.0	36	47.2	27	33.3
8 & 9	30	46.7	29	44.8	27	51.9	33	72.7	21	28.6	27	48.1	22	18.2
10 & 11					18	83.3	8	87.5	13	38.5	13	53.8	13	46.2
0–9	211	18.5	283	21.9	228	24.6	225	47.1	106	28.3	164	34.8	132	22.0
0–11					246	28.9	233	52.8	119	29.4	117	35.6	145	24.1
Group II La Ressource, La Pearl, Richefond														
0 & 1	12	8.3	24	12.5	15	6.7	15	6.7	38	23.7	14	14.3	14	0.0
2 & 3	21	14.3	33	12.1	21	9.5	24	16.7	31	25.8	21	9.5	16	6.3
4 & 5	32	18.8	30	30.0	22	9.1	29	24.1	34	17.6	14	14.3	23	8.7
6 & 7	15	13.3	23	30.4	22	22.7	24	37.5	45	31.1	17	17.6	23	26.1
8 & 9	10	10.0	19	26.3	11	18.2	18	27.8	23	47.8	17	23.5	19	21.1
10 & 11					10	50.0	5	0.0	6	50.0	15	13.3	20	30.0
0–9	90	14.4	129	21.7	91	12.1	110	23.6	171	28.1	83	15.7	95	13.7
0–11					101	15.8	115	22.6	177	28.8	98	15.8	115	16.5

[a] Number negative at first of two surveys.
[b] Percentage positive at second survey.

rates of new *S. mansoni* infections among 0–14-year-old children were generally greater than in the other three high transmission comparison settlements of Richefond, Le Pearl and La Ressource (Table 7.20).

The programme was a collaborative one: funds for additional units were provided by the Rotary Clubs of Castries and Guelph (Canada), with the Research and Control Department being responsible for siting the units and for their construction. Water was provided from the government distribution system and the Research and Control Department provided a new water storage tank; seven standpipes served the villages.

Four laundry and shower units were constructed in 1975 and became serviceable at the beginning of 1976, providing one shower and one laundry tub per 10 households (compared with 12.5 households in the south of the valley). Water contact studies were initiated in 1975 and repeated at the same times in 1976 when the effect of the new units on the extent of water contact was assessed. In 1977 the long term usage of units was investigated by a further series of studies. In the event, while observations were completed, drying of the rivers (see p. 218) resulted in inadequate water in the units and the return to the river of most of the women.

Owing to the inadequate water supply the scheme had to be amended, and in 1977 treatment was offered to all who had ever been known to have been infected. An alternative water source was found by the Central Water Authority and the standpipe water supply, supplemented with laundry and shower units, was investigated as a maintenance phase strategy after chemotherapy; this was relevant as many developing countries have, or plan to have, communal supplies, and chemotherapy plays an increasing role in schistosomiasis control.

In the remaining comparison villages, La Ressource, La Pearl and Richefond (high transmission) (Group II) and Au Leon, Gadette and Despinose (low transmission) (Group III), standpipe communal water supplies were available, but there were no laundry and shower units. In these villages treatment was offered in 1977 to all who were known to have been infected.

In all these former comparison villages transmission was monitored between 1977 and 1981 when the final survey was made and treatment was again made available. The final survey at Au Leon was abandoned owing to the very poor response of the community.

Parasitological findings

Incidence data between 1968 and 1975 and from 1975 to 1981 for the three groups of villages are shown in Tables 4.9, 7.20 and 7.21.

Table 7.21. *Richefond valley north: annual incidence of new S. mansoni infections before chemotherapy in 'old' comparison areas and during maintenance phase in three groups of villages*

Age at first of two surveys	1975–76		1976/77		1977–78		1978–79		1979–80		1980–81	
	No. neg.[a]	% inc.[b]	No. neg.	% inc.	No. neg.	% inc.	No. neg.	% inc.	No. neg.	% inc.	No. neg.	% inc.
Group I — Community water supplied & laundry shower units[c]												
0 & 1	32	3.1	21	0	10	0	6	16.7	11	0	10	0
2 & 3	53	20.8	49	10.2	35	0	24	0	22	0	14	0
4 & 5	30	30.0	38	13.2	51	2.0	32	6.3	33	0	28	0
6 & 7	35	25.7	27	29.6	27	11.1	50	4.0	36	2.8	38	5.3
8 & 9	32	40.6	25	20.0	23	8.7	22	13.6	25	16.0	35	14.3
10 & 11	27	44.4	20	15.0	22	4.5	28	14.3	16	6.3	22	9.1
0–9	182	23.1	160	14.4	146	4.1	134	6.0	127	3.9	125	5.6
0–11	209	26.3	180	14.1	168	4.2	162	7.4	143	5.6	147	6.1

Group II – Community water supplies; high transmission[b]

	No.[a]	%[b]	No.[a]	%[b]	No.[a]	%[b]	No.[a]	%[b]	No.[a]	%[b]	No.[a]	%[b]
0 & 1	16	0	10	10.0	5	0	2	0	2	0	3	0
2 & 3	25	4.0	25	8.0	14	7.1	11	0	7	0	10	10.0
4 & 5	21	14.3	21	9.5	17	5.9	22	0	18	0	13	7.7
6 & 7	19	31.6	16	12.5	21	9.5	24	0	28	5.0	20	20.0
8 & 9	18	22.2	21	42.9	16	12.5	11	18.1	20	0	18	22.2
10 & 11	15	40.0	11	72.2	10	0	16	0	19	0	13	23.1
0–9	99	14.1	93	17.2	73	8.2	70	2.9	75	1.1	64	15.6
0–11	114	17.5	104	23.1	83	7.2	86	2.3	94	1.4	77	16.9

Group III – Community water supplies; low transmission[e]

	No.[a]	%[b]	No.[a]	%[b]	No.[a]	%[b]	No.[a]	%[b]	No.[a]	%[b]	No.[a]	%[b]
0 & 1	33	0	26	0	14	0	19	0	10	0	5	0
2 & 3	68	1.5	58	1.7	40	0	27	0	24	0	14	0
4 & 5	59	8.5	71	7.0	73	0	59	0	38	0	19	0
6 & 7	74	10.8	60	10.0	64	1.6	64	1.6	56	0	31	0
8 & 9	70	17.1	61	14.8	61	3.3	47	8.5	35	0	23	4.3
10 & 11	47	17.0	53	11.3	54	7.4	46	4.3	28	0	12	0
0–9	304	8.6	276	7.6	252	1.2	216	2.3	163	0	92	1.1
0–11	351	9.7	329	8.2	306	2.3	262	2.7	191	0	104	1.0

[a] Number negative at first of two surveys.
[b] Percentage positive at second survey.
[c] Derniere Riviere, Belmont, Morne Panache II.
[d] La Ressource, La Pearl, Richefond.
[e] Au Leon, Despinose, Gadette.

Whereas incidence between 1968 and 1975 had generally been higher in the villages to have an upgraded standpipe system, once improvements had been made to the community water supply and laundry and shower facilities provided in 1975, incidence dropped from 23.1% to 14.4% (0–9-year-old children) between 1976 and 1977, lower than it had been at any time in the previous 8 years (mean 27.1%). In the villages of Richefond, La Pearl and La Ressource the incidence of 17.2% was similar to the mean incidence (18.4%) of the previous 8 years. Results from a single 12-month period are insufficient evidence alone on which to claim success, but the above findings do suggest reduced transmission with a community water supply and laundry and shower units. Further support for this was obtained from water contact studies (p. 228), which showed a 50% reduction in observed contacts compared with pre-control findings.

In chemotherapy campaigns in 1977 and early 1978 oxamniquine was offered to all persons in the three village groups who were known at some time to have been infected. Treatment was accepted by 796 persons in Group I villages and by 280 and 479 in Groups II and III villages respectively. Incidence declined in all village groups thereafter (Table 7.21).

At the time of treatment, blood spots were taken from 202 patients who had been found by stool survey to have been *S. mansoni* positive at some time during the previous 10 years: 70% were ELISA positive, probably indicating that the infection had spontaneously died out in some persons. One year later, blood was again taken from all 202 subjects: 34% were ELISA positive and 27% were positive on stool examination (Long, unpublished data).

After treatment there was no resurgence of transmission in Group I villages where laundry and shower units had been installed, although transmission continued at a low level. This was similar to findings in villages in Richefond south with individual household water supplies where, during evaluation of the maintenance phase, transmission continued at a low level.

Although incidence in the Group II villages remained low, and seemed to be steadily decreasing, there was a marked increase in 1980–81 involving La Pearl and Richefond (Table 7.22), villages which showed the highest prevalence and incidence in the original surveys (Table 4.7). The finding of a sudden change in incidence in these two settlements emphasises the focality of transmission and that transmission can change dramatically in some villages but not in others nearby. In Group III villages there was no evidence of a resurgence in transmission.

By 1981 prevalence and crude IPC had been lowered in all areas (Table 7.23), though less in Group II villages owing to the resurgence in

Table 7.22. *Richefond valley north – Group II villages: prevalence of* S. mansoni *amongst 0–14-year-old children before chemotherapy (1977 and 1978), and during maintenance phase; corresponding annual incidence of new infections between surveys amongst 0–11-year-old children*

Year of survey	Richefond				La Pearl				La Ressource			
	Prevalence		Incidence		Prevalence		Incidence		Prevalence		Incidence	
	No. exam.	% +ve	No. neg.	% inc.	No. exam.	% +ve	No. neg.	% inc.	No. exam.	% +ve	No. neg.	% inc.
1976	106	31			50	10			79	24		
1977	85	20	43	9.3	58	43	32	43.8	59	22	20	20.7
1978	85	18	29	2.6	44	30	14	35.7	60	2	30	0
1979	78	5	42	2.4	38	5	15	0	36	6	29	3.4
1980	92	4	55	1.8	29	0	20	0	37	3	19	0
1981	58	29	38	23.7	43	14	18	16.7	48	2	21	4.8

Table 7.23. *Richefond valley north – village Groups I, II, and III: changes in prevalence, intensity of infection and level of potential contamination*

Age group	1975 No. exam.	1975 Prev. (%)	1975 GM	1977 No. exam.	1977 Prev. (%)	1977 GM	1981 No. exam.	1981 Prev. (%)	1981 GM
Group I									
0–4	176	21	19	120	8	16	96	2	16
5–9	271	59	26	211	46	26	155	5	16
10–14	261	69	27	255	62	35	128	18	16
15–19	118	72	29	121	65	33	98	18	23
20–29	103	75	24	86	55	24	73	22	20
30–39	69	64	22	63	44	23	52	14	16
40–49	81	52	18	62	44	21	42	5	24
50–59	62	68	22	47	51	16	48	21	24
60+	60	50	24	48	21	16	44	21	24
0–14	708	53	26	586	45	31	379	8	16
15+	493	65	24	427	50	25	357	17	21
Crude IPC	12724			10047			2606		
% reduction	21%			21%			74%		
Cumulative reduction							80%		

Group II

									Mean for all age groups
0-4	68	7	16	55	5	14	29	7	
5-9	89	26	16	81	25	14	63	13	
10-14	93	52	23	66	48	26	57	26	
15-19	26	77	31	39	49	22	30	20	
20-29	33	67	24	29	69	29	20	15	
30-39	32	44	13	28	36	13	21	29	
40-49	24	58	16	26	35	18	17	0	
50-59	22	36	15	19	26	15	23	4	
60+	30	37	15	26	15	15	27	0	
0-14	250	30	20	202	27	20	149	17	19
15+	167	53	20	169	40	20	138	12	19
Crude IPC	8309				6460				2166
% reduction					22%		66%		
Cumulative reduction					22%				74%

Group III

									Mean for all age groups
0-4	187	4	14	138	1	13	52	0	
5-9	258	8	14	262	10	13	91	0	
10-14	195	26	18	198	19	19	63	5	
15-19	82	38	17	72	14	17	31	10	
20-29	97	49	18	82	32	20	26	4	
30-39	82	38	13	72	36	17	22	18	
40-49	52	21	16	49	16	20	24	0	
50-59	55	40	11	42	21	15	17	6	
60+	45	22	11	41	10	15	31	0	
0-14	640	12	16	598	11	16	206	1	18
15+	412	37	15	358	23	18	151	6	18
Crude IPC	3654				2779				774
% reduction					24%		72%		
Cumulative reduction					24%				79%

transmission. These findings are similar to those in Marquis where a community standpipe water system was not sufficient to prevent a resurgence of transmission in some settlements with high prevalence rates before chemotherapy. On the other hand, where prevalence was originally low (Group III settlements) no resurgence was noted within four years of treatment.

After the last survey in 1981 treatment was offered to all found infected.

Water contact studies

The seven main river contact points used by the communities of Derniere Riviere, Morne Panache II and Belmont were identified and observed one week in four on the same days in the first months of 1975, 1976 and 1977 (Jordan, unpublished data). The observer trained for the more extensive studies on the south side of the valley made the study.

The sex and age distribution of individuals observed are shown in Table 7.24. As so few males were observed further analyses were restricted to females. Owing to the presence of a standpipe water supply contacts for collecting water were rarely observed.

There was considerable daily variation in the number of observed contacts; Saturdays were the most popular for river activities, followed by Sundays and Mondays. The fewest contacts were seen on 'Banana days', when all segments of the population were harvesting bananas or carrying them to packing centres, but on these days contact through fording usually increased.

Table 7.24. *Richefond valley north: number of observed contacts by age and sex during the three study periods in Derniere Riviere, Belmont and Morne Panache II*

Age	Males			Females		
	1975	1976	1977	1975	1976	1977
0–4	60	14	94	88	33	72
5–9	165	52	138	261	144	193
10–14	100	57	123	337	166	365
15–19	13	11	26	256	92	265
20–29	4	7	11	170	103	319
30–39	5	3	1	162	116	223
40–49	5	1	5	127	51	144
50–59	11	10	0	56	42	70
60+	3	2	2	16	12	21
All ages	366	157	400	1473	759	1672

In 1975 there was little monthly variation in the number of contacts and such as there was could usually be related to school or public holidays, though results from June were inexplicably low (Table 7.25). Contacts by site varied depending on size, accessibility and popularity.

At the time of the 1976 study the laundry and shower units were in use and the number of observed contacts for males and females was approximately 50% lower than in 1975 (Table 7.24). Except for June, contacts for each month were fewer, all sites were affected and contacts for all activities were reduced.

Regrettably, the rains at the end of 1976 were poor and the 1977 dry season, the driest in 30 years, resulted in insufficient water for the piped supply and a gradual return of the communities to the river as the survey progressed (Table 7.25). In June and July of 1977 (at the end of the dry season when the water shortage was acute) observed contacts accounted for 38% of all contacts compared with 25% and 27% in the previous two years. The low number of fording contacts is a further reflection of the low state of the river which could be crossed without contact with water, but apart from this (and 'other contacts') the number of observed contacts for activities was greater than in 1975 and 1976.

While the inadequate water supply was disappointing, the contact studies of 1976 clearly demonstrate the influence of operational laundry and shower units on water contact: the importance of these findings is emphasised by the reverse findings when units become 'non-operational'.

Biological studies

These continued on the northern side of Richefond valley after the area was no longer being considered for comparison purposes. Studies continued at index sites but no snails were found after 1975. Additional sites were included for routine search but none revealed *B. glabrata* until 1977 when a roadside drain, fed by spillage from an outside domestic shower, was found to harbour a large colony in the drier months of the year. Snails disappeared in the middle of the year and were not found for the next two years until the dry season of 1980 when a small colony was present again for a few months.

Changes in the *B. glabrata* population in the area are difficult to explain, but are probably related to the changing agricultural practices, lower rainfall and deforestation referred to above. Whatever the reason, the limitations of surveys is apparent from the rapid increase in transmission recorded from La Pearl and Richefond in the 1980–81 period (Table 7.22). Some focus or foci of snails, undetected in spite of careful surveys, must have been responsible for this, but foci may have been only temporarily

Table 7.25. Richefond valley north – Derniere Riviere, Belmont, Morne Panache II: number of observed water contacts at seven major river sites, 1975, 1976, 1977

	1975		1976		1977	
	No. contacts	% of total	No. contacts	% of total	No contacts	% of total
Female contacts by the month						
January	260	17.7	109	14.4	162	9.7
February	183	12.4	53	7.0	150	9.0
March	206	14.0	76	10.0	290	17.3
April	245	16.6	132	17.4	209	12.5
May	221	15.0	185	24.4	221	13.2
June	143	9.7	144	19.0	307	18.4
July	215	14.6	60	7.9	333	19.9
Total	1473	100.0	759	100.0	1672	100.0
Female contacts by site						
A	457	31.0	29	3.8	333	19.9
B	148	10.0	100	13.2	157	9.4
C	139	9.4	128	16.9	291	17.4
D	58	3.9	23	3.0	154	9.2
E	328	22.3	251	33.1	302	18.1
F	195	13.2	115	15.2	157	9.4
G	148	10.0	113	14.9	278	6.6
Total	1473	100.0	759	100.0	1672	100.0

Female contacts by activity and age

Age in years	Total contacts[a]			Washing[a]			Bathing[a]			Playing[a]			Fording[a]			Other[a, b]		
0–4	88	33	72	0	0	0	23	12	28	57	18	38	7	2	6	1	1	0
5–9	261	144	193	43	15	19	41	31	65	110	56	84	58	35	16	9	7	9
10–14	337	166	365	143	72	153	52	6	80	57	32	93	77	53	31	8	3	8
15–19	256	92	265	161	72	200	32	1	34	18	8	29	45	11	2	0	0	0
20–29	170	103	319	117	91	270	20	3	14	9	7	31	23	2	1	1	0	3
30–39	162	116	223	132	84	190	11	3	9	7	12	16	10	13	7	2	4	1
40–49	127	51	144	96	34	114	10	2	10	7	5	11	13	8	9	1	2	0
50–59	56	42	70	39	28	51	1	4	6	9	6	5	4	4	8	3	0	0
60+	16	12	21	14	11	17	0	0	0	2	0	3	0	1	1	0	0	0
Total	1473	759	1672	745	407	1014	190	62	246	276	144	310	237	129	81	17	17	8

[a] Columns show figures for 1975, 1976 and 1977.
[b] Includes a small number of contacts for 'collecting water' and miscellaneous activities such as fishing, washing cars, horses or household articles from homes of dead persons.

present, such as the colony found in a roadside ditch (referred to above) for a few months in 1977 and 1980, but which was not present in the intervening years. (A similar finding of transmission in the apparent absence of snail colonies, was made in the Calypso north area – see below.) Results of sentinel snail exposures from 1975 to 1981 are shown in Table 7.26.

The reduction in the snail infection rate is a reflection of the reduced level of potential contamination brought about by the chemotherapy campaigns of 1977 and 1978.

The spontaneous decline in snail populations over much of the area and the interruption in water supplies make it difficult to assess accurately the long term impact of supplementing a public standpipe water system with laundry and shower units. However the water contact studies of 1976 provided a clear indication that such units are of value in reducing water contact and that this was associated with the lowest incidence of new infections for eight years, no such finding being recorded in the villages without laundry and shower facilities.

Summary and recommendations

Results from the earlier years of the study showed increased, then decreased, transmission, demonstrating how this can vary due to ecological factors – agricultural changes and rainfall probably being of most importance. Results also demonstrated that a water supply based on public standpipes is ineffective as a method of transmission control. However, when supplemented with laundry and shower units and selective population

Table 7.26. *Richefond valley north: results of sentinel snail exposures with human infection data and index of potential contamination amongst 0–14-year-old children.*

(*For data prior to 1975 see Table 4.13*)

Year	Sentinel snails			Human infection		
	No. examined	No. infected	% infected	Prevalence (%)	Intensity GM	IPC (% × GM)
1975	2723	1	0.04	47	25	1175
1976	2481	11	0.44	44	28	1232
1977	2579	11	0.43	41	29	1189
1978	2148	5	0.23	14	19	266
1979	1777	5	0.28	10	19	190
1980	2302	1	0.04	6	16	96
1981	1091	1	0.09	11	21	231

chemotherapy, transmission can be reduced and prevalence maintained at a low level.

No explanation can be provided for the marked increase in transmission in two settlements, Richefond and La Pearl, but the finding lends emphasis to results from Marquis where a resurgence of transmission occurred after chemotherapy in some high transmission settlements with only a community standpipe system. It is recommended to Government that adequate laundry and shower units be provided in all settlements and that this whole valley be given a high priority in terms of maintenance of the good water supply.

PART 2: CALYPSO AREA

(iii)   Individual household water with sanitation or with chemotherapy

Although proper disposal of human excreta is the most basic and theoretically simplest method of controlling schistosomiasis (and other intestinal helminths) it has rarely been seriously considered in control schemes.

Results of latrine campaigns in Egypt (Scott & Barlow, 1938 Weir *et al.*, 1952) are frequently quoted as having shown no effect on *S. mansoni* transmission. A critical review of the papers, however, suggests there was insufficient data for this conclusion, and in a short term study in villages in the Philippines the *S. japonicum* snail infection rate was higher in a village without latrines compared with the rate in a village with them (Pesigan *et al.*, 1958). However, Macdonald (1965) predicted that unless there was virtually 100% 'safe' disposal of excreta, latrines would not affect transmission, but this appears to have been based on the probably incorrect view that water bodies were 'saturated' with miracidia.

A number of factors limit the use of latrines for disease control in tropical countries, principally odour and fly problems associated with them, but even if satisfactory units are available their use in households is often restricted to adults as children soil them or fear they may fall in.

In spite of the discouraging past history of sanitation in schistosomiasis control, with the advent of new units more suitable for developing countries (Morgan & Mara, 1982) a trial to evaluate their effect was considered appropriate.

As any effect on transmission would be due to reduced contamination with *S. mansoni* ova of snail habitats (i.e. the same *modus operandi* of chemotherapy in transmission control), the project was designed to compare the efficacy of latrines and chemotherapy in two groups of villages each provided with individual household water supplies and laundry and shower units.

In the original plan, pre-control epidemiological and biological studies were to be conducted between 1974 and 1976, at which time it was planned that the water and latrine installations would be completed and chemotherapy would be offered to infected persons in the other area. There were serious delays, however, in the arrival of essential supplies, and community involvement was not as effective as had been hoped. The participation of the population in putting in water supplies gives them an investment in the scheme (if only in terms of energy expended), which should encourage better use and care of the facilities. In practice, the rate of digging pipe-lines and pits for latrines depended on the enthusiasm of the population and the time they had available for such work. Thus, although the scheme was not finally completed until early 1978 when water was eventually provided in the last village (with a low *S. mansoni* prevalence), evaluation was considered to date from the survey of 1977.

The study area

Prior to the control project, 7- and 8–year-old children attending one school in Desruisseau had been monitored annually since 1968 when 34% (39 of 114) were *S. mansoni* positive. Prevalence increased gradually over the years until 1973 when 57% were found infected (106 of 185 examined). As no biological studies were made at this time the reasons for this increase can only be surmised, but the period did coincide with one of low rainfall and therefore more stable river conditions conducive to transmission. During this period treatment had been given to patients referred from the Health Centre and others were treated in drug trials.

The two village groups are in the south-east of St Lucia between the Troumasse and Canelles rivers and separated by the Micoud or Ger river. A loop road (Calypso Road) passes inland from the coast and just south of the Troumasse river. At an altitude of 300 m, in the foothills of Mount Gimie, it swings south and east to run parallel and just north of the Canelles river (Fig. 7.11).

Villages on or near the northern side of the loop are Ti Rocher, Fond L'Or, Dugard and La Cour Ville. Four laundry and shower units were built and 349 individual households were provided with their own water supply and a water seal latrine (population approximately 13 00).

Villages on the southern side of the loop road, Anse Ger, Desruisseau and Blanchard, were provided with three laundry and shower units and 551 houses had an individual water supply (population approximately 2500).

Fig.7.11. Calypso area: map of study area showing villages and sites for biological study.

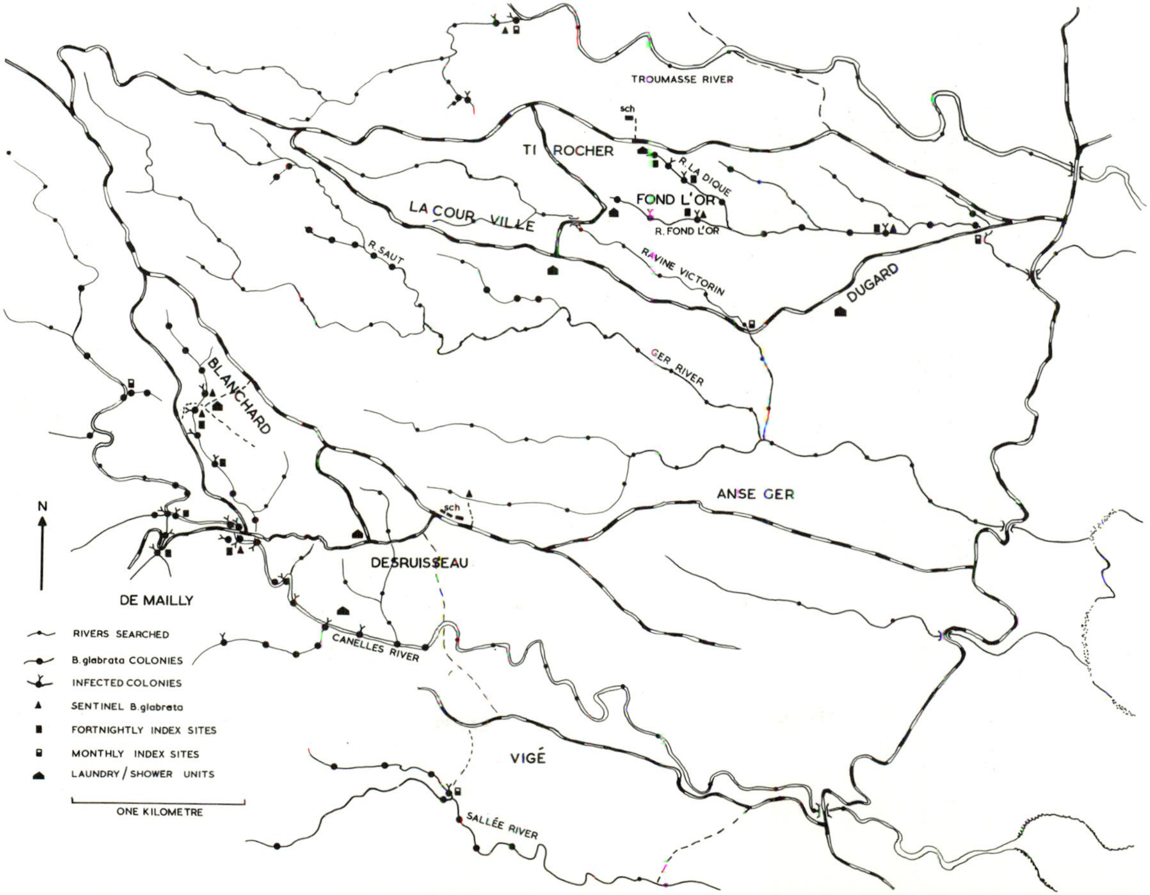

A few remote houses in both areas did not have water connections owing to the long pipe-lines that would have been required.

Prior to the control programme community standpipe systems provided limited water in each area but rivers were used for washing. In the northern area the Troumasse was little used owing to its inaccessibility, but the River Ger and its tributaries were used extensively.

The River Ger was used by some households from the southern area but the Canelles river provided the main washing sites. This is the longest flowing river in the area, with a dry season flow of 6–8 m³/min, increasing by two or three times towards the end of the wet season. Under stable conditions numerous quiet flowing sections occur, but heavy storms produced peak flows of over 100 m³/min or more. A small tributary, near Blanchard, provided a washing site with a slow rate of flow, but streams generally were precipitous with flow rates inimical to *B. glabrata*.

Pit latrines were commonly used for faeces disposal in St Lucia and were present in many yards where water seal latrine units were introduced. In 1977 a survey of sanitary facilities was made in the southern area; it probably gave an indication of the situation in the north prior to the water seal units being installed. Septic tanks were in use in 4% of households, pit latrines in 64% and 32% had no latrines or used an open pit.

There was limited contact between the northern and southern village groups, each of which has its own school. The only church and health centre are on the southern leg of the loop road, but people on the north receive religious and health care at facilities at Micoud (on the main coast road).

The main occupation is farming either on one of the larger banana plantations or on small holdings.

The water supply and latrines

The design of the water distribution system required extensive preliminary land surveying and mapping, with which a graduate and two students from the Sanitary Engineering School at Cali Columbia assisted.

A stream with good quality water was found on the lower slopes of Mount Gimie. As this is the highest point in St Lucia with an annual rainfall of nearly 4000 mm, a regular and adequate supply of water was assured. Maximum flow in the main 152 mm pipe-line was nearly 2 million l per day.

Distribution lines (101.6 and 50.8 mm) were installed by the Central Water Authority; distribution to individual houses was the responsibility of the Research and Control Department, which constructed laundry and shower units (financed by the Rotary Clubs of St Lucia and Guelph) in each village.

The involvement of the Research and Control Department in mainten-ance of the system terminated in 1978 when Government assumed full responsibility. (The Ministry of Community Development, Social Affairs and Sport is responsible for water supplies in St Lucia.) Problems arose with the intake and management of the distribution system, and abuse of the facilities was common with Fordilla taps being replaced by conventional outlets or vandalised to give a continuous flow of water to irrigate gardens. These factors affected the supply more in the northern villages and led to a return to washing in rivers and inadequate use of the water seal latrines.

The design of the water seal unit was based on local practices and preference. The material used was high impact polyethylene, the same material used for a similar unit manufactured in New Zealand for use in Fiji. The New Zealand unit was tried in St Lucia but was unsatisfactory under local conditions. Another design was developed to cater for the local preference for a riser with a seat which is associated with a higher standard of living, although for community use a squat, hole-type latrine is preferred. The unit (Fig. 7.12) is easy to transport and the smooth plastic makes it easy to clean and flush, using about 2 l of water; it incorporates the riser bowl and S-trap in two separate components which fit together

Fig.7.12. Calypso area – north: water seal units showing the two sections and how they fit together in construction. (Photograph by G. O. Unrau.)

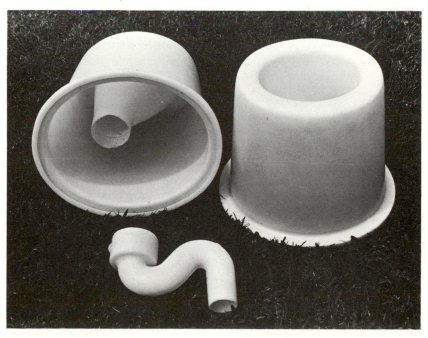

and are mounted on a 1.23 m by 1.23 m concrete slab over a pit usually about 2 m deep. The unit may also be used with an off-set pit where soil conditions warrant. This also has the advantage that new pits can be dug without disturbing the latrine. The pits were dug and the superstructure provided by householders as their contribution to the programme. In addition they also dug channels for the water supply pipe-line to individual houses. (The latrine units were provided by the Edna McConnell Clark Foundation. See Appendix 6.)

Although the construction of a water distribution system may take months or years, ideally in a research project such as this the whole distribution should be completed and 'turned on' in all villages at the same time; in practice this is not feasible. Thus, water became available in both areas over a two-year period, from early 1976 to early 1978. Similarly latrine installation on the northern side commenced at the end of 1976 but was not completed until early 1978 when the chemotherapy programme on the southern side of the project area was completed.

An intensive health education campaign was mounted to explain to the people the reasons for the facilities and how latrines should be used and maintained in order to get maximum benefit from them. The units were remarkably free of trouble and proved very popular with the villagers.

Chemotherapy

A single treatment campaign for all persons found infected at surveys in 1976 and 1977 (i.e. similar to Cul de Sac where treatment was offered to those found infected at the 1975 and 1976 surveys), was carried out and completed in January 1978. Oxamniquine at a dose of 15 mg per kg body weight was well tolerated. Post-therapy side effects were not specifically investigated. Eight hundred and seventy three patients were treated in field campaigns and 70 were treated in the ward representing a response rate of approximately 90 %. The 10–14-year age group showed the best compliance, 97%, while the least co-operative was the 20–29-year age group with 80% accepting treatment. The response rate of the two sexes was similar.

Parasitological findings

The first house census and survey was made in 1974. Children to the age of 14 were examined annually; thereafter, adults were re-examined in 1976, 1977 and 1980 (northern area) and 1981 (southern area).

Pre-control

Overall prevalence and incidence of new infections between pre-control surveys are shown for each village in Table 7.27.

Table 7.27. *Calypso area: overall prevalence by settlement at 1974 and 1977 surveys and incidence between surveys amongst children aged 0–11 years.*

Villages in order of incidence 1976–77

Settlement	1974 Overall prevalence (%)	1974–75 No. neg.[a]	1974–75 % inc.[b]	1975–76 No. neg.	1975–76 % inc.	1976–77 No. neg.	1976–77 % inc.	1977 Overall prevalence (%)
Southern settlements								
Desruisseau	59	139	39.6	144	16.7	190	15.3	33
Blanchard	46	179	21.2	221	11.8	291	13.1	27
Anse Ger	18	102	4.9	131	2.3	138	4.3	9
Northern settlements								
Fond L'Or	50	22	18.1	20	15.0	30	26.7	38
Ti Rocher	53	129	23.2	132	9.8	189	23.0	24
La Cour Ville	6	36	0.0	60	6.7	86	8.1	10
Dugard	19	57	7.0	54	5.6	56	1.8	12

[a] Number negative at first of two surveys.
[b] Percentage positive at second survey.

Incidence between 1975 and 1976 was lower than in the previous 12 months; it increased in northern settlements the following year but over the 1974–77 pre-control period prevalence declined in both areas. In the northern area there was little change among males (Fig. 7.13) but among females there was a significant drop (Z = 3.76, significant at the 0.01% level). Among all age groups of both sexes in the southern area prevalence was lower in 1977 than in 1974 (significant in both sexes at the 0.01% level; Fig. 7.14). The decline in prevalence could have been due to a number of factors associated with the work of the Department; the presence in the area of parasitological and biological survey teams required explanation which may have had some educating effect, and between 1974 and 1975, 93 persons in the south received treatment when referred from the Health Centre; in addition, the return of only uninfected snails to their habitat,

Fig.7.13. Calypso area – north: changes in *S. mansoni* prevalence among males and females between 1974 and 1977, pre-control, and in 1980 after water and sanitation.

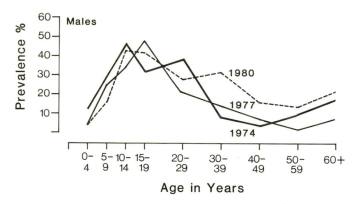

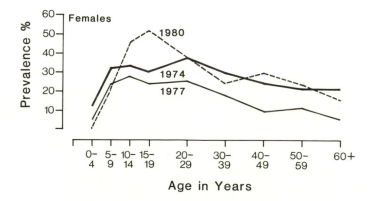

may have played a part. The gradual extension of available water supplies, and latrines in the north, may also have had some effect.

Parasitological data at the last pre-control survey are shown in Table 7.28. The response of the populations in the two areas was similar and typical of other areas. In each area the sexes were similarly infected but rates were a little lower in the northern area.

Fig.7.14. Calypso area – south: changes in *S. mansoni* prevalence among males and females between 1974 and 1977, pre-control, and in 1981 after chemotherapy and individual household water supplies.

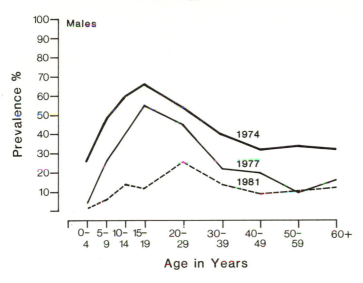

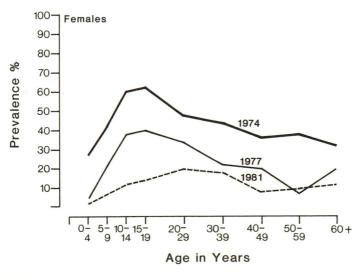

Table 7.28. *Calypso area: prevalence and intensity of S. mansoni infection with the corrected index of potential contamination (1977)*

Age in years	Males			Females			Both sexes				
	No. exam.	Prev. (%)	GM	No. exam.	Prev. (%)	GM	% of pop. (1)	Prev. (2)	Prev. (%) GM (3)	Corr. IPC	Relative % IPC
Southern settlements											
0–4	181	4	23	165	4	16	17.2	4	22	15	2
5–9	246	26	23	259	22	25	20.2	24	24	116	19
10–14	187	40	30	186	39	33	14.7	39	31	178	28
15–19	106	55	31	130	41	24	10.0	47	27	127	20
20–29	86	45	17	134	33	28	12.0	38	22	100	16
30–39	78	23	15	112	22	26	8.2	23	21	40	6
40–49	48	21	13[a]	80	20	19	7.0	20	16	22	4
50–59	74	11	13[a]	68	7	21[a]	5.3	9	11	5	1
60+	43	16	13[a]	55	20	21[a]	5.4	18	28	27	4
0–14	614	24	26	610	22	28	100.0	23	27	(630)	100
15+	435	32	21	579	27	24		29	23		
Northern settlements											
0–4	117	4	21[a]	87	5	22[a]	17.2	4	19	13	3
5–9	141	26	21[a]	134	24	22[a]	20.2	25	21	106	22
10–14	99	34	39	103	29	29[a]	14.7	32	30	141	30
15–19	47	49	32	49	24	18	10.0	37	27	100	21
20–29	58	22	15	80	28	16	12.0	24	16	46	10
39–39	40	15	26[a]	63	18	21[a]	8.2	17	23	32	7
40–49	29	7	26[a]	39	10	21[a]	7.0	9	22[a]	14	3
50–59	29	3	26[a]	39	13	21[a]	5.3	9	22[a]	10	2
60+	26	8	26[a]	43	7	21[a]	5.4	7	22[a]	8	2
0–14	357	21	28	324	20	22	100.0	21	26	(470)	100
15+	229	21	24	313	17	19		19	21		

[a] Means of combined age groups.

Table 7.29. *Calypso area: annual incidence of new S. mansoni infections amongst children prior to control (1974–77) and after*

Age in years	1974–75		1975–76		1976–77		1977–78		1978–79		1979–80		1980–81	
	No. neg.	% inc.	No. neg.	% inc.	No. neg.	% inc.	No. neg.	% inc.	No. neg.	% inc.	No. neg.	% inc.	No. neg.	% inc.
Southern settlements														
0 & 1	71	12.7	80	5.0	72	2.8	52	0	47	0	49	2.0	54	0
2 & 3	102	25.5	95	5.3	131	4.6	139	0.7	117	1.7	86	0	81	1.2
4 & 5	74	20.3	103	15.5	139	10.0	133	5.3	135	5.2	144	2.1	131	3.8
6 & 7	75	32.0	87	6.9	115	20.9	139	8.6	161	3.7	137	4.4	146	2.1
8 & 9	53	35.8	62	14.5	80	11.3	115	12.2	125	4.0	144	4.9	137	10.2
10 & 11	45	28.9	69	17.4	82	22.0	87	12.6	113	14.2	99	9.1	123	12.2
0–11	420	25.2	496	10.7	619	11.8	665	6.8	698	5.2	659	3.9	672	5.7
Northern settlements														
0 & 1	39	5.1	31	6.5	34	2.9	27	3.7	27	7.4	25	4.0		
2 & 3	53	11.3	59	3.4	65	3.1	67	6.0	70	5.7	53	1.9		
4 & 5	42	16.7	55	9.1	75	12.0	88	11.4	78	6.4	70	8.8		
6 & 7	42	21.4	47	4.3	76	32.9	61	21.3	66	10.7	89	9.0		
8 & 9	39	20.5	44	20.5	66	24.2	58	24.1	49	30.6	48	20.8		
10 & 11	29	20.7	30	13.3	45	15.6	50	36.0	41	24.4	36	16.7		
0–11	244	15.6	266	9.0	361	16.6	351	17.1	331	13.0	321	10.0		

Table 7.30. *Calypso area: prevalence and intensity of* S. mansoni *infection in South and North Canelles area*

Age	1974			1977			1981		
	No. exam.	% +ve	GM[a]	No. exam.	% +ve	GM	No. exam.	% +ve	GM
Southern settlements									
0–4	365	27	21	346	4	22	249	2	15
5–9	365	53	28	505	24	23	433	5	15
10–14	344	60	38	373	39	32	394	14	14
15–19	193	64	40	236	47	27	207	14	16
20–29	222	51	28	220	38	22	194	22	18
30–39	142	42	26	190	23	21	182	17	20
40–49	115	35	17	128	20	15	134	9	13
50–59	109	37	13	142	9	11	110	15	15
60+	92	33	27	98	18	28	118	14	15
0–14	1073	46	30	1224	15	27	1076	8	14
15+	873	47	27	1014	29	23	945	16	17
Crude IPC[b]	11378			5379			1813		
Reduction				53%			66%		
Cumulative change					53%			84%	

Age	1974			1977			1980		
	No. exam.	% +ve	GM	No. exam.	% +ve	GM	No. exam.	% +ve	GM
Northern settlements									
0–4	175	13	18	204	4	11	142	2	10
5–9	216	31	23	275	25	21	257	20	17
10–14	173	41	25	196	33	30	189	46	31
15–19	88	32	19	96	37	27	88	48	33
20–29	109	38	21	138	24	16	86	34	30
30–39	68	24	22	103	17	23	86	28	26
40–49	61	18	15	68	9	13	59	24	17
50–59	41	22	17	68	9	48	63	21	23
60+	43	21	13	69	7	16	47	19	17
0–14	564	28	23	675	21	26	588	24	24
15+	410	28	19	542	19	21	429	31	27
Crude IPC	4589			3994			6322		
Reduction				13%			increase 41%		
Cumulative change					13%			+38%	

[a] Geometric mean of e.p.ml faeces.
[b] Sum of produce of prevalence and GM for each age group.

Post-control

Southern settlements. From 1977 to 1981 incidence rates in the southern settlements were significantly lower than pre-control (Table 7.29) and by 1981 prevalence was reduced from 24% to 12%; intensity of infection also declined and the crude IPC was reduced by 66% (Table 7.30).

Northern settlements. The 1980 survey of children in the northern settlements showed little effect on transmission; annual incidence rates between 1977 and 1980 were no different from the pre-control data from 1974–77 (Table 7.29). (Although over the last three years of the project there was some evidence of declining transmission, i.e. incidence of 17.1%, 13.8% and 10.9%, this was probably only due to the high incidence between 1977 and 1978 (17.1%), greater than any of the pre-control figures).

In view of the impending closure of the Research and Control Department, evaluation was prematurely terminated after a final survey of adults which showed increased prevalence (Table 7.30).

This affected females above the age of 10 ($Z = 4.65$, significant at the 1% level) and males above the age of 30 ($Z = 2.57$, significant at the 1% level) (Fig. 7.13). Intensity of infection increased among adults and the crude IPC increased by 41%. Continuing transmission was confirmed by a cohort study which showed a high C/R ratio (3.00) among adults (Table 7.31).

Analysis of data from separate settlements (Table 7.32) showed that not only was prevalence unaffected by the latrines and water in any village, but that in two, Fond L'Or and La Cour Ville, there was a marked increase.

At the termination of the programmes chemotherapy was offered to all

Table 7.31. *Calypso area north: results of a 1977–80 cohort study showing change in status of* S. mansoni

		Age group	
		0–14	15+
No. examined		431	376
No. (%)	1977	96 (22)	49 (13)
Conversions		76	54
Reversions		27	18
C/R ratio**		2.81	3.00
No. +ve (%)	1980	145 (34)	85 (23)

** In both age groups difference between conversions and reversions was significant at 1% level.

Table 7.32. *Calypso area north: prevalence of S. mansoni amongst 0–14-year-old children and corresponding incidence of new infections between surveys amongst 0–11-year-old children*

Year of survey	Fond L'Or Prevalence No. exam.	% +ve	Incidence No. neg.	% inc.	Ti Rocher Prevalence No. exam.	% +ve	Incidence No. neg.	% inc.	Duggard Prevalence No. exam.	% +ve	Incidence No. neg.	% inc.	La Cour Ville Prevalence No. exam.	% +ve	Incidence No. neg.	% inc.
1974	65	51			310	38			120	17			69	1		
1975	59	39	22	18.2	287	36	129	23.3	94	17	57	7.0	83	2	36	0.0
1976	52	37	20	15.0	355	19	132	9.8	111	12	54	5.6	137	7	60	6.7
1977[a]	63	38	30	26.7	355	26	189	23.3	111	10	56	1.8	152	9	86	8.1
1978	58	24	27	14.8	323	32	175	21.7	92	8	59	6.8	134	20	90	15.6
1979	64	33	33	27.3	293	27	161	13.7	89	6	59	3.4	124	21	78	12.8
1980	64	47	35	25.7	287	25	141	11.3	98	7	65	2.9	139	23	80	6.3

[a] Commencement of control.

known to have been infected but untreated. In the northern settlements only 71% (274 of 388) accepted treatment, thus leaving a large reservoir of infection. In the southern settlements 87% (460 of 529) of infected persons were treated.

Biological studies

All streams and their feeder marshes were examined for populations of *B. glabrata*. Based on these surveys nine index sites (four in the northern area and five in the south) were selected for routine fortnightly sampling: a further five sites, chosen on the basis of observed human contact combined with the presence of a *B. glabrata* population, were sampled monthly. Both areas were re-surveyed at least annually. In addition, special surveys were carried out as needed, e.g. following parasitological evidence of a focus of transmission. Only uninfected snails found on survey were returned to their habitats.

Miracidial densities were monitored at seven sites by exposing sentinel snails. A 48-hour exposure was used in an attempt to increase the sensitivity of the method. Rainfall data were collected from two gauges, one each at the upper Canelles bridge at Ti Rocher. The gauges were read once weekly beginning in January 1976.

Results from the northern area are summarised in Table 7.33 and Fig. 7.15. Based on biological findings, the virtual absence of infected field and sentinel snails after 1977 would suggest latrines and water had been successful in reducing transmission. (The low number of sentinel snail infections in the northern area could be related to the human population there living further from the streams than in the south.)

Parasitological data, however, suggested otherwise and although extensive and intensive searches were made for transmission foci none was

Table 7.33. *Calypso area north:* S. mansoni *infection rates in sentinel snails*

Year	No. examined	No. infected	% infected
1974	1172	3	0.26
1975	1282	6	0.47
1976	1589	1	0.06
1977	1191	0	0.00
1978	943	8	0.85
1979	733	0	0.00
1980	727	0	0.00
1981[a]	583	0	0.00

[a] 6 months only.
Prentice, unpublished data.

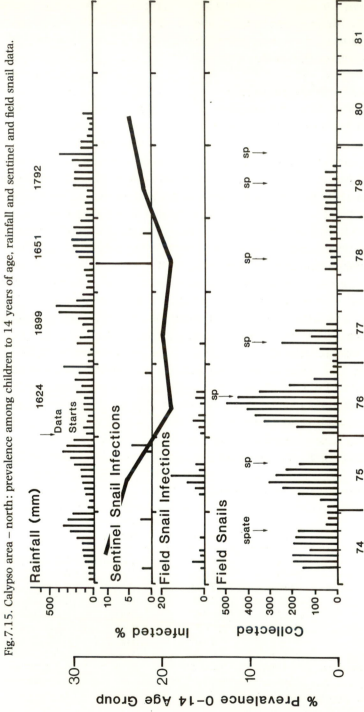

Fig.7.15. Calypso area – north: prevalence among children to 14 years of age, rainfall and sentinel and field snail data.

found. It must be assumed, therefore, that continued transmission resulted from sporadic snail infections in small, transient colonies distributed along the various ravines which meander through the populated area. Such colonies were located at various times but on only one occasion (in April 1981) were infected snails found. If this is the true explanation, then it points to the importance of relatively low numbers of infected snails distributed over a wide area and confirms the necessity of applying focal control measures to any snail-infested stream which passes through the inhabited area, irrespective of whether or not infections have been found.

Results of sentinel snail exposures from the southern area are summarised in Table 7.34 and Fig. 7.16. Until September 1975 numerous small localised snail colonies were found along the edge of the Canelles river – frequently associated with washing sites. These were, however, flushed out in September by heavy rains and never became re-established. It seems that increased cultivation on the steep valley sides may have allowed faster run off and more frequent severe flushes. Whatever the reason for the absence of colonies, the finding contrasts with the numerous colonies found in the river when observations were started. This coincided with the end of a series of dry years when more stable conditions would have favoured snail colonies in flowing water. A small focus of transmission was found in Blanchard stream – not only a favourite washing place but a stream crossing point. In 1974 amongst a collection of 163 snails 91 (56%) were infected (Table 7.35).

Sentinel and field snails were frequently found infected during the first few years of the study but numbers decreased from 1977, coinciding not only with completion of water supplies and the chemotherapy programme but rainfall conditions that decimated the snail populations that year.

Table 7.34. *Calypso area south:* S. mansoni *infection rates in sentinel snails*

Year	No. examined	No. infected	% infected
1974	1253	24	1.92
1975	1524	7	0.46
1976	1496	5	0.33
1977	1205	3	0.25
1978	985	5	0.52
1979	830	0	0.00
1980	1166	6	0.51
1981[a]	548	0	0.00

[a] 6 months only.
Prentice, unpublished data.

Fig.7.16. Calypso area – south: prevalence among children to 14 years of age, rainfall and sentinel and field snail data.

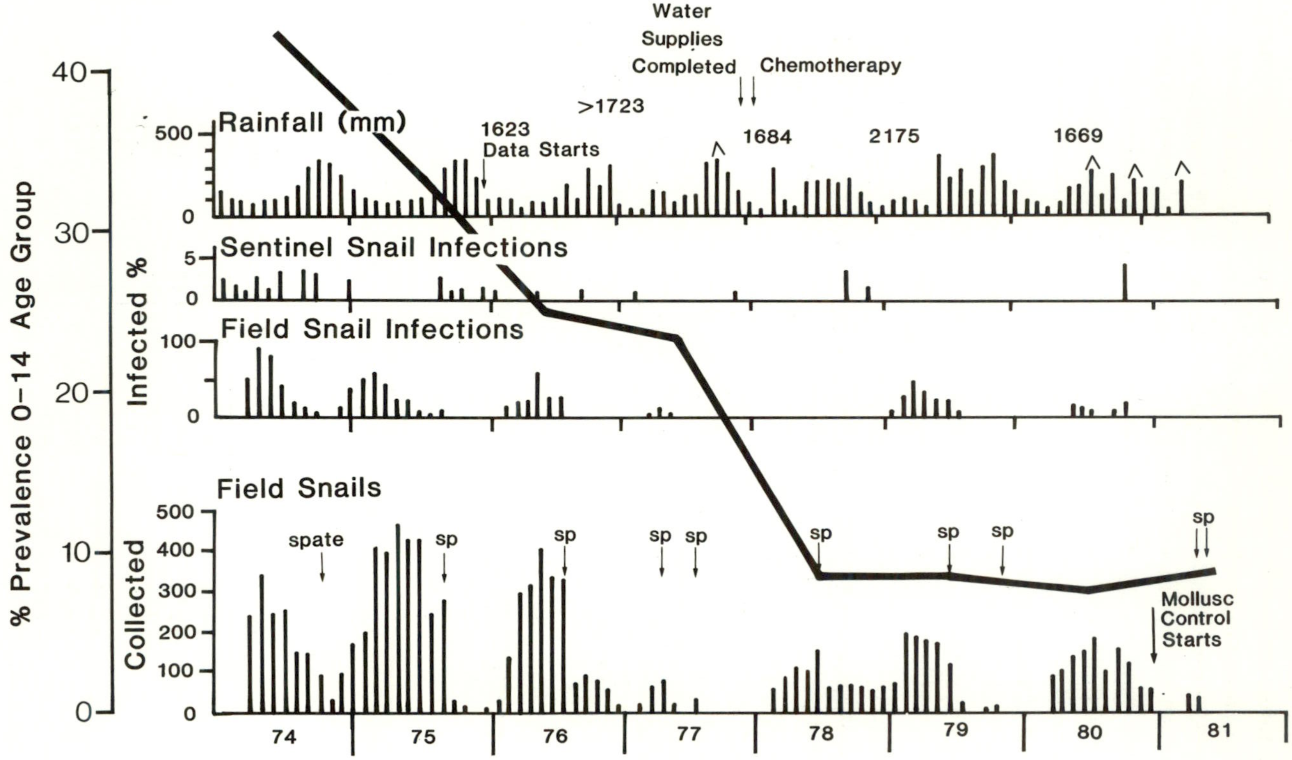

The presence of infected snails in the Blanchard stream in 1979 showed that in spite of chemotherapy the reservoir of infection was sufficient to continue transmission, but the low incidence of new infections reflects the success of the domestic water supplies and laundry and shower units in keeping the population out of the stream. It was observed, however, that when this leads to people abandoning their previous source of water there may be an increased use of the stream for sanitary purposes.

Routine focal control was started in April 1981 in sites known previously to have supported colonies of *B. glabrata*, and *T. granifera* were introduced into all areas. (See Chapter 12.)

Costs

Owing to the water supplies being installed in collaboration with Government it was not possible to cost these programmes, but the cost of the chemotherapy programme in the southern settlements was calculated: cost per stool examined US $1.27, per case detected $5.28, per person treated $9.86 and per person protected $3.72. All costs were higher than in Marquis valley (Table 5.13), due largely to the greater distance of the area from the laboratory and the longer time the survey team spent travelling – an hour compared with 15 minutes to reach Marquis.

The latrine units were custom made in the United States. As the order was for a limited number the unit cost of $36.12 was higher than it would have been had a larger number been ordered. Materials, labour and transporting slabs cost $7.96, making the total cost of an installed unit $44.08; pits for the units were dug by the householder.

Table 7.35. *Calypso area south:* S. mansoni *infections in field* B. glabrata *from the Blanchard stream index site*

Year	No. examined	No. infected	% infected
1974	823	295	35.8
1975	1165	121	10.4
1976	1795	54	3.0
1977	138	13	9.4
1978	531	3	0.6
1979	981	155	15.8
1980	1106	55	5.0
1981	Mollusciciding started in January		

Prentice, unpublished data.

Other health benefits

It was hoped that the provision of domestic water supplies would have health benefits other than reducing exposure to schistosome infection, and that the latrine facilities on the northern side of the valley would be accompanied by further advantages.

Detailed studies were made, therefore, of socio-economic conditions and benefits deriving from the water supplies in the Calypso south area, and from the water and latrines in the north. Findings were compared with data from Cul de Sac valley where there was a community standpipe water supply of limited distribution. Longitudinal investigations related mainly to the nutritional status of infants, height and weight increments, the frequency and duration of diarrhoeal disease, and prevalence of infection with *Ascaris* and *Trichuris*. Blood samples were also collected at regular intervals and examined for antibody titres to rotavirus by Dr Kapikian at the Laboratory of Infectious Diseases, National Institutes of Health, USA (Henry, 1981, and personal communication).

The impact of the water and latrines on the frequency and duration of episodes of diarrhoea in cohorts of infants was investigated by household visits, when the mother was asked to indicate, on a specially designed card, those days in each month when she considered the infant's stool was abnormally loose. Analysis of the data indicated a gradient in the percentage of children experiencing bouts of diarrhoea from a maximum of 23.5 % in Cul de Sac valley to 17.7% in Calypso south and 11.1% in the northern settlements (Table 7.36).

Although before the installation of sanitary facilities infant weights were similar in the three areas, and up to 6 months similar to the Harvard Standard, after water was available weights of infants from 6 to 24 months of age improved greatly in the Calypso area (more in the south than north) but showed no change in Cul de Sac, where infants were shorter than those from the other valleys: heights in Calypso north and south were similar.

Longitudinal studies were made of stools from cohorts of infants; they were examined by a quantitative formol-ether concentration technique. Results for *Ascaris* and *Trichuris* infections are shown in Table 7.37.

As treatment was given for *Ascaris* after each survey (in the three valleys) and high cure rates are obtained with piperazine, the figures for this helminth are considered to show the incidence of new infections since the previous survey. Incidence was significantly lower in both the Calypso areas compared with Cul de Sac; intensity of infection also tended to be lower.

Data for *Trichuris* represents prevalence at different surveys. There was

Table 7.36. *Calypso areas: distribution of diarrhoea by age in longitudinal study of infants compared with similar data from Cul de Sac*

Age of infant (months)	Cul de Sac (comparison)		Calypso South (water)		Calypso North (water and latrines)	
	No. infants studied	% with diarrhoea	No. infants studied	% with diarrhoea	No. infants studied	% with diarrhoea
<6	89	30.3	112	28.6	72	19.4
7–9	121	23.1	149	26.8	107	18.9
10–12	178	30.3	188	26.6	135	18.5
13–15	191	23.0	194	16.0	175	13.1
16–18	197	26.9	191	14.1	173	10.4
19–21	204	21.1	176	11.9	167	3.0
22–24	165	18.2	126	8.7	133	3.3
25–27	113	18.6	68	5.9	65	4.6
28–30	68	17.6	19	0.0	42	0.0
Total	1326	23.5	1223	17.7	1068	11.1

[a] Same infants studied at different ages.
F. Henry, personal communication.

Table 7.37. *Calypso areas: comparison of incidence of Ascaris and prevalence of Trichuris and intensities of infection after intervention compared with comparison area*

	Mean age in months	Cul de Sac (comparison)			Calypso South (water)			Calypso North (water + latrines)		
		No. exam.	% +ve	GM	No. exam.	% +ve	GM	No. exam.	% +ve	GM
Ascaris										
Dec. 1977	7	79	7.6	29.9	71	4.2	6.4	63	1.6	1
July 1978	14	78	34.6	15.8	71	18.3	22.6	60	21.6	12.6
Jan. 1979	20	77	53.2	20.7	70	45.7	25.9	61	27.8	7.9
Aug. 1979	27	70	40.0	41.4	62	33.9	19.3	59	23.9	12.6
Trichuris										
Dec. 1977	7	79	2.5	4.7	71	0	—	63	0	—
July 1978	14	78	12.8	21.0	71	7	12.4	60	10	8.7
Jan. 1979	20	77	26.0	19.0	70	25.7	7.5	61	24.6	5.8
Aug. 1979	27	70	58.6	35.4	62	30.6	5.8	59	33.9	9.5

F. Henry, personal communication.

little difference between findings from the intervention areas which were, however, lower than in Cul de Sac.

Evidence from Health Centres in the three valleys also supported the finding of improved health among the cohorts of infants over 18 months of age. The frequency of infants attending was established from their Health Passports; those with diarrhoea or vomiting, and skin diseases (conditions often associated with impure and inadequate water), were more frequently seen in Cul de Sac valley than in the Calypso areas. Complaints of respiratory infections and other minor ailments, not associated with water, were, however, similar in the three valleys (Table 7.38).

The rotavirus study was of particular interest and was probably the first longitudinal investigation of its kind. Perhaps surprisingly in view of the infection frequently accompanying diarrhoea which is often associated with impure water, there was no significant difference in infection rates in the three valleys.

It was gratifying that although in the northern settlements the water supplies and latrines failed to affect transmissions of *S. mansoni*, they did appear to be beneficial to infants in the area. The reason for the difference is probably due to the limited water that was available being used for the infants, but women continued to wash in the rivers when piped water was inadequate.

Summary and recommendations

It was disappointing that the water supplies in the northern area were irregular as this led to an unsatisfactory trial of water seal latrines in *S. mansoni* transmission control. The basis of this programme was to prevent (a) exposure (by water supplies), and (b) contamination (by latrines), but as both required water, when this was inadequate the scheme

Table 7.38. *Calypso area: frequency of complaints among infants in longitudinal study attending Health Centres for water-associated and other diseases compared with similar data from Cul de Sac*

	Cul de Sac (comparison)	Calypso South (water)	Calypso North (water + latrines)
No. children attending	72	61	54
% with diarrhoea/vomiting	34.7	27.8	18.5
% with skin diseases	20.8	4.9	3.7
% with respiratory infections	45.8	37.7	40.7
% with other complaints	6.9	1.6	3.7

F. Henry, personal communication.

was doomed. In retrospect, the use of the more conventional type of latrine (i.e. pit latrine with recent modifications to eliminate odour and fly problems) might have given better results.

While the increasing prevalence of *S. mansoni* in the northern settlements was disturbing, and the failure to locate transmission sites in spite of repeated surveys was frustrating, it was further confirmation of how difficult such sites can be to locate, particularly in areas where they are small and possibly only temporary. This area must be considered one of high risk for continued and perhaps increasing transmission.

In view of the failure to control transmission in the northern part of the Calypso area, results from the southern sector lose their full meaning. However, basically the area duplicated the findings of the last four years of the experimental water supplies in Richefond valley south, i.e. that after chemotherapy when household water supplies and laundry and shower units are available transmission appears to become stabilised at a much lower level.

Biological studies indicated the important finding that when piped water is available faecal contamination may increase on the banks of streams, previously the main source of water in a community. In the event of a breakdown in water supplies, resumed use of the stream may lead to renewed transmission which, because of increased contamination, may be at a higher level than previously. This suggests that when environmental improvement is planned in a developing area latrines dependent on water should not be used, as water supplies in such areas are notoriously liable to breakdown.

Recommendations to Government were that in view of the precarious state of water supplies they should not be the basis of future transmission prevention, although every effort should be made to improve intake, security of the main pipe-line and management of distribution system. Focal snail control should be maintained as the main measure to prevent transmission and should be carried out in actual and potential transmission sites. Eventually this may be unnecessary if *T. granifera* becomes well established to the exclusion of *B. glabrata*.

8

Schistosomiasis in other areas

School surveys

A number of schools outside the main control areas were surveyed as part of a search for undetected transmission foci in the island (Fig. 8.1). The home location of each child was identified and if more than 5% of children from one area were *S. mansoni* positive a village survey was carried out. If the village seemed suitable for a small research orientated control project, this was initiated, otherwise routine public health control was implemented. Results of school surveys are shown in Table 8.1. Small research schemes were also initiated at the Sulphur Springs, known to have been a focus of infection since 1924, and at La Caye.

It is apparent that prevalence had spontaneously declined in the coastal urban areas since the 1961 survey by Pannikar. Reasons for this are discussed in Chapter 1. The lack of any decline at Laborie is due to children from the inland village of Banse and others nearby attending the school.

Schemes with a research background

Monier

In 1974, of 131 10–14-year-old children at school at Grande Riviere (Gros Islet), 11 (8.4%) were found *S. mansoni* positive on stool examination: 8 of the 11 came from the small settlement of Monier where, in a village survey, 31 of 91 (34%) inhabitants were found infected; 23 accepted treatment and routine mollusciciding was started. After two subsequent surveys and treatments, all but four of the inhabitants present at the time of the 1976 survey had been treated.

Although index sites were kept free of *B. glabrata*, they were present in swamps. As the snail infested area was small, an attempt was made at snail eradication. In March and April 1977 marshy areas were intensively sprayed and drip feeds were used to treat flowing habitats; watercress beds and seepage areas were treated with 5% sand granules (Prentice & Barnish, 1980). The sites remained snail-free for six months, but all sites dried up in August. However, by November 1977 sites had refilled with water, *B. glabrata* were detected in the main watercress bed, and by December they were widely distributed.

Biological control with *H. duryi* was then unsuccessfully tried but within two years of seeding the two upper seepage areas with *T. granifera* in May 1978, *B. glabrata* were eliminated (see Chapter 12). A final parasitological survey in 1981 gave no evidence of a resurgence of transmission; 5 of 108 persons were *S. mansoni* positive and all were treated.

Fig.8.1. Location of schools surveyed and areas where research orientated or public health control schemes were initiated.

SCHOOLS

1   Monchy
2   Corinth
3   Castries
4   Ciceron
5   Anse La Raye
6   Canaries
7   Bouton
8   Mon Repos
9   Les Etangs
10   Choiseul
11   Laborie
12   Vieux Fort

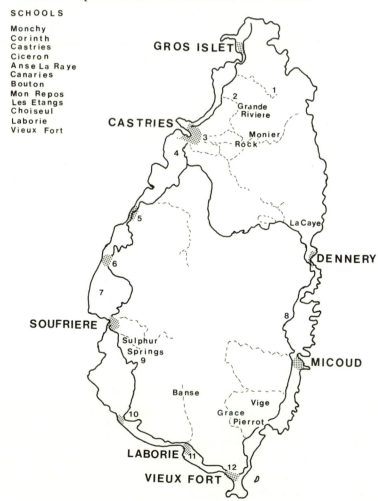

Sulphur springs

This isolated community of approximately 120 persons lives on the southern hillside of a small valley near Soufriere. The main stream arises in an area of flat marshy ground surrounded by steep hills, and flows 250 m until it forms a waterfall before flowing a further 50 m where it is joined by hot sulphurous water from the fumeroles of a 'drive-in volcano', one of the main tourist attractions in the island. Snails were found in the header marsh, a dasheen marsh, in numerous ditches in the valley and in a small tributary that joined the stream above the falls. Infected snails were frequently found in a washing site above the falls and in a pool below it. (See also p. 350.)

Near the waterfall, baths had been built and supplied with sulphurous water, claimed to have beneficial medicinal effects. After taking a bath, bathers washed off the sulphurous water under the falls and, in 1924, this led to the first reported case of schistosomiasis in the island. Later, three tourists became infected at the site (Most & Levine, 1963).

Table 8.1. *Prevalence of* S. mansoni *found at school surveys*

School	Year of survey	Map reference	Prevalence		Pannikar (1961)
			No. exam.	% +ve	
Marchand[a]	1967		451	15 ⎫	Castries
	1974		788	2 ⎬	23%
La Clery[a]	1967		221	3 ⎭	
Vieux Fort	1974	12	127	5	15%
Grande Riviere[b]					
(Gros Islet)	1974		131	8	
Anse La Raye	1975	5	199	1	36%
Laborie[b]	1975	11	887	14	17%
Monchy	1976	1	406	<1	
Ciceron	1976	4	248	5	
Canaries	1976	6	349	<1	64%
Choisel	1977	10	393	2	
Pierrot[b]	1978		47	13	
Grace[b]	1978		110	7	
Bouton	1979	7	50	6	
Mon Repos	1979	8	585	2	
Les Etangs	1979	9	158	<1	
Sans Soucis	1979		44	2	
SDA[a]	1979		19	11	
Corinth	1979	2	57	5	

[a] Schools in Castries.
[b] Followed by village surveys.

The small community above the falls was surveyed in 1974; 79% (86 of 115 examined) were found infected; 27 had egg counts greater than 50 e.p.ml faeces. These high egg excretors were treated with hycanthone, 2 mg/kg body weight, when it was calculated the contamination potential would have been reduced by 80%. The effect on transmission of this targeted treatment was to be assessed.

As a preliminary, snail populations were controlled for three months to allow maturation of any worms in the human population, but, following therapy, colonies were to be allowed to build up prior to examination for infections.

The whole ecology of the area was disturbed, however, by geothermal drilling in the area, including in the stream bed, and the targeted chemotherapy project had to be abandoned before evaluation was possible. At a re-survey in January 1976 after treatment of high egg excretors, overall prevalence was 56%; all infected persons were then offered treatment. In all, this was given to 95 of the 112 persons in the village – those uninfected included 5 children aged 0–4, 6 aged 5–9 and 4 adults; one child and one adult were infected (10 and 20 e.p.ml faeces respectively), but were not treated. While these were the only two known positives potentially likely to lead to infected snails, it must be accepted that a low proportion of those treated would also still be excreting a few eggs.

An attempt was then made to eliminate snails from the complex of streams, pools and marshes. Two slow-release formulations were used – 5% niclosamide wheat flour granules (Chapter 11) in flooded dasheen plots, stagnant ditches and marshes; and 5% niclosamide sand granules were left as depots at the source of seepage-fed ditches. The main stream was treated with a drip feed.

After four treatments at 14-day intervals no *B. glabrata* could be found. A few snails were found sporadically over the next few months in spite of further local treatments, and from June the area was re-treated by conventional spraying techniques to the end of the year. The efforts to eradicate the snails from this small focus by granules and later spraying were unsuccessful. The persistence of the snails in the face of prolonged molluscicide pressure may be due to a few being buried in the soft mud by cows, farmers (or spraymen!) moving in the area, later to be returned to the surface through agricultural activities.

In December 1976 control operations ceased and the snail population left to recover in order to provide natural index sites for snail population and cercariometric study to monitor the long term effects of the chemo-therapy. Re-population was rapid, and extensive colonies built up in the stream, the dam built by the geothermal drilling team, and many of the marshy areas. The dam formed a new potential transmission site: it had been built on a previously snail free stream to provide water for the drilling team and left as a washing facility in place of sites destroyed by drilling. Infected snails were found with increasing frequency throughout the area between 1977 and 1979 (Table 8.2), associated with a gradual increase in the prevalence of human infections (Table 8.3). *B. glabrata* appeared in the new dam in late 1978, and were found consistently until 1980; however they were infected only between January and April 1979 (16 of 1041 snails, 1.5%), a finding emphasising that sites can be infected only temporarily.

In November 1979 the valley was seeded with *T. granifera*; during the wet season of 1980 they became more numerous than *B. glabrata* whose

Table 8.2. *Sulphur Springs*: S. mansoni *infection in field* B. glabrata

	Streams and ditches			Dams and pools		
Year	No. exam.	No. +ve	% +ve	No. exam.	No. +ve	% +ve
1977	7379	9	0.12	1313	1	0.08
1978	8453	10	0.12[a]	908	2	0.20
1979	3757	18	0.48	2001[b]	16	0.80
1980	3918	14	0.36	811	0	0.00
1981[c]	805	0	0.00	233	0	0.00

[a] Lower limit only: a qualitative rapid screening method was used. It detected infected colonies quickly but could only determine that one or more infected snails were present.
[b] New dam became infected; it silted up in 1980 but remained free of *B. glabrata* thereafter.
[c] 6 months only.

Table 8.3. *Sulphur Springs: results of parasitological surveys*

	1974		1977		1978		1980		1981	
Age group	No. exam.	% inf.	No. exam.	% inf.	No. exam.	% inf.	No. exam.	% inf.	No. exam.	% inf.
0–9	28	57	15	13	14	14	12	8	12	0
10–19	35	80	28	7	22	14	18	22	15	40
20–39	8	100	9	0	7	14	6	17	6	33
40+	41	83	37	0	34	0	20	0	25	4
Total	112	77	89	4	77	8	56	11	58	16

numbers began to decrease, but the 'sponge' effect of *Thiara*, as well as the reduction in *B. glabrata*, may have contributed to the reduced snail infection rate in the final phases of the programme (Table 8.2) (Lavacuente, Brown & Jobin, 1979). Infected snails were not found throughout 1978, but cercariometric measurements were consistently positive (Fig. 8.2). In 1979 infected snails were sometimes present but cercariae were not detected; however stream flow was much reduced by drought conditions when cercarial loss would have been exceptionally high.

Analysis of the past history of the nine human infections found in 1981 indicates that apart from one, an immigrant from Soufriere, all had been found previously infected: only one had not been treated. All nine had quantitative egg counts of 10 or 20 e.p.ml faeces.

In spite of intensive treatment it is apparent that, in the absence of a maintenance phase strategy, prevalence increased and reached 22% in the 10–19-year age group by 1980, four years after therapy, and 40% by 1981, but intensities of infection were low. All nine found infected in 1981 and three of the six positive at the 1980 survey were treated.

La Caye

Stools from this village of approximately 500 population were used for a community based comparative study of the Kato and Bell quantitative stool examination techniques and for evaluating the RIA and ELISA sero-diagnostic methods (Chapter 3).

In 1978 treatment with 15 mg/kg oxamniquine was given to 89% of

Fig.8.2. Sulphur Springs: number of infected *B. glabrata* and their correlation with positive cercariometry findings from index sites (Prentice, unpublished.)

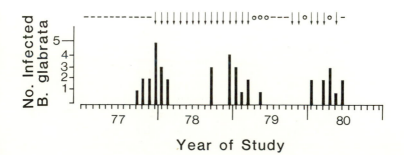

o   **Cercariometry–ve**

↓   **Cercariometry + ve**

–   **Not Done**

those found *S. mansoni* positive on examining three Bell filter papers. A re-survey was made two years later when prevalence (again based on three Bell filter paper examinations) had fallen from 67.7% (412 examined) to 16.6% (337 examined): the 'cure' rates among those under and over 14 years of age were 80 and 90% respectively. Blood spots were also collected from 293 persons: 53% gave a positive ELISA compared with 71% of 405 before treatment (Long, unpublished data) (Fig. 8.3).

While there was a marked drop in ELISA positivity after treatment, it was not as great as in Richefond north, where amongst 202 persons treated ELISA positivity fell from 70% to 34% in 12 months (Chapter 7). The greater decline there was probably due to examination of treated persons only and the community having a good water supply with better control of transmission.

Pierrot and Grace

As a result of surveys of school children, foci of infection were located at Pierrot (13% positive) and Grace (7% positive) (Table 8.1). Village surveys were carried out and low overall rates of infection were found – 9.4% and 11.6% at Grace and Pierrot respectively. Blood spots were collected for comparing parasitological results with the ELISA sero-diagnostic test (Fig. 8.4) The prevalence, calculated for probable missed *S. mansoni* cases, is also shown. At Grace the low prevalence found among persons below the age of 20 years compared with higher rates in

Fig.8.3. La Caye: comparison of parasitological (– – –) and ELISA (——) survey results in 1978 and two years after treatment.

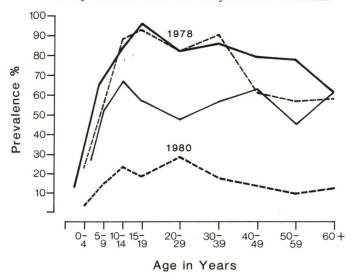

the older age groups probably indicates transmission had been much reduced in recent years. Treatment with oxamniquine was offered in both villages to those found parasitologically infected and was accepted by 68 (of 73 infected) and 63 (of 71) at Pierrot and Grace respectively.

Colonies of *B. glabrata* were found in both areas, in Ravine Bois Flot and Ravine St Urbain. Molluscicing was carried out and a laundry and shower unit was built at Pierrot (donated by the Rotary Clubs of St Lucia (Vieux

Fig.8.4. Pierrot and Grace: comparison of parasitological and ELISA survey results and calculated prevalence (△) allowing for cases missed on stool examination.

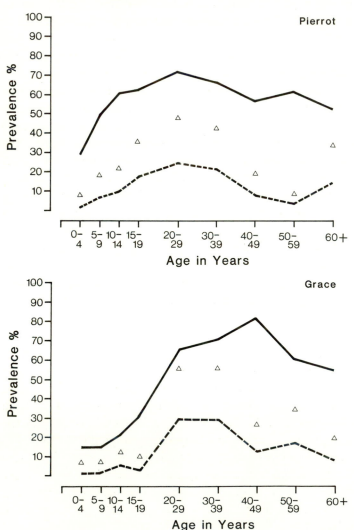

Fort branch) and Guelf in Canada). Regrettably the unit was little used as the water supply was inadequate.

Rock

The compatibility of *P. glauca* and *B. glabrata* was investigated in a marsh/stream complex on the western side of Marquis valley. This is described in Chapter 12.

Public health control

Soufriere township

The first schistosomiasis survey in St Lucia was made among school children at Soufriere in 1931, when 10% were found infected. As indicated elsewhere (Chapter 2), no control was instituted (it would have been difficult at that time), but a laundry unit was constructed in 1954. In 1961, Pannikar found 27% of the population below 20 years of age and 51% of the 20–40-year-olds infected. Although few *B. glabrata* were found near the town, 40% infection rates were reported from areas inland (presumably near Fond St Jacques). However, during a detailed snail survey of the area in 1968, infected *B. glabrata* were found in 11 of 17 sites around the town; the river was then re-aligned and canalised in 1972, and although two small colonies of *B. glabrata* were later found near the town (one in a small canal supplying water to a coconut oil factory, and one in a roadside ditch on the Fond St Jacques road), they were unlikely to have been transmission sites.

In 1973 school children were examined and 34% were found infected. Further analysis showed a prevalence of 26% among those living in Soufriere township compared with 53% amongst those living on the edge of town, in Fond Beniere, Palmiste and Wingsville, many of whom had to ford the Soufriere river to get to school.

Infected *B. glabrata* were found in unimproved sections of the river in 1974, but the area was heavily polluted by effluent from the oil factory and there was little human contact. It seems likely that the environmental changes associated with canalisation had drastically affected the snail habitat, and that any snails found had probably been washed down from the Fond St Jacques area. Snails continued to be found regularly in the canal supplying water to the factory, but only occasionally in the river.

In 1975 colonies were treated with molluscicide as a public health control measure, such treatment being repeated at monthly intervals. *B. glabrata* were last found in the river in June 1976, and in the oil factory canal in May 1977. In January 1981 monthly searches were changed to a 6-week cycle.

In October 1976, 74 of 1004 (7.4%) 5–14-year-old children were found infected; 68 were treated with oxamniquine.

Realignment and canalisation of the river just above the town was probably the largest factor in reducing *B. glabrata* populations and transmission, although later, vegetation at the sides of the river appeared and provided suitable habitats for snail colonies. Their non-appearance may be due to the use of molluscicide higher up the river at Fond St Jacques (Chapter 6); thus, although the cost per head of population of snail control there was comparatively high, cessation of control would probably lead to a recurrence of transmission in Soufriere township.

The last survey made by the Department in 1981 was to assess the situation in Soufriere school children, just 50 years after the first survey; 2.9% were found to be excreting *S. mansoni* eggs.

Rural areas

Public health control was also carried out in a number of rural areas. The school survey at Laborie (14% positive) suggested a focus of infection to the north of the town. In three villages, Banse, La Grace and Berange, a prevalence rate of 39% was found in 1975. Treatment was offered then and after surveys of 1978 and 1979. Mollusciciding was carried out from 1975 to 1977, after which nine index sites were selected for checking during 1980 and 1981. No infected *B. glabrata* were found among nearly 500 examined. At a final survey in 1981 only 17 of 494 (3.4%) of the population were found infected – all were treated.

Vige is a settlement south of the Canelles river and adjacent to the Calypso south control area. At a survey in 1974, 57% of the population were infected and offered treatment. The Government water supply was found to be non-operational and was repaired by the Department. There was a further survey and treatment in 1977. At the final survey in 1980, 12 of 157 were infected (8%) with no infections in the 0–4-year age group. All found infected were treated.

Results of a school survey at Grande Riviere (Gros Islet) identified Monier as a small focus of transmission, but also suggested there was some transmission in Grande Riviere; a village survey revealed 88 of 725 (12.1%) were *S. mansoni* positive. The age prevalence curve, however, indicated that while in the past transmission had been high (40% prevalence in the 20–29-year age group), it had fallen with only 2% of the 0–14-year age group being infected. Treatment was offered to all found infected, but no further action was taken.

Residual infections

Although final surveys at the end of the four-year maintenance phase strategies in the main control areas showed that overall prevalence varied between 4 and 14%, and treatment was offered to those found infected, the true rate was inevitably higher for reasons discussed elsewhere. Residual infections were also present in other areas where treatment was not always accepted but control had reduced prevalence and intensity of infection to low levels.

In all these rural areas there was, therefore, a potential for renewed transmission. In some areas snail populations appeared to be declining, whether temporarily or permanently it is impossible to assess, but large populations were present elsewhere. The biggest reservoir of infection remaining in the island was, however, thought to be in Castries amongst the immigrants who had moved from rural areas for work. A radio and newspaper appeal was therefore launched for these people to come forward for examination, but only one person responded, and he was infected.

In an attempt to find and treat these people, stools from hotel employees and those employed in various trades and light industries were examined. Over 500 stools were examined, of which 12% were *S. mansoni* positive. All were treated, but it was considered that a large population of infected persons remained in the city.

Recommendations for future control

When the Department closed at the end of 1981, recommendations were made to Government that continued snail control was necessary in some of the main control valleys and also in areas where research or public health control schemes had been initiated. *A Guide for the Control and Surveillance of Bilharzia Transmission on Saint Lucia, West Indies: a Consolidation Phase Strategy* was prepared for Government and for the three-man team who had been trained for the work. The Guide gives, in simple text, details of the molluscicide to be used, the equipment and how to maintain it, and a recommended day-to-day work schedule with drawings of all areas to be searched for snails and treated. In addition, recommendations were made to monitor infection in school children by ELISA carried out on finger prick blood specimens.

9

Comparison of control strategies

The Research Control Department began work at the end of a period of low rainfall, during which time transmission was probably at a higher level than in the first six years of operations when above average rains were consistently recorded (Fig. 1.3). This could well have been a factor in the decreased prevalence and intensity of infection noted, particularly in Cul de Sac valley, during the pre-control phase of operations. However, from 1971 to 1974 when the major control programmes were operating, rainfall was again low and transmission would normally be expected to be at a high level – as it was in the uncontrolled northern side of Richefond valley. In later years, from 1976 to 1981, rainfall was near average for the island, when transmission would probably have been steady.

Parasitological evaluation of comparison and control areas
Differential changes in prevalence by age and sex
Results of the different projects were based on the presence of *S. mansoni* ova in faecal samples collected from all ages of both sexes of the population. It was, however, apparent that while the response to a request for samples was initially high, it generally decreased as the number of surveys increased, suggesting that pre-control studies should be kept to a minimum.

Spontaneous changes in transmission that affected prevalence were noted in the two untreated comparison areas, but while in Roseau valley prevalence declined among children it increased among adults, although later it fell (Chapter 4). Spontaneous changes in Group I settlements on the northern side of Richefond (Chapter 4) showed a different pattern with increased prevalence among adults, followed by an increase among children, but in Group II villages prevalence increased among adults while the younger age groups showed no change. In these three areas the changes were the same among males and females. In the northern Calypso area water supplies and sanitation failed to prevent an increase in prevalence in males above the age of 30, and in females above the age of 10 years.

In view of these spontaneous changes, that surprisingly tended to affect adults more than children, it appears necessary to study indices of infection in all age groups of the population in the evaluation of schistosomiasis control programmes.

It was apparent also that the sexes may be affected differentially; with domestic water supplies the fall in prevalence among male children was greater than among other segments of the population, and where routine focal mollusciciding was evaluated in Fond St Jacques the fall in prevalence among males was greater than among females. However, with the area-wide snail control in Cul de Sac, and with chemotherapy in the Marquis valley, changes in prevalence were similar in all age groups of both sexes. All age groups and both sexes should therefore probably be used when evaluating intervention methods.

Parasitological efficiency

Changes in parasitological findings in the comparison area on the northern side of Richefond valley and in the initial phase of the various control schemes are summarised in Table 9.1.

The overall pattern of change in the comparison area does not reflect the rise then fall in indices of infection that occurred between 1970 and 1975, but the change in incidence (as in the failed water with sanitation programme in Calypso north) was substantially less than in any of the control schemes. Prevalence was higher in 1975 than in 1970, but the intensity of infection and the contamination potential were lower.

The chemotherapy programme in Marquis valley resulted in the greatest fall in incidence, with an overall decline of 87.3%. Prevalence also showed the greatest decline, 88%, as did the contamination potential, 90%; parasitologically, the best results were obtained from this strategy.

In the snail control schemes, area-wide in Cul de Sac valley and focal control in Fond St Jacques, overall declines in incidence and prevalence were similar, but intensity was reduced more with area-wide control – possibly due to the higher levels of infection in Cul de Sac at the commencement of the programme.

Results of the environmental control programme (individual household water supplies in the southern part of Richefond valley) would probably have been better if the area of control had included the northern side of the valley, as a high proportion of children from the control area went there

Table 9.1. *Summary of parasitological results of different pilot control schemes*

	Incidence[a]			Overall prevalence			Overall intensity			Contamination potential		
	From (%)	To (%)	Reduction (%)	From (%)	To (%)	Reduction (%)	From (%)	To (%)	Reduction (%)	From (%)	To (%)	Reduction (%)
Richefond (north) Untreated (1970–75)												
High transmission	25.1	20.8	17	49	53	(+8)	31	24	23	15713	11332	28
Low transmission	10.4	8.7	16 (16)[b]	28	37	(+32)(+20)	23	15	35 (29)	8288	3676	56 (42)
Marquis valley Chemotherapy (1973–76)												
High transmission	22.2	3.9	82	41	4	90	20	14	30	8201	462	94
Low transmission	5.1	0.4	92 (87)	14	2	86 (88)	20	15	25 (27)	2613	360	86 (90)
Snail control *Cul de Sac valley* Area wide (1971–75)												
High transmission	23.2	5.7	76	45	24	47	34	22	35	15061	5560	63
Low transmission	4.7	2.3	51 (64)	13	7	46 (46)	22	17	23 (29)	2888	1365	53 (58)
Fond St Jacques Focal (1976–80)												
High transmission	15.1	7.6	50	43	22	49	22	21	5	8867	4703	47
Low transmission	5.7	1.2	79 (65)	9	5	44 (46)	14	10	29 (17)	1218	484	60 (53)
Richefond (south) Environmental control (1970–75)	22.6	13.1	42	56	38	32	34	17	50	20053	6411	68
Calypso (south) Water+therapy (1976–81)	10.4	5.7	45	33	12	64	21	16	24	5581	1813	68
Calypso (north) Water+sanitation (1977–80)	9.4	10.0	(+6)	20	27	(+35)	23	23	0	3994	6322	(+41)

[a] Among 0–9-year-old children. [b] Overall % reduction.

Table 9.2. *Summary of results of maintenance phase strategies after chemotherapy*

	Years followed	Incidence[a] From (%)	To (%)	Overall prevalence From (%)	To (%)	Overall intensity From (%)	To (%)	Contamination potential From (%)	To (%)	Reduction (%)
Focal snail control										
Cul de Sac	1977–81	0.4	0.5	5	4	14	18	819	944	(+15)
Water supplies										
Household + L/S units										
Richefond (south)	1977–81	6.4	1.0	13	9	17	17	2083	1399	33
Calypso (south	1977–81	6.8	5.7	21	12	25	16	5379	1813	66
Community + L/S units										
Richefond (north; GRP I)[b]	1977–81	4.2	6.1	47	12	25	19	10047	2606	74
Community										
Marquis	1976–80	4.9	7.2	3	6	14	20	822	2037	(+148)
Richefond (north; Grp II)[b]	1977–81	8.2	15.6	33	14	19	19	6460	2166	66
Richefond (north; Grp III)[b,c]	1977–81	2.3	1.0	15	4	17	10	2779	774	72

[a] Among 0–9-year-old children.
[b] Chemotherapy not completed until 1977.
[c] Low transmission area.

to school; nevertheless, a substantial reduction in all indices of infection was recorded. Results of the programme where water supplies were combined with chemotherapy (Calypso south) should have been better than the separate schemes of water (Richefond south) and chemotherapy (Marquis), but in the event they were not, and the additional chemotherapy led to only marginally better incidence results than those from water alone. A number of factors were probably responsible – more treatment campaigns in the Marquis valley, a higher compliance rate, and the use of the more effective hycanthone in the first two treatments. The reduction in prevalence (64%) in the Calypso area, double that in Richefond, was due to the immediate effect of chemotherapy.

The results from Calypso north, with water and sanitation, showed an increase in all indices except intensity of infection, which was unaltered. It is stressed again that the sporadic water supply, when it was needed for the proper functioning of the latrines, did not provide an adequate evaluation of this control approach.

Table 9.2 summarises changes in the maintenance phase after chemotherapy campaigns in all areas.

In general, the best results were obtained where focal snail control or individual household water supplies and laundry with shower units were available: incidence and prevalence remained low or showed a decrease, although intensity of infection showed little change.

Results from Richefond north are less clear as the reduced prevalence in these village groups is largely due to chemotherapy which was not completed until after the 1977 survey. Although there was an apparent paucity of snails in Richefond valley, incidence increased slightly in village Groups I and II and in the Marquis valley, with significant increases in two of three Group II villages (Table 7.22) and in two of four high transmission villages in the Marquis valley (Table 5.6). No increase was noted in the low transmission Group III villages, and minimal increases occurred in other villages in Marquis valley.

It appears, therefore, that community water supplies alone are unlikely to prevent a resurgence of transmission in all villages, but this is less likely if adequate laundry and shower units supplement the system as reduced water contacts were recorded (Table 7.25). Individual household water supplies with laundry and shower units were effective in maintaining a high level of transmission control.

Comparative costs
Single approach to control

In view of the escalating prices towards the end of the Department's operations, for comparing the cost of later control projects with

Table 9.3. *Comparison of actual and amended costs (standardised to 1970–75) of single approach control schemes.*
Correction factor based on Cost of Living Index (Fig. 3.8)

| | Water supplies (Richefond) | Snail control | | Chemotherapy (Marquis) |
		Area-wide (Cul de Sac)	Routine focal (Fond St Jacques)	
Years of control	1971–75[a]	1970–75[b]	1976–80	1973–76
Population	2000	5000	1300	3000
Costs:				
Capital	72266	2727[c]	1760[c]	
Cost/person/year	1.81[d]	0.12	0.34	
Operational	23943[e]	74338	14938	11904
Cost/person/year	2.99	3.24	2.87	1.0
Total cost/person/year	4.80	3.36	3.21	1.0
Correction factor	Nil	Nil	2.0	1.14
Amended cost	4.80	3.36	1.60	0.88

NB Salaries of senior staff and freight charges have not been included. All items were imported into St Lucia duty-free.

[a] Based on 4-year period from time four of five villages had water.
[b] Scheme extended 55 months (Table 6.24).
[c] $\frac{2}{3}$ of actual cost of equipment and supplies as still in use at end of period.
[d] Capital cost amortised assuming 20-year life of system.
[e] Maintenance costs (Table 7.12). Cost for 1971–72 counted as the same as for following year.

earlier schemes some adjustment of actual expenditure was necessary. For comparing the cost of area-wide and routine focal snail control, chemo-therapy and household water supplies, adjustments were made, (Table 9.3) as described in Chapter 3.

It is apparent that the provision of water supplies was the most costly control programme, although the operational cost (i.e. cost of maintaining the system – $2.99 per person) was less than for the area-wide snail control. As has been stressed, this was an experimental scheme where the use of different water sources was investigated, and if a gravity-fed system had been utilised, recurrent costs (for electricity) would have been elimi-nated. The cost of installing any water system will depend on availability of water, and its cost-effectiveness will be increased in densely populated areas where distribution costs per family are low. Apart from the obvious social and medical benefits of water, the system provided a continuing maintenance phase control strategy that, to the end of the programme, prevented a resurgence of transmission after chemotherapy. Foreign currency was necessary for 59% and 47% of capital and maintenance costs respectively. (Transportation charges, all equipment and supplies for the water systems, power lines and electricty charges were included in this calculation.)

The question of providing free water is often raised. In the present scheme, where a houseowner requested an indoor tap (rather than the outlet being in the yard outside the house), a meter was installed and the Government rate for water was charged. However, the collection of a nominal water charge from all with a yard supply would probably be neither politically acceptable nor feasible to implement.

When the project started in 1965 it was essential that maximum effort be made in all strategies evaluated. If they were a success less intensive measures could be considered. Area-wide snail control was, therefore, necessary as the value of chemical control in reducing transmission had not been demonstrated conclusively. When this approach was shown to be effective – but too costly for public health control – the less intensive routine focal control was introduced in Fond St Jacques. The method was effective, and 52% less costly than the area-wide control in Cul de Sac. It has, however, been pointed out that the topography of the two areas is very different, and a better comparison of the two methods was their use in Cul de Sac valley when the cost of focal snail control was less than a tenth the cost of area-wide control, based on standardised costs (Table 6.24). Focal control may not be feasible in all endemic areas, but where well defined water contacts points are identified it should prove effective. It is, however, more costly in terms of the proportion of foreign currency needed for molluscicide (55%) than area-wide control (12%) in the overall cost of the scheme, although actual expenditure may be less. In this respect the surveillance/mollusciciding programme may be preferred where only 3.5% of costs were for chemical (Table 6.24). Continued application of molluscicide is required to prevent snail colonies being re-established and these recurrent costs are unlikely to diminish.

The four chemotherapy campaigns in Marquis valley constituted the cheapest scheme and were parasitologically the most effective; the cost of drugs that required foreign currency amounted to 16% of the total cost. As indicated elsewhere (Chapter 5), the scheme would have been much less expensive if the Kato stool examination technique had been available at the commencement of the programme. Probably two surveys would have sufficed to detect the same number of cases as were detected by the four surveys of the campaign. On this assumption, and that the time spent on stool examination would thus be halved, and using oxamniquine, the cost of the scheme would probably have been reduced by 33% to US $0.30 per head per year.

Maintenance phase

Chemotherapy is now assuming the major role in control programmes, but in most, for a variety of reasons, a reservoir of infection inevitably remains. Transmission is thus likely to continue at a low, but probably increasing, level (as in Marquis valley and elsewhere) (Prentice & Barnish, 1981) unless a supplementary control strategy is present. Thus, after chemotherapy in Cul de Sac valley, routine focal snail control prevented a resurgence of transmission, as did the domestic water supplies with laundry and shower units in the southern parts of Richefond valley and the Calypso area.

Table 9.4. *Actual costs in consolidation phase of control in three valleys*

Valley	Control	Years	Cost (/person/year)	
Richefond (south) (Pop. 2000)	Domestic water			
	Amortised capital	1971–81	$1.81	
	Running/maintenance	1977–81	$9.28	$11.48
	Supplementary therapy	1975–81	$0.39	
Cul de Sac (Pop. 5000)	Focal snail control	1977–81	$0.65	$1.04
	Supplementary therapy	1975–81	$0.39	
Marquis (Pop. 3000)	Chemotherapy	1973–80	$0.50	

The costs of different consolidation phase strategies are summarised in Table 9.4. As these followed chemotherapy campaigns, the cost of the latter has been spread over the period of the study. Thus, as there was no control supplement in Marquis valley, the actual cost of the four treatment campaigns has been spread over the eight years of the study, and in the Richefond and Cul de Sac valleys the actual cost of the two chemotherapy campaigns of 1975 and 1976 has been spread over these two years plus the four year follow-up period. (At the time therapy was offered in Cul de Sac and Richefond south, there had been control for four years, and prevalence had been lowered so that fewer persons needed treatment than would have been the case earlier.)

The extremely high maintenance cost of the water supplies was due to the increasing cost of generating electricity (Table 7.12). Although focal snail control was much less costly than area-wide control and appeared to be effective in preventing renewed transmission, it seems likely that, in spite of a resurgence in some villages in Marquis valley after chemotherapy, re-treatment of children after three to four years would probably be the least expensive method in a consolidation phase strategy in St Lucia.

Follow-up and recommendations

In addition to the recommendations to Government outlined in the different chapters on control, the monitoring of the human population by two methods was advocated. Stools from in- and out-patients are regularly examined at Victoria Hospital (Castries) and St Jude's Hospital near Vieux Fort. It was recommended that monthly records be kept of results, giving particular regard to age and home location of all persons examined in an attempt to identify areas where any resurgence of transmission occurred.

It was further recommended that blood spots should be collected annually from 5–14-year-old children at school in areas where transmission had occurred. These would be subjected to the ELISA at the Ross Institute in London.

It was also suggested that periodic visits be made to the island by senior staff of the Research and Control Department in order to review the situation and to make such further recommendations as necessary.

These recommendations were accepted by Government. It was also emphasised that every endeavour should be made to maintain water supplies in working order, that they should be expanded, and more laundry and shower units be built.

Recommendations were also made in respect of the potential hazard of *S. mansoni* transmission recurring in Roseau valley with the construction of a dam in the upper reaches of the watershed, where *B. glabrata* and a low level of *S. mansoni* remained. As a result of discussions with construction engineers, the more isolated of two possible sites was chosen for the dam. Other recommendations included the examination of any communities near the dam, and the resulting impoundment, and treatment of any infected with *S. mansoni*; examination and treatment of all labourers at the construction site; biological surveillance of the impounded river above and below the dam wall; and measures to prevent human settlements near, and with access to, the impounded water. The need for a reliable and adequate piped water supply in nearby villages was stressed. While there is a potential danger of transmission, it is thought this is not great, as *B. glabrata* in St Lucia do not appear to colonise large bodies of water; furthermore, in the sites proposed, impoundment would lead to a steeply sloping profile, with consequent deep water, and a shore line unattractive for settlement. It was also suggested that consideration be given to the introduction of weed-eating fish, in anticipation of them keeping the edges of the lake clear of water weeds and hopefully inimical to *B. glabrata*.

Requirements and effects of control strategies

The different technical requirements, demographic characteristics and effects of the control strategies evaluated are summarised in Table 9.5.

The pre-control investigation of transmission patterns is a prerequisite for effective and economical snail control and should probably be assessed over a year at the least. Trained and competent local field workers should be capable of the work if working under supervision. If focal snail control is used, a knowledge of water contact sites infested with the snail intermediate host is essential.

When chemotherapy is employed in control, and infected persons only are to be treated (selective population chemotherapy), case detection is of paramount importance and requires good microscopists, a quality control system and reliable record clerks. Random prevalence surveys can be made to detect areas of high prevalence where all persons might be treated. Some knowledge of the transmission pattern might be useful in the timing of chemotherapy which, if possible, should be given during the low or non-transmission season for maximum effect. In large scale schemes, however, such timing may not be feasible.

Few pre-control investigations are required for water supplies apart from locating a suitable water source for supplying an adequate and reliable supply, but detailed planning is required for developing and maintaining the system.

A high degree of public awareness is necessary in chemotherapy

Table 9.5. *Comparison of relevant technical requirements and demographic characteristics of different control strategies*

	Snail control	Chemotherapy	Water
Pre-control investigations	Transmission patterns	Case detection/sample surveys	Available water sources
Personnel	Public health workers	Technicians Paramedics	Engineers Artisans
Health education and community participation	+[a]	+ + + +	+ + + +
Supervisory requirements			
Initial	+ + +	+ +	+ + + +
Maintenance	+ +	+	+ +
Population protected	All using water bodies treated	Those treated; untreated may be exposed less to infection	Those using water supplies
Effect	Slow	Rapid	Slow
Other benefits	Minimal	Patients cured Pathology reversed	Improved health Social benefits
Immigration	Little effect	Significant	Little effect
Foreign exchange	Chemicals	Drugs Diagnostic tools	Pipes, fitting, pumps, tanks etc.

[a] Level of involvement: + least; + + + most.

campaigns to ensure the fullest community participation possible, both in detecting infected persons and in accepting treatment. Health education is also necessary where water is provided so that communities make the best use of it. Intensive campaigns may be required to encourage the use of laundry and shower units.

In contrast, community participation is of little importance in snail control schemes, although in some areas the community may assist in weed clearance in snail habitats; the public must, however, be made aware of what is happening.

Supervisory requirements: Once the transmission patterns have been determined and the appropriate methods of mollusciciding have been developed for routine application, there should be less need for ongoing supervision if field staff are reliable, but periodic checks are needed to ensure the programme is being effectively carried out. As mollusciciding may be necessary on a 6-weekly cycle, operational areas for a snail control team may of necessity be comparatively small.

While investigation of the transmission pattern is a prerequisite for effective mollusciciding, it is not a requirement for the initiation of schistosomiasis control. In most endemic areas there is sufficient information on the transmission to aid timing of chemotherapy which, for optimal effect, should be given in the low transmission season. If transmission is known, or thought, to be year round, then snail control may be useful if it precedes the chemotherapy campaign.

For chemotherapy campaigns specially trained nurses and other health workers can administer the drugs now used in control schemes. After treatment there should be plans for the difficult task (impossible in some areas) of recording the arrival of immigrants, their examination and treatment, but this should not prevent treatment teams moving to new areas, to return at a later date when re-treatment is required. Since the aim of modern control strategies is a reduction in morbidity rather than the interruption of transmission, re-treatment will be required before prevalence and intensity of infection reach levels predisposing to hepatosplenomegaly. This contrasts with snail control where regular, 6-weekly mollusciciding may be required so that operational areas for control teams may not be large.

The planning and installation of water supplies require a high level of professional involvement, and maintenance by artisans *must* be regular and effective; where a breakdown occurs repairs must be made immediately. (Evidence from the St Lucia project suggests that when piped water is available there is greater faecal contamination of surface waters as they are no longer used for domestic purposes, so that a high level of transmission may occur if the population resumes using snail infested water.)

The population affected by the different control strategies varies: with effective snail control all those previously using cercarial infested water will be protected, but when piped water is available only those using it, to the exclusion of contacting infested water, will be safe from infection. In chemotherapy schemes those treated will receive maximum benefit, but if community participation is at a high level, cercarial infection rates in snails will be lowered so that untreated persons will be less exposed to further infection.

The effect of chemotherapy is rapid; prevalence and intensity of infection are reduced, incidence of new infections declines, those with early organomegaly may be cured and in others the disease process may be halted. In contrast, while both snail control and water supplies reduce the incidence of new infections and there is a slow reduction in prevalence of infection, the effect on morbidity may be only slowly apparent and disease processes minimally affected. Water supplies have additional health and social benefits but no other benefits are apparent from snail control, although if the snail intermediate host of *Fasciola hepatica* uses the same habitat as the intermediate host of schistosomiasis some control of liver fluke may be attained.

Immigration of infected populations has little effect on snail control or on control by water supplies if these are available for the new arrivals. However, infected immigrants can seriously jeopardise results of chemo-therapy campaigns as they may form a significant reservoir of infection after communities have been treated. To counter this, some form of registration and examination (for subsequent treatment) of immigrants is theoretically desirable, but in large scale operations, such as the Blue Nile Health Scheme, this is unlikely to be practicable, so that some form of snail control may be necessary.

Foreign exchange requirements vary with the availability of different items in the country, but in most instances molluscicide and drugs must be purchased from Europe. In some developing countries components for water supplies will be available, but in most they would need to be imported.

The St Lucia project and the global schistosomiasis problem

The St Lucia project was originally designed to compare three methods of controlling transmission. It was shown that preventing infection by controlling snail populations or reducing exposure to infected water resulted in similar slow declines in prevalence and intensity of infection that would only slowly affect morbidity and disease; the cost-benefit of both approaches is greatest in areas of high population density. Community based chemotherapy, on the other hand, resulted in a rapid reduction in indices of infection that would prevent the development of clinical manifestations, and furthermore was the cheapest method of control. It may also be the best approach in widely dispersed populations who can assemble for treatment.

Studies in St Lucia confirmed a Brazilian observation that morbidity and hepatosplenic disease are related to intensity of infection. The use of newly developed drugs, suitable for community use, led to reduced organomegaly and the concept of direct and rapid disease control rather than control of transmission that was considered appropriate in 1965. This new strategy is now generally accepted, as is the fact that a low prevalence will remain, but that the intensity of infection is unlikely to be associated with serious disease unless renewed transmission occurs.

The new drugs are being used in large scale control schemes in Brazil, Egypt and many other countries. The schemes were however, undertaken with little or no previous investigation of consolidation phase control strategies, which became a feature of the final four years of the St Lucia project, when it was shown that the reservoir of infection remaining after intensive chemotherapy was sufficient for transmission to continue at a low but probably increasing rate, this latter depending on local epidemiological conditions. However, where routine focal snail control is practicable, its use may prevent or delay a resurgence of transmission. This was also prevented by domestic water supplies and laundry and shower units and probably also when these supplemented a community standpipe water supply. The importance of community involvement and co-operation and health education in schemes involving chemotherapy and water supplies became apparent, and contrasted with the need for a community to accept snail control only once they had been assured water and crops would not be adversely affected.

No endemic area of schistosomiasis, whether involving *S. mansoni* or *S. haematobium* or *S. japonicum*, can be considered a 'typical area', owing to variations in ecology, transmission patterns and sociocultural characteristics of the population. There will, therefore, probably never be a blue print for an effective control protocol applicable for all areas, but principles of control are common to all areas as the requirements for transmission – a low level of sanitation, and a suitable snail intermediate host in water used by the population – are always present. Evidence suggests that, in spite of widely different cultures, the acquisition of infection through domestic water contact, and the man–parasite and parasite–disease relationships, are similar in different areas. The main difference appears to be in the transmission patterns relative to the habitat of the snail intermediate host, which may be flowing or static, large or small water bodies and associated with different seasonal transmission patterns that depend largely on variations in temperature or rainfall or both. The effect of control of exposure (i.e. by provision of adequate water facilities) and control of the parasite (i.e. by chemotherapy), both requiring little pre-control study, are thus likely to be similar in different endemic areas. The variations in transmission patterns from one area to another (largely dependent on local ecological and epidemiological characteristics of the snail intermediate host) necessitates their clarification in an area for preparing a suitable strategy for the economic and effective use of molluscicide.

While it is apparent that chemotherapy is now the main component of schistosomiasis control, the effectiveness of the drug delivery system and the extent of population compliance will largely determine the reservoir of infection remaining. Other factors include the methods used for case detection (unless the whole population is treated), the 'cure rate', the incidence of new infections, and the extent of immigration of infected persons. In most endemic areas where control is needed (i.e. areas of high prevalence and intensity), renewed transmission can be expected unless chemotherapy is supplemented by other methods of intervention. The alternatives appear to be:

(1) Where water is available for community use it must be plentiful, easily accessible and the system efficiently maintained and supplemented with adequate laundry and shower facilities. If supplies are not available, considerations should be given for their installation, not primarily for the control of schistosomiasis but as an amenity for the community and for their other health benefits. There is, however, some evidence that these may be minimal in communities at the lower end of the socio-economic scale (Shuval, Tilden, Perry & Grosse, 1981). Water supplies are being provided in many areas but laundry and shower units are not usually included. Health education is an essential integral part of these facilities to ensure that the best use is made of them.

(2) Where infected immigrants are a major concern attempts to control their movement should be considered as well as their examination and treatment, but such programmes are often impossible to implement. Some form of snail control, if possible based on a routine focal application of molluscicide, should therefore be considered.

Notwithstanding the addition of the above control measures, prevalence of infection amongst children should be periodically determined and treatment given as required.

(3) Whether or not supplementary intervention methods are possible, future treatment programmes may be required. The reservoir of infection remaining after the initial treatment campaigns has been discussed

elsewhere (Chapter 5), and the extent of this, combined with local epidemiological factors, will affect a resurgence of transmission and the rate at which prevalence and intensity of infection increase. It may be necessary to re-treat children only when prevalence among the 5–14-year-old age group reaches about 25–30%, which may not be for four to five years after well-attended intensive campaigns, and infected immigrants are not a problem.

With our present knowledge and the tools available much can now be achieved in the way of schistosomiasis control; low prevalence and intensities of infection can quickly be obtained but not easily maintained, and continued vigilance is required; to further reduce a low level of infection may be difficult, costly and probably unnecessary as far as schistosomal disease is concerned. Intensive application of initial intervention may be required by specialist groups, but thereafter every effort should be made to involve Primary Health Care (PHC) workers in the consolidation phase.

Although the annual cost of the maintenance phase may be less than a dollar per head of population, for many of the Third World countries this figure is completely unrealistic for disease prevention when the Central Government expenditure on health per head of population may be only one or two dollars.

The global schistosomiasis problem, the government health budgets and the financial allocation for schistosomiasis control were reviewed recently (Iarotski & Davis, 1981). Data on the total health budgets, as a proportion of the national budget, vary from that given in other sources (Cumper, 1984; Anon., 1982b), but the pattern is clear. As a per cent of the national budget, health expenditure varies but is rarely greater than 10%. Health expenditure per head of population, however, varies with the GNP/*caput*. Data from three sources are shown in Table 9.6; it is apparent that where progress has been made with schistosomiasis control, those countries have high incomes with a GNP/*caput* greater than $1000.

A few of the larger countries with middle incomes (GNP/*caput* $250–1000) such as the Sudan, Egypt and the Philippines, have schemes supported financially by outside agencies; however, little in the way of effective control is carried out in countries with a GNP/*caput* of less than $250, and Chad with 86% of its population at risk (second only to the Sudan, 89%) and Mali and Malawi, each with 59% at risk, are among the worst affected nations.

Progress in the control of schistosomiasis will depend on the priority rating given by the health authorities to the infection. Emphasis is now being placed on PHC as a means of attempting to reach the goal of 'Health for all by the year 2000'. The use of PHC facilities in Third World countries,

Table 9.6. *Extent of schistosomiasis problem in different countries and expenditure on health*

Country	GNP/caput ($) a	Population (millions) a	% at risk a	Health budget % of national budget		Expenditure/caput ($)		
				a	b	a	b	c
Low income countries								
GNP/caput $ <250								
Mali	103	6.0	59	—	6.9	—	—	1
Ethiopia	104	28.9	31	—	4.5	—	—	1
Upper Volta	104	6.1	?	—	12.0	—	—	1
Chad	121	4.2	86	—	—	—	—	1
Malawi	183	6.0	59	4.0	4.1	1.6	—	2
Tanzania	183	16.1	19	10.0	7.1	3.7	6.1	3
Sierre Leone	190	3.5	?	—	5.2	—	—	3
Middle income countries								
GNP/caput $250–1000								
Kenya	250	14.3	42	—	8.2	—	7.5	5
Mauritania	255	1.5	25	—	—	—	—	3
Sudan	272	17.0	89	—	—	—	6.7	1
Togo	272	2.3	83	—	5.8	—	7.9	—
Egypt	279	38.7	46	3.0	3.2	5.1	—	8
Yemen AR	299	5.2	38	4.0	—	1.8	—	—
Cameroon	313	7.7	48	—	4.8	—	—	3

Ghana	374	10.3	49	8.8	7.4	10.8	17.0	4
Liberia	413	1.5	47	—	7.9	—	—	7
Philippines	416	45.0	9	3.3	5.1	2.7	11.5	2
Zambia	455	5.1	?	—	7.0	—	15.2	11
Morocco	517	18.2	?	—	3.0	—	—	7
Dominican Republic	791	5.0	6	18.0	8.9	16.7	—	15
Tunisia	799	6.0	3	7.0	6.9	19.7	—	22
Syria	826	7.8	?	—	0.9	—	—	3

High income countries
GNP/caput $1000

Brazil	1299	112.2	27	2.8	6.5	2.8	—	21
Iraq	1387	12.2	44	7.0	1.7	12.9	—	—
Iran	2059	34.4	>1	4.0	2.9	30.0	50.2	23
Puerto Rico	2305	3.3	63	9.0	—	52.0	—	—
Venezuela	2536	12.7	>1	—	4.6	39.6	100.4	35
Saudi Arabia	4422	7.0	14	2.0	—	106.5	—	—
Libya	5961	2.4	8	—	3.2	—	136.9	—

[a] 1976 data from or calculated from Iarotski & Davis (1981).
[b] 1976 data from or calculated from Cumper (1984).
[c] Anon. (1982).

particularly if a *selective* primary health care approach is adopted (Walsh & Warren, 1980), could be the basis for a concerted effort to prevent schistosomal disease in those countries where high prevalence and intensities of infection are found. Personnel could be trained to perform simple investigations and control procedures that would materially affect schistosomal morbidity among children. Health education of the population would need to be an integral part of such an approach and, for *S. mansoni* endemic areas, parasitological diagnosis would be needed, but advances in stool examination techniques have made possible the rapid screening of large numbers of children – particularly those with high intensities of infection and liable to develop disease. Single-dose treatment, however, even with special low prices for large scale purchases for National Control Programmes (Oxamniquine $0.89 per 25 kg child, and praziquantel $1.04), are not inexpensive.

PHC morbidity control of *S. haematobium* is, however, more feasible. While metrifonate is not ideal (owing to the three treatments required) it costs only $0.13 to treat a 25 kg child, and is highly effective in reducing egg output to a low level. Case detection is relatively easy and treatment can be given to all children with obvious haematuria or when detected by the use of simple urine dipsticks (when purchased in bulk these may cost as little as $0.05 per strip). The parasite will not be eradicated, but if used over a number of years prevalence and intensity of infection (and the associated morbidity) would be markedly reduced. Additionally, as children are responsible for excreting a very high proportion of *S. haematobium* eggs in the community, some reduction in transmission may result.

The effect of these disease specific control measures will be much increased if measures against the snail intermediate host can be undertaken and improvements in sanitation and water supplies are undertaken – the latter being in the forefront of PHC activities.

The principles of schistosomiasis control are now fairly well established, but the constraints that prevent their application are not only financial, but include also the lack of motivated health administrators and trained personnel, an effective infra-structure and, in many cases, logistical problems. In many areas these will not be overcome in the foreseeable future and it is problematical what advice can be given to these countries, although external aid for supporting control schemes is not diminishing. However, our better understanding of the development of schistosomal disease, the development of simplified diagnostic techniques and the development of drugs for field use on a community basis make it possible to view the future of schistosomiasis control with greater optimism than 25 years ago.

Part II: Complementary investigations

10

Drug trials

In 1918 tartar emetic was introduced as a treatment for schistosomiasis. Later, other antimonial preparations were available, but it was not until 1935 that the first oral treatment with lucanthone became available. This drug, and niridazole, developed in the early 1960s, required several days of treatment, had unpleasant side and toxic effects, and they were thus unsuited for large community based chemotherapy campaigns. Between 1965 and 1975, however, three new drugs – hycanthone, oxamniquine and praziquantel – became available for the treatment of *S. mansoni*, and trials were conducted to assess their effectiveness in St Lucia. All were given in a single dose, hycanthone by intramuscular injection (now infrequently used), the others orally.

Hycanthone mesylate

This drug, an active metabolite of lucanthone, was introduced in 1965 (Rosi *et al.*, 1965). Initially, doses of 2 or 3 mg/kg body weight were administered orally for 5 days to patients with *S. mansoni* in Brazil, and resulted in 'cure' rates of about 80% at 4 months (Katz *et al.*, 1968). Later, using a single intramuscular injection of 3 mg/kg b.w., a 96% 'cure' rate was obtained in 30 patients (Katz, Pellegrino & Oliveira, 1969). Similar good results were obtained in Rhodesia in urinary and intestinal schistosomiasis (Clarke, Blair & Weber, 1969). As the drug appeared to be the first effective single dose schistosomicidal drug it was evaluated in St Lucia (Cook & Jordan, 1971)

Initial trials

The 103 patients treated had been referred to the outpatient clinic or had been found infected during school surveys; 69 were below the age of 14 years, 34 above. Hycanthone was given by injections into the gluteus minimus muscle at a dose of 3 mg/kg b.w; side effects were monitored over the next 3–4 days. All patients were treated in the Research Ward.

Pre-treatment investigations included quantitative evaluation of the *S. mansoni* egg output based on three stool specimens, a general clinical examination when liver size was recorded as the number of centimetres below the xiphoid in the mid-sternal line and below the costal margin in the mid-clavicular line; splenic enlargement was recorded as the number of centimetres below the costal margin. A variety of laboratory tests were made including complete blood counts, urinalysis, bromsulphalein (BSP) excretion, and electrocardiogram. (Patients were excluded from the trial if the BSP excretion was abnormal.) The ECG was repeated at 24 hours after treatment in the first 50 patients and again at six weeks in the first 25. Blood counts and urinalysis were repeated at six weeks and six months. Stool examinations, qualitative and quantitative, were repeated (three specimens per patient) at six weeks, four and six months post-treatment. Hatch tests were carried out at the six month follow-up.

Side effects. Vomiting was the most frequently reported effect, occurring in 48 (47%) patients. Thirteen patients vomited more than four times, but in only two was it considered severe. Although fewer children less than 10 years of age vomited, the difference between this and older patients was not significant. Thirty-three other patients complained of mild anorexia, nausea, or abdominal pain, but these are frequently noted in untreated patients (Cook, Jordan, Woodstock & Pilgrim, 1977). Three patients developed fever – in two it was associated with an upper respiratory tract infection, but no cause could be found for the third case where leucocytosis of 33 000/mm^3 with 61% eosinophils was recorded. No jaundice was seen and no history was obtained of its developing at follow-up. ECG tracings were normal apart from T-wave inversion at 24 hours in one child; the tracing was normal at 48 hours.

Parasitological effects. The 'cure' rate (no eggs detected in three stools by any method used) among 94 followed to six months is shown in Tables 10.1 and 10.2. The 'cure' rate was similar in children and adults (Table 10.1) and although a little lower amongst the most heavily infected patients (Table 10.2), there was no significant difference between groups. The overall reduction in egg output was high, 97%, and was not related to age. Of 91 stools tested at six months miricidia were hatched from 14.

Expanded study – 2-year follow-up

In addition to the patients in the above study, others were treated in the Research Ward or as out-patients. No side effects were noted among 38% of 260 ambulatory patients compared with 21% of 173 treated in hospital, but the frequency of vomiting was similar in the two groups (Cook, Woodstock & Jordan, 1974).

Parasitological effect. Results of follow-up examinations at 6, 12 and 24 months are shown in Table 10.3. Extremely good results were maintained to 12 months and were only minimally diminished at 24 months. Results from older patients were a little better than from 0–14-year-olds (Table 10.4); similarly, lightly infected persons showed better results than those heavily infected (Table 10.5). There is little evidence from these studies that

Table 10.1. *Results of hycanthone trial, showing age distribution of 103 patients treated, pre-treatment levels of egg excretion, incidence of vomiting as a side effect,'cure' rate and percentage decrease in egg excretion levels at six months*

| Age group (years) | No. of patients treated | Mean no. of eggs excreted per ml of faeces before treatment | Results at six months | | |
			No. of patients followed	No. considered cured (%)	Decrease in no. of eggs excreted (%)
<10	24	185.2	20	4 (20)	95.5
10–14	45	168.7	44	14 (32)	98.5
15–19	20	129.4	20	4 (20)	96.2
>20	14	154.4	10	4 (40)	99.5
Total	103	168.5	94	26 (28)	96.9

Adapted from Cook & Jordan, 1971.

Table 10.2. *Analysis of 'cure' rate in 94 patients treated with hycanthone according to pre-treatment levels of egg excretion and followed to six months*

No. of eggs excreted per ml of faeces before treatment	No. of patients followed to six months	No. considered cured (%)
<50	34	10 (29)
50–200	34	10 (29)
>200	26	6 (23)
Total	94	26 (28)

From Cook & Jordan, 1971.

the hepatic shift of *S. mansoni* in man is not long lasting, as is claimed to be the case in mice (Rogers & Bueding, 1970).

Re-infections, defined either as a rise in egg excretion to greater than pre-treatment levels or a substantial rise after negative examinations, were more frequent in the 0–14-year age group and amongst patients from areas where no control was being carried out. Despite this, the intensity of infection among 143 followed to 24 months was 95% lower than before treatment.

The effect of hycanthone on liver and spleen enlargement is shown in Table 10.6.

In general, a decrease in the size of the spleen occurred more frequently than did a reduction in liver size; it also occurred more rapidly, but changes were less frequent among adult patients. These changes were similar to those found in a controlled trial of hycanthone and placebo, in which the changes in serum enzyme levels reflecting liver and muscle damage and changes in symptoms after treatment were also investigated (Cook *et al.*, 1977).

Trial of hycanthone and placebo

Children were treated with 2.5 mg/kg b.w. hycanthone or an injectable vitamin placebo similar in appearance to it.

Children were admitted to the Research Ward in groups and allocated to a 'treatment' group by the spin of a coin. All investigations were made 'blind'. In addition to parasitological evaluation, enzyme determinations – creatine phosphokinase (CPK), lactic dehydrogenase (LDH), serum glutamic oxaloacetic transaminase (SGOT), serum glutamic pyruvic transaminase (SGPT) and alkaline phosphatase – were made. Changes in the alkaline phosphatase levels were minimal in both groups; minor increases occurred

Table 10.3. *Effect of hycanthone treatment on* S. mansoni *egg excretion*

Months after treatment	No. patients treated	No. eggs by any method (%)	No. viable eggs[a] (%)	Total reduction in egg excretion (%)
6	340	179/340 (53)	274/308 (89)	98
12	223	118/223 (53)	175/202 (87)	98
24	198	97/198 (49)	119/172 (69)	86

[a] Denominator is not constant because hatch tests could not be done on each patient at each follow-up visit, whereas qualitative and quantitative examinations were always done.
From Cook *et al.*, 1974.

Table 10.4. *Analysis by age group of results of hycanthone treatment in 143 patients followed in detail to 24 months*

Age group (years)	No. patients	Time after treatment	No. eggs by any method (%)	No. viable eggs[a] (%)	Re-infected (%)	Total reduction in egg excretion M78(%)
0–14	84	6 wks.	46/84 (55)	Not done	0	98
		6 mos.	37/84 (44)	61/74 (82)	0	98
		12 mos.	35/84 (42)	60/71 (85)	2 (2)	97
		24 mos.	37/84 (44)	57/79 (72)	15 (18)	85
⩾15	59	6 wks.	34/59 (58)	Not done	0	98
		6 mos.	38/59 (64)	45/51 (88)	0	99
		12 mos.	35/59 (59)	47/53 (89)	0	99
		24 mos.	36/59 (61)	44/54 (82)	7 (12)	90
Total	143	6 wks.	80/143 (56)	Not done	0	98
		6 mos.	75/143 (53)	106/125 (85)	0	99
		12 mos.	70/143 (49)	107/124 (86)	2 (1)	98
		24 mos.	73/143 (51)	101/133 (76)	22 (15)	87

[a] Denominator is not constant because hatch tests could not be done on each patient at each follow-up visit.

From Cook *et al.*, 1974.

Table 10.5. *Analysis by intensity of infection of hycanthone treatment in 143 patients*

Intensity of infection	No. patients	Geometric mean, egg excretion	Hepatomegaly (%)	Splenomegaly (%)	No viable eggs[a]		
					6 months (%)	12 months (%)	24 months (%)
Light (0–50)[b]	66	12.2	11 (17)	5 (8)	45/53 (85)	51/56 (91)	54/62 (87)
Moderate (51–399)	64	134.8	22 (35)	11 (17)	51/59 (86)	49/59 (83)	40/59 (68)
Heavy (≥400)	13	629.5	6 (46)	2 (15)	10/13 (77)	7/9 (78)	7/12 (58)

[a] Denominator is not constant because hatch tests could not be done on each patient at each follow-up visit.
[b] e.p.ml faeces.
From Cook et al., 1974.

Table 10.6. *Therapeutic effect of hycanthone on liver and spleen enlargement*

Clinical state	Age group (years)	No. patients	Mean extension below costal margin (cm)		Significant decrease[a]	Normal	Unchanged	Time to max. decrease
			MCL[b]	MSL[c]				
Hepatomegaly	0–9	14	2.5	5.6	12	9	2	14 mos.
	10–14	18	2.4	7.1	18	10	0	16 mos.
	≥15	7	3.1	8.8	6	2	1	18 mos.
			Mean Hackett grade					
Splenomegaly	0–9	2	2.0		2	2	0	6 mos.
	10–14	11	1.8		10	5	1	6 mos.
	≥15	5	2.4		3	2	2	12 mos.

[a] For liver, decrease of > 2 cm or regression to normal. For spleen, decrease of one Hackett grade.
[b] Mid-clavicular line.
[c] Mid-sternal line.
From Crook et al., 1974.

in the other enzyme levels with mean maximum elevations 2–4 days after 'treatment', returning to normal in most patients by the 7th day and in all by day 14. Elevation was greatest in CPK (common in skeletal muscle), least in SGOT (a more specific hepato-cellular enzyme) and intermediate in SGOT and LDH (common in liver and muscle). The findings suggest that the observed changes were due to muscle damage at the site of the injection rather than an effect on the liver, although raised SGOT and SGPT levels have been reported by other workers.

Six months after 'treatment' an enquiry was made into symptoms in the two groups, but in general there was neither a difference between pre- and post-treatment findings nor between groups. All patients gained weight with the mean increase for the hycanthone group being greater by 1.2 kg. At the conclusion of the study the placebo group patients were treated with hycanthone.

Dose response

It was apparent from these studies that hycanthone at a dose of 3 mg/kg b.w. was a highly effective schistosomicidal drug; however although side effects were accepted in hospital and clinic patients, they were unpleasant and may be unacceptable in community treatment campaigns. Trials were made, therefore, to assess the side effects and parasitological response to doses of hycanthone lower than the 3 mg/kg dose initially tried (Cook, Jordan & Armitage, 1976).

The trials with the lower doses followed sequentially the initial trials; patients were referred to the Department by district or hospital medical officers; they were treated in the Research Ward or as out-patients, but were not randomly assigned to the different regimes of treatment.

Side effects from treating 173 patients with 3 mg/kg b.w. formed the

Table 10.7. *Side effects of hycanthone treatment in hospitalised St Lucian patients infected with* S. mansoni

Dose (mg/kg)	No. of patients	Vomiting (%)	Minor side effects (%)	None (%)
3.0	173	88 (51)	48 (28)	37 (21)
2.5	105	17 (16)	23 (22)	65 (62)
2.0	102	14 (14)	13 (13)	75 (73)
1.5	65	4 (6)	8 (12)	53 (82)
1.0	95	3 (3)	8 (8)	84 (89)

From Cook *et al.*, 1976.

Table 10.8. *Effect of hycanthone treatment on S. mansoni egg excretion in hospitalised and ambulatory patients seen at six months after treatment*

Dose (mg/kg)	No. of patients	Egg excretion before treatment[a]	No eggs by any method (%)	No viable eggs (%)	Total reduction in egg excretion (%)
3.0	143	51.2	75/143 (52)	106/125 (85)	97
2.5	88	93.1	49/88 (56)	73/84 (87)	98
2.0	103	80.3	53/103 (51)	74/95 (78)	98
1.5	99	64.1	57/99 (58)	70/87 (81)	98
1.0	88	42.0	35/88 (40)	69/83 (83)	89

[a] Geometric mean, eggs/ml faeces.
[b] Denominator is not constant because hatch tests could not be done on each patient at each follow-up visit, whereas qualitative and quantitative examinations were always done.
From Cook *et al.*, 1976.

standard with which effects from doses ranging from 2.5 mg to 1.0 mg/kg b.w. were compared. In hospital-treated patients they declined markedly with lower doses, with vomiting occurring in only 3% of patients given 1.0 mg/kg compared with 51% of those given the 3.0 mg/kg dose (Table 10.7).

Parasitological results. Results of stool examinations six months after treatment are shown in Table 10.8. Doses of 1.5 mg/kg to 3 mg/kg gave similar results, with no eggs being found in 51–58% of patients in the different groups and the total reduction in egg excretion being 97 or 98%. Results from the 1.0 mg/kg were less satisfactory, with no eggs being found in only 40% of patients and an 89% reduction in egg excretion level.

Further detailed logit regression analysis allowing for initial egg output, dose and age of patient showed that results were significantly affected ($P < 0.001$) by each factor, the percentage success rate being greater with the higher doses, with low levels of egg excretion among adults.

The decrease in liver enlargement was similar with all doses of hycanthone used, and ranged from 34–44%. The numbers of patients in different groups with splenomegaly were too small for an accurate assessment of any differential effect, but there was evidence that a decrease in spleen size by one Hacket grade occurred more frequently with the higher dose of drug.

The effect of intensity of infection on cure rates has been known for some time (Jordan, 1969), but the effect of age on outcome of chemotherapy is not so widely recognised. Although this may in part be due to the higher egg excretion levels commonly found in younger age groups, the presence of immature worms in this segment of the population may also be responsible as treatment of infections of two to three months standing was less satisfactory than treatment of infections of a year's duration (Katz, 1971).

Absence of liver toxicity

Although hycanthone is an extremely effective drug, there were potential problems in respect of its mutagenicity in *in vitro* systems (Hartman, Berger & Hartman, 1973; Hetrick & Kos, 1973), though not in mammalian tests (Russell, 1975). Apart from these doubts, acute liver necrosis was reported in approximately 1 in 15 000 persons treated. With the introduction of orally administered oxamniquine, hycanthone treatment ceased in St Lucia, but a review was made of the 2723 patients who had received the drug (Cook & Jordan, 1976).

All patients had a brief medical history taken and an abdominal examination. The drug was not given to children weighing less than 15 kg and chronic diseases such as hypertension, diabetes, chronic pulmonary disease, congenital heart disease, sickle cell anaemia and arteriosclerotic cardiovascular disease were more fully evaluated prior to treatment. Pregnant females were not treated (excluded by urine HCG slide test). Two females received treatment close to the time of conception and delivered normal offspring.

Initially patients were treated in the Research Ward and observed for 5–7 days; those treated as out-patients returned 48–72 hours after treatment, and those treated in the field were visited by a nurse daily until no further side effects were noted.

Repeat treatments were given to 92 patients at least six months after the first injection. Two patients had uncomplicated infectious hepatitis with jaundice three and five months after treatment, but no jaundice or serious side effects were noted in any of the 2723 patients treated.

Oxamniquine

Oxamniquine was first used in Brazil in 1972 but the early injectable formulations led to considerable local swelling and were unsatisfactory although parasitological results were good (Prata, 1978); in 1974 orally administered preparations became available.

Oxamniquine *versus* hycanthone

A comparative trial with oxamniquine, hycanthone and a placebo was undertaken (Cook, unpublished data). As age and pre-treatment egg output had been shown to affect results of hycanthone, only patients with *S. mansoni* egg excretion levels greater than 50 e.p.ml faeces were admitted for trial within two age groups (below and above 15 years of age) and randomly allocated to have oxamniquine, 15 mg/kg b.w., hycanthone, 2.0 mg/kg b.w., or placebo.

Four to eight patients were admitted to the Research Ward at a time and assigned a study number to which a treatment had been randomly assigned. Placebo (lactose) capsules were identical in appearance to oxamniquine so that the treatment given was known only to a physician taking no further part in the trial. Patients assigned to the hycanthone group and requiring an injection were obviously known to all. Except for these patients, monitoring of side effects, clinical examinations and laboratory examinations were carried out without knowledge of the treatment given. All patients were seen for follow-up approximately 90 days after treatment when those who had received placebo were treated with oxamniquine.

Three separate stool specimens were collected from each patient before treatment and at follow-up. They were examined qualitatively, quantitatively and by hatching of *S. mansoni* eggs. A variety of laboratory tests were made including complete blood counts, urinalysis and SGOT.

The age distribution of patients in each group was similar and indicated that randomisation was successful.

Side effects are shown in Table 10.9. They were generally more frequent among those given hycanthone. The absence of complaints of dizziness (a usual side effect) in the oxamniquine treated group may be accounted for as treatments were usually given after a heavy noon meal. Fever (100–101 °F) was found in a few patients with both drugs. It was usually accompanied by eosinophilia and frequently a white blood cell count greater than 10 000/mm³, but this was not reflected by mean values which showed no consistent change. Eosinophilia was common at days 3 and 7 with both drugs – and, surprisingly, with placebo, suggesting the possibility of technician bias. Side effects were not related to age.

Table 10.9. *Frequency (%) of side effects in patients after hycanthone (2 mg/kg b.w.) and oxamniquine (15 mq/kg h.w.)*

	Hycanthone	Oxamniquine	Placebo
Number treated	30	34	29
No side effect	50.0	79.4	79.3
Vomiting	13.3	—	—
Anorexia	26.7	—	—
Abdominal pain	26.7	11.8	20.7
Diarrhoea	—	2.9	—
Headache	3.3	—	10.3
Fever	13.3	17.6	—

Table 10.10. *Parasitological results at three months post-therapy*

	0–14 years			15+ years		
	Hyc.	Oxam.	Plac.	Hyc.	Oxam.	Plac.
Number treated	15	15	14	15	19	15
No. (%) 'cured'	3 (20)	3 (20)	0	3 (87)	13 (68)	0
Egg excretion:						
Before treatment	124[a]	140	119	91	82	96
% reduction	97.5	94.8	7.3	97	97	34

[a] Geometric mean of e.p.ml faeces.

Urinalysis results were not remarkable. Mean SGOT levels among hycanthone treated patients increased above 40 on days 1 and 3 in children and adults respectively, but were within normal limits by day 7. Five children given oxamniquine showed raised levels (range 52–71) on day 1 after treatment, but mean values were within normal limits.

Parasitological results three months post-treatment are summarised in Table 10.10. Results with the two drugs were similar and although there were high percentage reductions in egg output, 'cure' rates among children were poor.

Single *versus* split dose

In view of the low 'cure' rate among children, reported above, field trials were undertaken to assess the effect of 15 mg/kg b.w., given in two doses 6–8 hours apart.

Children in the water supply area of Richefond valley were used for the trial in 1975. They were asked to attend the Richefond Health Centre where they were assigned a study number to which a treatment group had previously been randomly assigned – 49 were treated in each group.

Treatments were given after noon (the time of their heaviest meal), and those to receive a second dose were given it and asked to take it after their evening meal or before retiring.

Three stool specimens were examined qualitatively and quantitatively before treatment and at six weeks post-therapy. A nurse visited the local school, or the children's home, the day following treatment in order to assess side effects. These were similar with the two regimes – 88% had no complaints, 4% complained of dizziness, 8% (split dose) and 4% (single dose) complained of abdominal pain, and in each group one of the 49 children complained of diarrhoea, headache and malaise.

Six weeks after treatment, 93 of those treated provided three stool specimens for assessment – 33 of 46 (72%) having the single dose were 'cured' compared with 15 of 47 (32%) of those having the split dose.

Pre-treatment egg output in the two groups was low (22 e.p.ml faeces) and at six weeks showed similar reductions – 90% (split dose) and 94% (single dose). (The low pre-treatment egg count reflects the effect of household water being available during the preceding 3–4 years.)

As the 'cure' rate with the single dose was obviously the better regime of treatment, no further trials with a split dose were made.

Praziquantel
Comparison of effects in children and adults

A study was designed to compare the tolerance and efficacy of praziquantel in the treatment of children and adults with *S. mansoni*. As the drug was known to be highly effective at a dose of 40 mg/kg b.w., a low dose was given (25 mg/kg b.w.) to facilitate detection of any differential effect in the two age groups (R. W. Goodgame, unpublished data).

One hundred and forty nine patients were treated in the Research Ward: 69 adults, ages 15–64 years (mean age 24), and 80 children ages 6–14 (mean age 10). Before therapy, three stools were examined quantitatively, all patients were clinically examined and the following laboratory tests were made – haemoglobin, white cell count and differential, SGOT and SGPT, alkaline phosphatase, total and direct bilirubin and blood urea nitrogen. Laboratory tests were repeated 24–48 hours after treatment. Patients were observed for 48 hours, when vital signs were taken and side effects monitored twice daily by the response to the question 'Are you having any trouble?' A detailed examination was undertaken if a positive response was elicited. Results of laboratory tests are shown in Table 10.11.

Mean values were significantly different only for the differential white cell count which showed an increase in neutrophils and a reduction in lymphocytes and eosinophils. Neutrophilia occurred in two-thirds of patients, being more frequent in those with higher egg loads. Changes in the level of eosinophils were not related to egg excretion, but decreases in the percentage of lymphocytes were greater in patients with high egg loads.

The mean SGOT decreased after treatment, although in 8 patients there was a rise from below to above 50 units: 9 patients showed a similar rise in SGPT (of whom 5 also had a raised SGOT). There was evidence that a rise in enzyme level was associated with high egg counts.

Table 10.11. *Laboratory results in adults and children given a single oral dose of praziquantel, 25 mg/kg*

Test (no. examined)	Pre-treatment	24–48 h post-treatment
Haemoglobin (146)	12.1 g/dl	11.8 g/dl
White blood cells (143)	7704/mm³	8110/mm³
Differential (143)		
Neutrophils ⎫	41	52[a]
Lymphocytes ⎬ (%)	46	38[a]
Eosinophils ⎭	14	10[b]
SGOT (127)	28.4 units	29.9 units
SGPT (128)	19.4 units	21.3 units
Alkaline phosphatase (126)	10.9 units	12.5 units
Urea (49)	14.1 mg/dl	14.5 mg/dl

[a] Significant change from pre-treatment by the paired t-test, $P < 0.001$.
[b] $P < 0.01$.

The frequency of side effects is shown in Table 10.12.

The most common complaint was mild, low-epigastric abdominal pain, occasionally colicky, which occurred among children and adults 2–6 hours after taking the drug and rarely persisting 24 hours; similar complaints were later reported in trials in East Africa (McMahon, 1981; Smith, Highton & Robert, 1981) and Brazil (da Silva *et al.*, 1981). Fever occurred in 11% of all patients and was more common in children. It occurred 24–48 hours after treatment; the highest recorded temperature was 102 °F. In a Brazilian trial of praziquantel in mainly adult patients with hepatosplenic schistosomiasis, fever was reported in 28% of patients (da Silva *et al.*, 1981), but in only a small number in the East African trials. In the St Lucian trial dizziness was reported in one patient and urticaria in two, both side effects being reported infrequently elsewhere.

A 27-year-old female who had a normal medical history, physical and laboratory examination pre- and post-treatment, presented four months later with typical acute myeloblastic leukaemia and died three weeks later from sepsis. Immediate notification of Bayer Pharmaceuticals revealed this to be an isolated case.

Side effects in relation to different levels of intensity of infection (based on pre-treatment egg count) are shown in Table 10.13. Abdominal pain was over twice as frequent in those patients with infections greater than 100 e.p.ml compared with those with a very low intensity of infection. The frequency of other gastrointestinal symptoms, with the exception of diarrhoea, were also related to egg output.

The finding that fever and abdominal side effects are related to the intensity of infection rather than the dose of drug (in contrast to the

Table 10.12. *Frequency (%) of children and adults with side effects from a single oral dose of praziquantel, 25 mg/kg b.w.*

Side effect	Children	Adults
Number treated	80	69
Vomiting	3.8	5.8
Anorexia	10.0	5.8
Abdominal pain	43.8	42.0
Diarrhoea	2.5	8.7
Headache	6.3	10.1
Fever > 100°F	16.3[a]	5.8[a]

[a] Difference between adults and children is significant by chi-square test, $P < 0.05$.

hycanthone trial, Table 10.7) are difficult to explain. Although abdominal symptoms are not uncommon when patients with *S. japonicum* are treated with praziquantel, they are infrequently reported in the treatment of *S. haematobium*, and neither abdominal nor 'total side effects' were related to the dose given (Davis, Biles, Ulrick & Dixon, 1981).

Stools of patients who initially had a pre-treatment egg output level greater than 50 e.p.ml faeces were re-examined at three and six month follow-up examination; pre-treatment, the geometric mean of *S. mansoni* egg output for children and adults were 137 and 106 e.p.ml respectively. Results of follow-up examinations are expressed as the mean reduction in

Table 10.13. *Frequency (%) of side effects related to intensity of infection*

Side effect	Intensity of infection[a]		
	1–49 e.p.ml (35 patients)	50–99 e.p.ml 51 patients)	Above 100 e.p.ml (63 patients)
Vomiting	0.0	5.9	6.4
Anorexia	0.0	9.8	11.1
Abdominal pain	25.7[b]	37.3[b]	55.6[b]
Diarrhoea	2.9	7.8	4.8
Headache	2.9	5.9	12.7
Fever 100 °F	0.0[c]	7.8[c]	20.6[c]

[a] e.p.ml faeces.
[b] Differences are significant by the chi-square test, $P < 0.02$.
[c] Differences are significant by the chi-square test, $P < 0.01$.

Table 10.14. *Parasitological response to praziquantel therapy (25 mg/kg b.w.) at 3 and 6 month follow-up examinations – number (%) of those examined showing different levels of reduced egg output*

% Reduction in egg output	3 months		6 months	
	Children 60	Adults 43	Children 56	Adults 36
100 ('cure')	27 (45.0)	27 (62.8)	31 (55.4)	24 (66.7)
98–99.9	15 (25.0)	7 (16.3)	9 (16.1)	7 (19.4)
95–97.9	5 (8.3)	5 (11.6)	5 (8.9)	2 (5.6)
90–94.9	5 (8.3)	2 (4.7)	8 (14.3)	—
80–89.9	4 (6.7)	1 (2.3)	2 (3.6)	3 (8.3)
< 80	4 (6.7)	1 (2.3)	1 (1.8)	—
Mean % reduction	94.7	98.0	97.6	98.2

egg output (Table 10.14). Although there was a suggestion of better results among adults, neither the higher 'cure' rates nor egg reductions were significantly different from the children.

The initial intensity of infection did not affect the parasitological result – egg reductions of 98.4% and 97.3% were found in patients with pre-treatment egg counts above and below 100 e.p.ml respectively, similar to results of trials in Tanzania (McMahon, 1981).

Evaluation of side effects in double-blind study

Because of the apparently high frequency of abdominal pain encountered during the above treatment of 149 patients, a double-blind study was designed to evaluate side effects among a further 120 patients (53 adults and 67 children) with levels of egg excretion of 30–40 e.p.ml. Four regimens were administered: praziquantel 25 mg/kg b.w., praziquantel 50 mg/kg b.w., and oxamniquine 15 mg/kg b.w., and placebo in 'matched colour' capsules.

Patients were not informed that there were any differences in treatment, and side effects were elicited as before by a physician who was unaware of the treatment received by patients. Those who received placebo were subsequently treated prior to discharge from the Ward.

Abdominal pain was found more frequently in praziquantel treated patients (16 of 60, 26.6%) than with either oxamniquine or placebo (3 of 60, 5%), and nausea and short-lived vomiting occurred only in the praziquantel groups. Side effects were not related to the dose of praziquantel used and in no patient were they severe enough to require medication.

Table 10.15. *Number of patients with side effects in double-blind study: 30 patients in each group*

Side effect	Praziquantel 25 mg/kg	Praziquantel 50 mg/kg	Oxamniquine 15 mg/kg	Placebo
Fever 100 °F	3	5	1	1
Abdominal pain[a]	10	6	1	2
Nausea	1	4	0	0
Vomiting[b]	0	3	0	0
Dizziness	1	1	3	0
Diarrhoea	1	0	1	0
Headache	1	1	1	0
Anorexia	0	1	0	0
Urticaria	1	1	0	0

[a] $P < 0.01$ by chi-square test.
[b] $P < 0.05$ by chi-square test.

Table 10.16. *Effect of anthelmintic drugs on S. mansoni egg excretion and hatching*

		Days post-treatment					
		−3-1	+1-3	+4-6	+7-9	+10-12	+13-15
Niridazole	Number of specimens	20	26	28	24	31	26
7 patients	Mean egg excretion	189.8	167.6	53.0	47.7	35.6	5.6
(25 mg/kg × 7 days)	Mean % hatching	53.5	27.0	14.2	8.4	1.5	1.3
Hycanthone	Number of specimens	21	22	22	25	22	20
7 patients	Mean egg excretion	213.0	333.3	401.0	105.2	44.9	6.6
(1.5–2.5 mg/kg)	Mean % hatching	51.9	23.1	18.5	22.9	10.7	2.0
Pyrantel	Number of specimens	15	14	13	8		
5 patients	Mean egg excretion	250.3	459.9	340.0	238.3		
(5 mg/lb)	Mean % hatching	50.1	26.5	30.2	32.1		
Levamisole	Number of specimens	12	9	11	18		
4 patients	Mean egg excretion	137.3	124.1	145.1	178.7		
(120 mg × 2 days)	Mean % hatching	64.3	27.2	32.0	22.7		
Piperazine	Number of specimens	15	19	11	17		
5 patients	Mean egg excretion	308.4	384.7	232.4	151.4		
(30 ml × 2 days)	Mean % hatching	48.5	20.4	13.3	15.8		
Bephenium	Number of specimens	11	14	13			
4 patients	Mean egg excretion	79.2	103.2	68.5			
(5 g × 2 days)	Mean % hatching	57.0	28.4	33.8			

The double-blind study confirmed results of the previous one that side effects are likely to be greater in patients with high levels of egg excretion compared with low levels. Thus they may be more frequent in initial chemotherapy campaigns in areas of high *S. mansoni* prevalence, but probably of less severity in re-treatment campaigns when the intensity of infection may be lower.

Anthelmintic drugs and *S. mansoni* hatching

Miracidial movement was observed to be sluggish on several occasions when stools were used to obtain miracidia for various studies. It was discovered that the sluggish miracidia came from stools of patients who had received piperazine for treatment of *Ascaris* infection on the day before collection. Because of this observation, a small study was undertaken to determine the effect of various anthelmintics on *S. mansoni* egg hatching. Thirty-two patients were studied. All stool specimens were collected for three days before treatment and up to 15 days after treatment for quantitative egg excretion and determination of the rate of hatching. The results are summarised in Table 10.16. The rate of hatching before any treatment varied from 48.5 to 64.3%, mean 53.6%. All drugs caused a fall in the hatching rate 1–3 days after administration. With the two antischistosomal drugs, niridazole and hycanthone, egg excretion levels and the hatching rate fell to very low levels 13–15 days after treatment, but with other anthelmintic drugs the mean egg excretion rates showed little change. Depression of hatching rates, however, continued throughout the observation period, but patients were not followed long enough to determine the duration of this effect on hatching (Upatham & Cook, unpublished data).

11

Molluscicide trials

In the course of biological work in St Lucia, overgrown marshes and swamps were frequently found to harbour *B. glabrata*, and although there may be little human contact with such habitats they provide a reservoir of snails that seed other water bodies. Direct application of molluscicide from sprayers to these situations is frequently impossible and aerial application only becomes feasible if the area is large and free of hazards for planes; however results of this approach might be improved if heavy granules, pellets or brickettes could be used to penetrate vegetation. Alternatively, granules might be applied when these sites are dry to release chemicals when they refill and the aestivating snails emerge and become susceptible to control. Apart from swampy areas, small trickles of water at the head of natural drainage systems are often too small and too numerous to be treated with automatic dispensers, yet their flows are often sufficient to wash away molluscicide applied by hand sprayers before it has time to affect snails (Sturrock, 1974*a*). There is, therefore, a need for other formulations of molluscicide.

Niclosamide granule formulations

Although Bayer AG and Shell Chemicals developed granular formulations for their molluscicides they were never successfully marketed; an experimental gelatin-based granule containing niclosamide was produced by Croda Polymers Ltd (London, England), and successfully tested in St Lucia, but development ceased in 1974 (Upatham & Sturrock, 1977). When applied to simulated banana drains at a dose of 5 mg/l active ingredient (a.i.), the molluscicidal effect lasted for almost six weeks compared with one or two weeks when the emulsifiable concentrate of niclosamide was used at the same concentration. When granules were exposed to various combinations of climatic factors the molluscicidal activity varied. The rate of release of the chemical was found to be accelerated by rain and high humidity, probably due to softening of the granule. However, at higher temperatures and low humidity the granules retained their activity for eight weeks, possibly due to hardening of the capsule.

Niclosamide sand granules were developed for the control of *B. choano-mphala* in deep water near the edges of Lake Victoria in Uganda and were used against *B. pfeifferi* in vegetation along lake edges (Prentice, 1970). In an attempt to improve on this formulation niclosamide (70% wettable powder) was combined with gelatine, wheat flour and sand (Prentice & Barnish, 1980). In field trials wheat flour and sand granules containing 5% niclosamide were effective in marshes, seepages and ditches at less cost than conventional sprays. Sand granules were easily made and less costly, and were for most purposes the preferred formulation. If residual properties can be exploited hardened gelatine granules may be preferable (see Appendix 7).

Persistence of niclosamide
On mud surfaces

Niclosamide is gradually inactivated by light (especially UV light) and is absorbed onto organic material, and its combination with mud is irreversible by ordinary means (Gönnert & Strufe, 1961). However, in control schemes it would sometimes be logistically useful if dry snail habitats could be treated with molluscicide rather than to delay treatment until they are refilled.

Experiments were therefore carried out to determine the persistence of niclosamide on mud surfaces in St Lucia (Sturrock, 1974*b*). Banana drains were simulated in 20×30 cm enamel pans 5 cm deep and half filled with clay from field sites. Natural spring water was added to each pan and allowed to evaporate, leaving a smooth, dry clay surface. Niclosamide was sprayed over the mud surface as was routinely done in field-spraying operations. The pans were protected from rain and midday sun; the temperature ranged from 20–30 °C and relative humidity from 70–95%. The toxicity of molluscicide at different times after application was assayed by filling pans with spring water, and adding 5–10 snails. After 24 hours these were removed, transferred to fresh water and mortality assessed after a further 48 hours. Despite several cycles of wetting and drying, the mud surfaces remained molluscicidal for over 12 months.

This finding in St Lucia appears to differ from other reports of mud detoxifying the chemical. A number of factors may be responsible for this. The spring water used in the St Lucia experiments had a pH of 7.5, total hardness 50 p.p.m as $CaCO_3$ and total alkalinity 70 p.p.m. as $CaCO_3$, whereas hard (408 p.p.m. total hardness as $CaCO_3$), alkaline (448 p.p.m. at $CaCO_3$) water caused rapid detoxification (Meyling, quoted by Sturrock, 1974 *b*). Sturrock (*loc. cit.*) discussed the possibility that alkaline or acid waters might alter niclosamide ions so that they react with complementary ions on the surface of mud particles to produce insoluble non-toxic salts.

However, in tests with British muds, organic matter was more important than non-colloidal inorganic materials in detoxifying niclosamide. If chemi-sorption takes place, detoxification would be irreversible, but if physical adsorption took place it would be reversible. There is some evidence, however, that at pH 7.3 or less the chemical would precipitate on to the mud substrate to re-dissolve when water was added (Meyling & Pitchford, 1966).

On vegetation

Field observations were made in banana drains in which emergent vegetation, mainly *Panicum pupurascens* and *Ludwigia erecta*, had been sprayed with a mixture of niclosamide e.c. and 15% diesel fuel. Foliage samples, with and without visible chemical, were collected, subsamples were tested for residual molluscicide at weekly intervals for eight weeks using the standard bioassay. No diminution in snail toxicity occurred in samples stored in the laboratory or exposed to outdoor tropical conditions for over a year (Sturrock, 1974 *b*).

Slow-release copper

For some situations slow-release molluscicides have advantages over conventional formulations in that they should be easy to transport, handle and to disperse in different habitats. Additionally, they may be toxic to cercariae and miracidia.

A slow-release compound composed of 50% copper sulphate monohydrate in an inert elastomer was made available for laboratory and field testing against *B. glabrata* by Prof. N. Cardarelli of the Creative Biology Laboratory, Akron, Ohio (Christie, Prentice, Upatham & Barnish, 1978).

In laboratory trials different concentrations of molluscicide were tested; a pellet formulation gave 100% kill of snails at a concentration of 8 mg/l active ingredient (a.i.) and the granule formulation, which acted faster, at 4 mg/l a.i. At 50 mg/l a.i. pellets produced complete mortality in four days when there was no change of water, but with a daily water change 100% mortality only occurred after 25 days. Added mud and algae were found to cause copper concentrations to fall markedly after six days.

In field experiments with granules, concentrations of 25, 50 and 100 mg/l a.i. were evaluated in four banana drains. Only at 100 mg/l a.i.

was complete mortality obtained at 16 weeks, but this concentration had no effect on *B. glabrata* when introduced into a marsh. In both field situations the chemical adversely affected the *Potamopyrgus coronatus* and *Dreponotrema surinamensis* present.

Effect of low copper levels on infection of B. glabrata

At concentrations less than required to kill snails, slow-release molluscicides may affect the ability of miracidia to infect snails. This was investigated in a series of experiments using copper sulphate (Christie & Upatham, unpublished).

Table 11.1. *Effect on snail infection rate and the number of sporocysts ( ) of pre-treating miracidia with copper (mean of two replicates)*

Copper p.p.m.	Time (mins.) of exposure of miracidia to copper					
	30		60		90	
	No. snails exam.	% infected	No. snails exam.	% infected	No. snails exam.	% infected
0.00					58	53.4
					(45)	
0.01	57	33.3	56	42.9	52	32.7
	(32)		(53)		(42)	
0.10	53	26.4	58	13.8	56	16.1
	(35)		(27)		(15)	
1.00	56	16.1	44	11.1	53	11.3
	(35)		(20)		(14)	

Table 11.2. *Effect on snail infection rate and the number of sporocysts ( ) of pre-treating snails with copper (mean of two replicates)*

Copper p.p.m.	Time (mins.) of exposure of snails to copper					
	30		60		90	
	No. snails exam.	% infected	No. snails exam.	% infected	No. snails exam.	% infected
0.00					52	63.5
					(47)	
0.01	56	25.0	52	26.0	55	21.8
	(30)		(28)		(31)	
0.10	51	17.6	44	13.6	50	24.0
	(21)		(64)		(18)	
1.00	49	16.3	47	12.8	48	25.0
	(23)		(47)		(18)	

The effect on snail infection rates and the number of developing sporocysts was investigated by exposing either the miracidia, snails or both to varying concentrations of copper for 30, 60 or 90 minutes prior to their being placed together in water containing no copper. In all experiments 35 8–10 mm B. *glabrata* were mass exposed for an hour to 5 miracidia each.

Table 11.3. *Effect on snail infection rate and the number of sporocysts (in parentheses) of pre-treating miracidia and snails with copper (mean of two replicates)*

	Time (mins.) of exposure of snails and miracidia to copper					
	30		60		90	
Copper p.p.m.	No. snails exam.	% infected	No. snails exam.	% infected	No. snails exam.	% infected
0.00					60	53.3 (38)
0.01	53 (35)	20.8	44 (50)	22.2	55 (30)	21.8
0.10	48 (29)	22.9	52 (36)	15.4	59 (29)	10.2
1.00	49 (21)	10.2	49 (0)	0.0	52 (0)	0.0

Table 11.4. *Effect on snail infection rate and the number of sporocysts (in parentheses) of pre-treating miracidia and snails with copper and exposing together in a copper environment of same concentration (mean of two replicates)*

	Time (mins.) of exposure of miracidia and snails to copper					
	30		60		90	
Copper p.p.m.	No. snails exam.	% infected	No. snails exam.	% infected	No. snails exam.	% infected
0.00					58 (38)	51.7
0.01	54 (28)	18.5	52 (32)	13.5	52 (26)	21.2
0.10	50 (40)	8.0	52 (32)	11.5	55 (80)	1.8
1.00	55 (0)	0.0	58 (0)	0.0	55 (0)	0.0

Results are shown in Tables 11.1, 2 and 3. In a final experiment miracidia and snails treated with copper were subsequently brought together in water containing the same concentration of copper, a situation that would occur with a slow-release compound in the field. Results are shown in Table 11.4. The results were analysed by an analysis of variance with an arcsine transformation of data. Differences shown were analysed further using either Student's 't' or 'Q' test.

Results from all the copper treatments of miracidia were significantly different from the control but at the 0.10 and 1.00 p.p.m. copper levels, results did not differ from each other. The number of sporocysts, though not analysed statistically, was lower at the two higher concentrations in the 60 and 90 minute treatments.

Pre-treating snails with copper resulted in a significantly lower infection rate than the control but there was no difference between the effect of the different copper concentrations. After exposure for 90 minutes lower numbers of sporocysts were recovered.

With pre-treatment of miracidia and snails, analysis of variance showed that copper levels and time were significant. All values for the different treatments were significantly different from the control. The numbers of sporocysts tended to be lower with higher copper concentrations after 30 and 60 minutes exposure.

All values from the different levels of copper differ significantly from the controls, but the number of sporocysts were unaffected.

Although copper sulphate gave satisfactory results in the laboratory as a molluscicide and, even at sublethal doses, reduced the infective capacity of miracidia, its field performance was unsatisfactory. In common with earlier studies by other workers, it was found that substantially higher doses were required for satisfactory kills than those needed in the laboratory. The estimated dose of 100 mg/l would be uneconomic. In view of its poor performance as a molluscicide, it also seems unlikely that it would have much effect on miracidia in field conditions. Where prolonged treatments are required, slow release with tributyl tin oxide (TBTO) promises to be more effective if TBTO can be shown to be safe.

Slow-release tributyl tin oxide

Preliminary studies were made of the effect on *B. glabrata* populations of different doses of rubber pellets containing 6% TBTO (Biomet SRM) (Christie & Prentice, unpublished data).

Trials were made in isolated marshes in the upper part of Canaries valley; three were seasonal with water levels and *B. glabrata* populations fluctuating with rainfall. One marsh served as a control, the others were treated with 5 or 10 g/m² of pellets in September (in the wet season) of 1977. *B. glabrata* remained absent for 20 weeks in the swamp treated with the lower dose and did not return to pre-treatment levels for a further 16 weeks. *B. glabrata* rapidly disappeared in the marsh treated with 10 g/m² and were not subsequently found as the marsh dried.

Trials were made in a permanent marsh fed from a seepage area and where *B. glabrata* populations were fairly constant. A second similar marsh served as a control. Pellets at a dose of 20 g/m² were applied in September, 1977. Snails were moribund the following day and the marsh remained free of *B. glabrata* for 13 months; numbers did not reach pre-control densities for a further 3–4 months. In the untreated marsh *B. glabrata* numbers remained high throughout the period.

In a further trial, TBTO at a dose of 10 g/m² was effective in reducing marsh snail populations, and in an effluent stream *B. glabrata* were undetected in the 10 months that studies were made following application.

Results suggest TBTO would be an extremely effective molluscicide in St Lucia marshes; control for over 12 months with a single application of 20 g/m² in an area with over 3800 mm of rain annually is a remarkable result and the cost would be comparable with monthly applications of niclosamide. The chemical appears to be a most promising molluscicide, but until further toxicological data are available and the long term cumulative effects in the aquatic environment have been investigated the use of the chemical (and related substances) cannot be recommended. The most recent investigations of TBTO, both in the laboratory and field, are discussed in the following sections which have been contributed by Christie *et al.*[*]

As already mentioned studies in other geographical areas indicated that slow-release formulations of bis(tri-*n*-butyl) tin oxide (TBTO) showed promise as a means of lowering intermediate host populations (Duncan, 1980); the potential of a 6% TBTO slow-release formulation was therefore investigated in laboratory and field experiments.

Laboratory investigations

For the laboratory work, a model ecosystem was designed (Fig. 11.1). Filtered river water was supplied at a rate of 6 l/day via a drip feed to duplicate tanks. The flow was split into halves by means of an Archimedean clock device. The upper trays, which simulated marshes, contained 1 kg of washed mud and 3 l of filtered river water. Overflow from the upper tanks dripped into other containers, which simulated rivers and contained 1 kg of washed, coarse sand and 3 l of filtered river water. The overflow from these latter trays dripped into a disposal pipe. Pellets

---

* Workers involved in this research were J. D. Christie, E. S. Upatham, L. R. Sherman, T. L. Carlson & N. F. Cardarelli.

containing 6% TBTO (M & T Chemicals Co.) were added at levels of 2, 5, 10 or 20 g of pellets/m² of marsh surface. Every two weeks, 20 *P. reticulata*, 20 *B. glabrata* and 20 *P. coronatus* were added to each 'marsh', and 20 *P. reticulata*, 20 *B. glabrata*, 10 *Macrobrachium faustinum* (shrimp) and 10 *P. glauca* to each 'river'. Control ecosystems containing no molluscicide were treated in the same manner as tanks which contained pellets. The time required for 100% mortality of each group of organisms at each dose of pellet was determined; if 100% mortality had not occurred within two weeks, the number of animals dying within that time period was recorded.

Laboratory experiments were also conducted using 6% TBTO slow-release pellets containing the chemical labelled with C^{14} at the butyl-one position (New England Nuclear, Inc.). These pellets, at a dose of 2 g/m² of bottom area, were added to trays containing various combinations of filtered river water (3 l), sand (1 kg), mud (1 kg) and organisms. At pre-determined intervals, 2 ml of water were removed and added to 8 ml of liquid scintillation 'cocktail' (Aquasol; New England Nuclear, Inc.). The d.p.m. was determined by the appropriate correction of c.p.m. obtained by counting beta emissions from water and 'cocktail' in a Beckman LS 100 C scintillation spectrometer.

Differences were detected among means and proportions by analyses of variance, Student's *t* test, χ^2 test with correction for continuity, or if variances were statistically different, by the *t'* test (Snedecor & Cochran, 1967). Differences among variances were compared by Bartlett's χ^2 test and equalities of slope and *y*-intercept of different regression equations were assessed by analyses of co-variance.

Effects on B. glabrata and P. reticulata. Where 100% mortality occurred in two weeks, time required for this event in the 'marsh' was generally less

Fig.11.1. Schematic diagram of mock ecosystem with upper tray representing 'marsh' and lower tray representing 'river'.

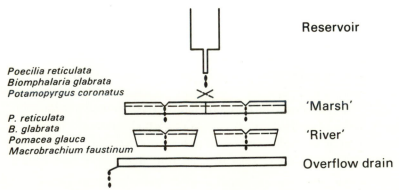

Poecilia reticulata
Biomphalaria glabrata
Potamopyrgus coronatus

Reservoir

'Marsh'

P. reticulata
B. glabrata
Pomacea glauca
Macrobrachium faustinum

'River'

Overflow drain

Fig. 11.2. Effect of various doses of slow-release pellets containing 6% TBTO placed in the 'marsh' of the mock ecosystem on *B. glabrata* exposed in the 'marsh' of that ecosystem. The solid bars represent time required for 100% mortality in replicate experiments. If 100% mortality was not reached in 14 days, the open bars represent the per cent mortality of that time. The arrow represents removal of the pellets from the 'marsh'.

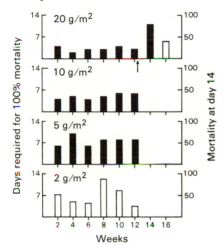

Fig.11.3. Effect of various doses of slow-release pellets containing 6% TBTO placed in the 'marsh' of the mock ecosystem on *B. glabrata* exposed in the 'river' of that ecosystem. The solid bars represent time required for 100% mortality in replicate experiments. If 100% mortality was not reached in 14 days, the open bars represent the per cent mortality at that time. The arrow represents removal of the pellets from the 'marsh'.

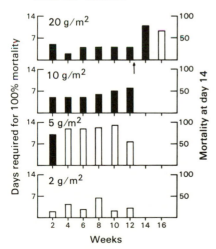

Fig.11.4. Effect of various doses of slow-release pellets containing 6% TBTO placed in the 'marsh' of the mock ecosystem on *P. reticulata* exposed in the 'marsh' of that ecosystem. The solid bars represent time required for 100% mortality in replicate experiments. If 100% mortality was not reached in 14 days, the open bars represent the per cent mortality at that time. The arrow represents removal of the pellets from the 'marsh'.

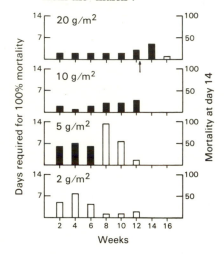

Fig.11.5. Effect of various doses of slow-release pellets containing 6% TBTO placed in the 'marsh' of the mock ecosystem on *P. reticulata* exposed in the 'river' of that ecosystem. The solid bars represent time required for 100% mortality in replicate experiments. If 100% mortality was not reached in 14 days, the open bars represent the per cent mortality at that time. The arrow represents removal of the pellets from the 'marsh'.

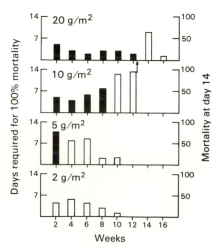

than or equal to the time required for the same phenomenon in the 'river' (Figs. 11.2–11.5; Table 11.5). The only exception to this generalisation is at the dose of 20 g/m² where guppies lived significantly longer in the 'marsh' than they did in the 'river'. Similarly, in groups where complete mortality was not observed, whether comparing the proportion of survivors against week of exposure or dose, a greater percentage was found alive in the 'river' than the 'marsh' (Tables 11.6 and 11.7).

Differences in mortality and survival of the two species of freshwater fauna were noted; in 'river' animals with 100% mortality within 2 weeks, guppies and *B. glabrata* died at the same time (Table 11.5). However, in the 'marsh', at doses of 5 and 10 g of molluscicide/m² *B. glabrata* lived significantly longer than did *P. reticulata*, while the opposite was found at the highest concentration of pesticide. In comparing points where survivors were found at the end of 2 weeks, guppies had a higher percentage of survivors than *B. glabrata* (Tables 11.6 and 11.7). The only exception to this observation was seen when comparing the percentage of survivors of the two species at 4 weeks in the 'marsh' and at 6 weeks in the 'river' (Table 11.7).

Table 11.5. *Days required for complete mortality of* B. glabrata *or* P. reticulata *in the 'marsh' or 'river' of a mock ecosystem in which the 'marsh' is treated with various doses of slow-release pellets containing 6% TBTO.*

The times are the means of values obtained at different weeks of exposure in replicate experiments

| | Days required for 100% mortality | | | |
| | B. *glabrata* | | P. *reticulata* | |
Dose of molluscicide	'marsh'	'river'	'marsh'	'river'
20 g/m²	3.1**[a] (0.2, 12)[b]	3.8** (0.3, 12)	2.2* (0.1, 12)	3.0** (0.3, 12)
10 g/m²	4.8 (0.1, 12)	5.9+ (0.4, 12)	2.5* (0.3, 12)	5.8+ (0.6, 8)
5 g/m²	7.6 (0.4, 12)	10.5++ (0.7, 2)	6.3+ (0.2, 6)	10.5++ (0.7, 2)

[a] The values marked with the same symbol are not statistically different from each other at the 0.05 probability level.
[b] The numbers in parentheses represent standard error of the mean and number of values respectively.

In comparing the percentage of *B. glabrata* and *P. reticulata* which survive, (Table 11.7), among guppies the survivorship increased with week of exposure in both 'marsh' and 'river' samples, while the same relationship did not hold for the *B. glabrata* samples. Moreover, in guppies, this relationship between week of exposure and percentage of survivors was satisfactorily expressed by linear regression equations, while in *B. glabrata* no such linearity was evident. Additionally, the two regression equations linking survivorship of *P. reticulata* and week of exposure for 'river' and 'marsh' samples were identical except for the y-intercepts which were significantly different at the 0.05 probability level (Bartlett's χ^2 for equality of variance = 1.02 with 1 degree of freedom; for equality of slope, $F = 0.50$ with 1 and 8 degrees of freedom; for equality of y-intercept, $F = 17.00$ with 1 and 9 degrees of freedom). With a common slope of 3.0, the y-intercept for the equation for 'marsh' guppies was 2.0, while the y-intercept for the equation for 'river' guppies was 12.0. What is not apparent from the data is that, in both species, regression of percentage of survivors in the 'river' as the dependent variable against percentage

Table 11.6. *Percentage of* B. glabrata *or* P. reticulata *surviving after 14 days of exposure in 'marsh' or 'river' of mock ecosystem which had had various concentrations of slow-release pellets containing 6% TBTO added to the 'marsh'.*

The percentages represent per cent survival at various doses for all weeks of exposure in replicate experiments

Dose of molluscicide	Per cent surviving			
	B. glabrata		*P. reticulata*	
	'marsh'	'river'	'marsh'	'stream'
20 g/m²	00.0*[a] (0/240)[b]	00.0* (0/240)	00.0* (0/240)	00.0* (0/240)
10 g/m²	00.0* (0/240)	00.0* (0/240)	00.0* (0/240)	2.5* (6/240)
5 g/m²	00.0* (0/240)	16.3** (39/240)	23.3** (56/240)	60.0+ (144/240)
2 g/m²	52.9+ (127/240)	75.4++ 181/240)	75.8++ (182/240)	78.8 (189/240)

[a] The values marked with the same symbol are not statistically different from each other at the 0.05 probability level.
[b] The numbers in parentheses represent the number of survivors compared to the number of animals exposed.

survivors in the 'marsh' as the independent variable yields two linear equations which are statistically identical (Bartlett's χ^2 for equality of variance $= 2.09$ with 1 degree of freedom; for equality of slope, $F = 0.33$ with 1 and 8 degrees of freedom; for equality of intercept, $F = 1.00$ with 1 and 9 degrees of freedom).

Radioisotope levels in water. Water samples from tanks containing water, water and mud, water and sand, or water, mud and organisms (10 *B. glabrata*, 10 *P. reticulata* and 10 *P. glauca*) were assayed for the presence of C^{14}-label two and four days after the addition of slow-release pellets containing C^{14}-TBTO. At both time intervals, the amount of label detected in the water was in the following order: water $>$ water $+$ sand $>$ water $+$ mud $>$ water $+$ mud $+$ organisms (Fig. 11.6). Moreover the radioisotope level at day 4 was greater than the level at day 2 in all corresponding tanks.

Additionally, except for the means of label in water from tanks containing water alone at day 2 and tanks containing water $+$ sand at day

Table 11.7. *Percentage of* B. glabrata *or* P. reticulata *surviving after 14 days of exposure in 'marsh' or 'river' of mock ecosystem at various times after different doses of slow-release pellets containing 6% TBTO have been added to the 'marsh'.*

The numbers represent survival at various weeks for all doses in replicate experiments. The coefficients of determination (r^2), slope, and y-intercept are given for regression equations linking week of exposure and percentage survivors.

| Week of exposure[a] | Per cent surviving | | | |
| | B. glabrata | | P. reticulata | |
	'marsh'	'river'	'marsh'	'river'
2	12.5*[b]	21.3**	16.9**	17.5**
4	16.9**	21.3**	11.3*	26.9+
6	17.5**	23.8+	17.5**	27.5+
8	3.1	16.9**	24.4+	41.9++
10	10.0*	23.1+	34.4***	47.5++
12	19.4**	31.3***	44.4++	51.3++
r^2	0.00	0.36	0.84	0.96
Slope	0.0	0.8	3.1	3.5
y-intercept	13.3	17.3	3.4	10.9

[a] The numbers of animals exposed in all cases was 160.
[b] The values marked with the same symbol are not statistically different at the 0.05 probability level.

4, the geometric means of label in water from all trays were significantly different from each other at the 0.05 probability level. When comparing tanks containing only water at day 2 and tanks containing only water at day 4, radioisotope emitted in the time interval of days 2–4 was 69% of that emitted in the interval of 0–2. However, assuming that the difference in C^{14} levels between water from tanks containing only water, and tanks containing water + mud was due to absorption by the mud, the amount of label absorbed by the mud in each time interval was similar: 66 124 d.p.m. in days 0–2 and 71 213 d.p.m. in days 2–4. In measuring the amount of radioactivity absorbed by sand or mud and organisms in these two time intervals, there was no similarity in loss of label such as measured in water from the tanks containing water and mud. If it is assumed that the difference between the amount of label detected in water taken from trays containing water + mud and trays containing water, mud + organisms is due to removal by the three species, there was no similarity in removal in the two time intervals.

Fig.11.6. Radioactivity expressed as d.p.m. in the water from containing 2 g/m² of slow-release pellets with C^{14}-labelled TBTO at 2 or 4 days after addition of the pellets. The tanks contained water; water and mud; water and sand; or water, mud, and organisms.

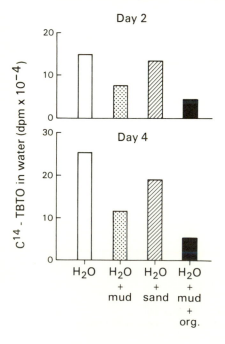

Field investigations

In field experiments, three 'seasonal' and two 'permanent' marshes were each sampled for 45 man-minutes for B. *glabrata* and other molluscan fauna at bi-weekly intervals for 18 months prior to adding any molluscicide. TBTO pellets were then added at doses of 5 and 10 g/m² to two of the 'seasonal' marshes and at a dose of 20 g/m² to one of the 'permanent' marshes. The remaining two untreated marshes served as controls. The areas were sampled at bi-weekly intervals for the next 18

Fig.11.7. Numbers of B. *glabrata* in marshes which have been treated with 5, 10, or 20 g of slow-release pellets/m² of surface area. The arrows represent addition of molluscicide.

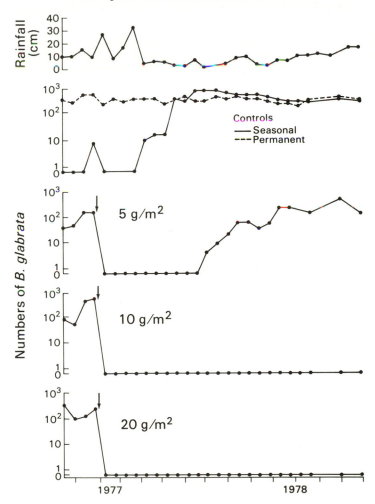

months. Prior to and during control, samples were taken of water and mud of the treated 'permanent' marsh, and water and sand of a ravine into which water from the marsh emptied directly. After storage in 4% formalin and extraction with hexane, organotin levels of the samples were determined using a modified phenylfluorone method (Sherman & Carlson, 1980).

The numbers of intermediate host snails found during the 18 months of pre-control sampling were similar to those depicted for a portion of the period (Fig. 11.7). After application of the molluscicide to the various marshes, numbers of intermediate host snails dropped to zero in all three control areas. In the 'seasonal' marsh treated with 5 g/m² of pellets, *B. glabrata* re-appeared after five months, their numbers approaching pre-

Fig.11.8. Organic tin levels in water and mud of a permanent marsh treated with 20 g of slow-release pellets/m² of surface area and in water and sand of a ravine into which the water from the marsh empties. The middle graph represents organic tin levels in sand and mud while the lower graph represents organic tin levels in water from the marsh and ravine. The solid line and circles represent samples taken from the ravine, while the open circles and interrupted line represents samples taken from the marsh. Each point is the geometric mean of 5 values.

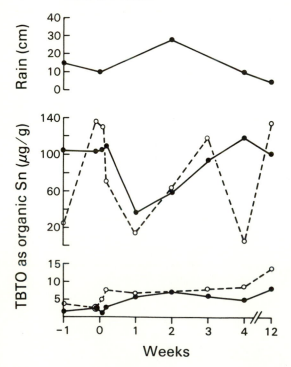

control values within seven months. In the 'seasonal' marsh treated with 10 g/m² of molluscicide, host snails did not re-inhabit the marsh until one year after application of the pesticide. In the 'permanent' marsh treated with 20 g/m² of slow-release material, *B. glabrata* did not re-appear until 18 months after treatment.

Organic tin concentrations in the mud of the marsh and sand of the ravine fed by the marsh waters did not change in any meaningful way after application of molluscicide (Fig. 11.8). Levels varied throughout the three month sampling period so that statistical correlation with treatment was impossible. Indeed, organic tin levels in the soil seemed to depend on rainfall which caused flooding and scouring of the surface soil of the marsh and ravine. On the other hand, increases were detected in the levels of organic tin in water from the marsh and ravine after application of the pellets. Prior to, and one day after, adding molluscicide to the 'permanent' marsh, the mean organic tin level was 3.0 µg/g of water. From one week after addition of pellets, to the termination of sampling three months later, organic tin levels increased significantly from 3.0 µg of tin/g of water to a mean of 6.43 µg/g of water. Furthermore, three months after the start of control, organic tin levels in the marsh water had increased to 13.42 µg of tin/g of water, which was significantly different from the level of 6.43 µg/g at the 0.05 probability level. Finally, throughout the experiment organic tin levels in ravine water were always less than concentrations in marsh water.

Cost of treatment. The assumptions used in calculating the cost of treating this 'permanent' marsh for one year by conventional means using an emulsifiable concentrate of niclosamide and with slow-release TBTO pellets

Table 11.8. *Assumptions involved in comparing the cost of marsh treatment with slow-release TBTO pellets* versus *the cost of treatment with niclosamide emulsifiable concentrate*

Marsh area	900 m²
Costs	
TBTO pellets	US $22.00/kg
Niclosamide	US $8.80/l
Wages	US $0.50/hour
Vehicle Cost	US $0.50/mile
Round-trip mileage	40 miles
Treatment schedule	
TBTP pellets	1/year
Niclosamide EC	2/lunar month

are listed in Table 11.8. Using these assumptions, treatment of this marsh with 6% TBTO slow-release pellets at a dose of 20 g of pesticide/m² of marsh surface area costs US $419.00 *versus* US $632.32 using conventional technology and niclosamide. The major cost associated with slow-release treatment is the expense of the chemical, while the major cost associated with conventional mollusciciding using niclosamide is transportation (Table 11.9).

Discussion

It is apparent that slow-release technology using TBTO as the active ingredient is successful in controlling marsh populations of *B. glabrata* for a period of 18 months. Furthermore, in the mock ecosystem, higher mortalities were found of *B. glabrata* than of *P. reticulata* at low doses of slow-release TBTO, i.e. 2 and 5 g of pellet/m² of 'marsh'. These results are in agreement with the data published by Upatham (1975) and Shiff and his colleagues (1974, 1977) who, in field trials with slow-release organo-tins, demonstrated killing of snail intermediate hosts without substantial damage of fish. However, if it is assumed that the levels of organic tin found in ravine water in the field trials are due exclusively to TBTO, then these concentrations are obviously greater than the value of 28 μg of TBTO/g of water, which is the 24-hour LC_{50} value for the cichlid, *Sarotherodon mossambicus* (Matthiessen, 1974).

One of the questions which remains unanswered is whether *B. glabrata* and *P. reticulata* absorb the molluscicide from the water or the substrate. Indeed, if the two animals have different sources of the molluscicide, this difference might explain differences in mortality. While the experiments with C^{14}-labelled TBTO suggest that TBTO is taken up by mud in fairly constant amounts over time, the regression analyses of the survivorship data suggest that perhaps the guppy is absorbing TBTO from the water, while the intermediate host snail absorbs TBTO from the soil. Both

Table 11.9. *Cost analysis (in US dollars) of marsh treatment with 6% TBTO pellets or niclosamide*

	6% TBTO pellets	Niclosamide
Chemicals	396.00	34.32
Labour	1.50	39.00
Driver	1.50	39.00
Transportation	20.00	520.00
Totals	419.00	632.32

equations regressing survivorship of *P. reticulata* against week of exposure in the 'marsh' and 'river' had high coefficients of determination with positive slopes, which were statistically identical. Moreover, the equations differed only in the value of the *y*-intercepts. These results indicate that the guppy is encountering an environment which is fairly uniformly laden with TBTO whose concentration may be decreasing as the length of the experiment is progressing. Using the snail mortality data, the regression of percentage of survivors against week of exposure is not satisfactory. As most of the *B. glabrata* survive at lower pesticide levels, they are probably encountering an environment which is uneven with respect to TBTO concentrations. Results of unpublished experiments with C^{14}-labelled TBTO suggest that such a patchy environment is offered by the mud, as radio-activity in this substrate is very variable depending on the distance away from the slow-release pellet at which samples are taken. Furthermore, at a dose of 20 g of molluscicide/m² in the mock ecosystems, a small zone (2 cm in diameter) was noted of inhibition of algal growth around the pellets, indicating limited diffusion of TBTO into the surrounding soil. Thus, the guppy is removing the pesticide from the water, while the snail may be obtaining the chemical from the mud or sand, where the concentration of the pesticide is very uneven.

If *B. glabrata* is absorbing TBTO from the mud, and if other organisms are capable of absorbing TBTO from this substrate, obviously the whole question of environmental persistence of the chemical or its toxic breakdown products in the soil becomes important. Unfortunately, measurement of organic tin levels of mud and sand in the field experiments do not offer any clues about absorption and persistence of TBTO in the environment. As inorganic tin in water or soil does not extract with hexane and is not measured by the modified phenylfluorone method (Sherman & Carlson, 1980), it is doubtful whether the high levels of organic tin measured in the sand and mud samples are due to contamination by inorganic metal. However, in Chesapeake Bay a species of *Pseudomonas* was found capable of methylating inorganic tin (Jackson, Blair, Brinckman & Iverson, 1982). Perhaps such microbial methylation is responsible for the high levels of organic tin observed in the mud and sand samples. These high levels obscured any addition of TBTO to the soil substrates by the slow-release pellets. There are indications from the mortality experiments in the mock ecosystems and unpublished experiments with radio-labelled TBTO that the pesticide is removed by flowing water fairly quickly and that any pesticide absorbed to mud is not released into water. When the pellets are removed from the 'marsh' treated with the highest dose of the molluscicide, within two weeks mortality of both *B. glabrata* and *P. reticulata* falls greatly.

Furthermore, in such a mock ecosystem, levels of radioactivity due to C^{14}-labelled TBTO fall to background within 16 days. Additionally, no radioactivity can be detected in alcohol washes of mud from these ecosystems, indicating that the C^{14}-labelled TBTO or its breakdown products are strongly bound to the mud.

Both slow-release TBTO and conventional mollusciciding are relatively expensive, and costs would be cut by applying molluscicide during the transmission season only. In the case of slow-release TBTO, a dose of $5g/m^2$ of snail habitat would protect for five months and levels of TBTO would be that much lower. Additionally, low levels of TBTO escaping into water can act as an inhibitor of miracidia and cercariae (unpublished observations by J. D. Christie and E. S. Upatham). The cost analysis does not include the expense of supervision of the workers applying the molluscicide or the cost of preliminary epidemiological and ecological surveys which allow optimal utilisation of any control method. Furthermore, the assumption is made that, when applying conventional molluscicides, the field workers always have transportation available to them, which, regrettably, is not always so. Thus, when the limited costs of supervision and transport needs are considered, in certain control situations, slow-release TBTO may be the more economical treatment.

12

Biological control

Chemical control of the snail intermediate host has been shown to be effective in reducing transmission of schistosomiasis but it requires continued applications which may have undesirable effects on the environment, and is costly. Biological control of snails has been advocated for many years, but results of various field trials have generally been unsatisfactory (Ferguson, 1977). There are reports in the literature of a number of snails competing with *B. glabrata* and this was studied in the field in St Lucia with *T. granifera*, *Helisoma duryi* and *Pomacea glauca*.

In the laboratory, predation of *B. glabrata* by the freshwater shrimp *Macrobrachium faustinum*, and predation of cercariae by the guppy *Poecilia (Lebistes) reticulata* and freshwater shrimps, were investigated.

Field studies
Thiara granifera
This snail was introduced into Florida, USA from South East Asia sometime in the early 1940s. It reached Puerto Rico around 1953 and spread into the Caribbean, being found in Antigua, Guadeloupe, Dominica, Martinique and Grenada. Populations of *B. glabrata* in Puerto Rico appeared to decline when sites became habitats for *T. granifera* and as it appeared that natural spread to St Lucia was inevitable a controlled study was made of its compatibility with St Lucian *B. glabrata* (Prentice, 1983*a*).

The snail is ovoviviparous and parthenogenetic, feeding on diatoms, algae and detritus rather than eating growing vegetation. The young snails are reared in a brood pouch and are approximately 2 mm in size when released into the environment. The snail breeds prolifically and large numbers can be maintained for a prolonged period of time in a given habitat. The snail can grow to about 30 mm in length, is streamlined with a heavy, high spiral shell and an operculum and is able to withstand flash floods and desiccation (Fig. 12.1)

T. granifera were obtained from the island of Dominica, reared in the laboratory and released in a marsh/stream complex at Monier in May 1978. Within 18 months they were widespread in the 0.3 hectare site and after two years *B. glabrata* had been eliminated and were not subsequently seen in this complex (Fig. 12.2).

T. granifera were later collected from this site and introduced into two other small marshes, Ravine Claire (near Fond St Jacques) and Ravine Victorin (in the Calypso area), and a more extensive stream site, Ravine Saut, also in the Calypso area. The populations built up rapidly, became the dominant species, and within a year no *B. glabrata* could be found in the three sites. *T. granifera* were also introduced into the Sulphur Springs area. Numbers increased rapidly, and although at the end of the programme *B. glabrata* had not been eliminated, their numbers were declining. (p. 261).

In two further sites *B. glabrata* populations were falling (although conditions were stable) when *T. granifera* were introduced. The numbers of the latter snail, however, increased, indicating that whatever was affecting *B. glabrata* (food shortage, disease or poisoning by agricultural chemicals) did not affect *Thiara*.

Fig.12.1. *T. granifera*. (From Prentice, 1983a.)

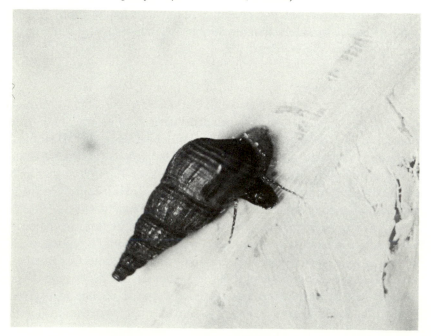

Other studies were made to investigate the ability of *T. granifera* to survive in semi-permanent habitats in Cul de Sac valley (M. A. Prentice, unpublished data). In January 1980 six banana drains containing *B. glabrata* were selected and alternate drains were seeded with 200 *T. granifera* each. Within three weeks of seeding all the drains dried out but for a period of ten weeks remained damp or had some pools after rain. They were then totally dry for a further period of 12 weeks. When the rain finally came in July, *Thiara* promptly reappeared and began to multiply. *B. glabrata* also survived this period but the population failed to build up to the expected numbers in either the experimental or control drain. In December 1980 the drains again dried out until April, when *T. granifera* appeared suddenly in large numbers following heavy rain. At this time the control drains were also invaded by *T. granifera* (Table 12.1). Under these particular circumstances *T. granifera* survives at least as well as *B. glabrata* but it failed to survive drying of a ditch at Sulphur Springs although *B. glabrata* did so. Its ability to survive under more rigorous circumstances (i.e. in unshaded dry ditches) remains to be fully assessed.

The results of these field studies were encouraging, but it was pointed out by Prentice (1983*a*) that 'the pendulum may swing back in favour of *Biomphalaria* at some time in the future, as happened when *Marisa cornuarietis* was introduced into a stream on St Kitts (Ferguson, 1977)'.

Fig.12.2. Numbers of *T. granifera* and *B. glabrata* from seven sites in a marsh/stream complex at Monier, plotted as means of samples collected over two months. (From Prentice, 1983*a*.)

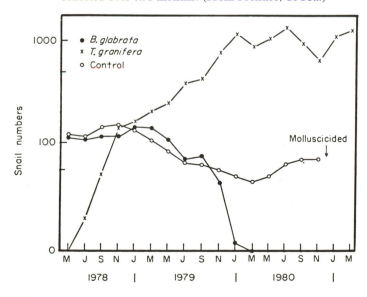

Table 12.1. *Numbers of B. glabrata and T. granifera in experimental and control banana drains in Cul de Sac valley*

		Experimental drains		Control drains		Condition of drains
		B. glabrata	T. granifera	B. glabrata	T. granifera	
1980	January	1806	—	1321	—	Pools
	February	1129	0	1040	—	Damp
	March	850	2	623	—	Damp and pools
	April	124	0	164	—	Damp
	May	8	0	0	—	Dry
	June	0	0	0	—	Dry
	July	0	0	0	—	Dry
	August	2	15	0	—	Pools
	September	3	27	0	—	Pools
	October	17	94	8	—	Pools
	November	15	146	18	—	Pools
	December	3	25	13	—	Damp
1981	January	3	2	0	—	Dry
	February	18	88	23	—	Pools
	March	0	0	0	—	Dry
	April	0	266	0	—	Floods
	May	22	981	30	931	Pools
	June	8	187	2	500	Damp

Marisa, however, is susceptible to the flushing action of flash floods whereas *T. granifera* colonises many different types of habitat including torrential streams; once established it usually maintains such large numbers that even if *B. glabrata* are not eliminated, *T. granifera* may reduce *S. mansoni* through the miracidial sponge effect (Lavacuente, Brown & Jobin, 1979). The snail rapidly colonises long stretches of stream and has been observed spreading upstream at the rate of about 100 m per month.

How, or why, *T. granifera* replaces *B. glabrata* is not known, but results from St Lucia suggest the effect becomes manifest when *T. granifera* numbers reach approximately double those of *B. glabrata*. Massive inoculation into *B. glabrata* habitats with thousands of *T. granifera* is possible as, once established in a site, vast numbers are usually present and can be readily collected.

Prentice also suggests the possible use of molluscicide to depress populations of *B. glabrata*: *T. granifera* are less susceptible to niclosamide and survived routine molluscicidal treatment. Laboratory investigations showed even hatchlings survived at concentrations twice that at which *B. glabrata* were killed.

To test whether *T. granifera* (or *B. glabrata*) secretes a chemical which inhibits egg laying or subsequent development, *B. glabrata* were exposed to water from a *T. granifera* and a *B. glabrata* colony.

Fifteen 150 ml crystallising dishes each containing three *B. glabrata* were divided into three groups. The first and second groups received a daily change of water taken from a crowded colony (400 in 1.5 l of water) of *T. granifera* and *B. glabrata* respectively. The third (control) group received a daily change of spring water. All were fed on boiled dasheen. Results are shown in Table 12.2.

Although the number of egg masses and eggs were lower when *B. glabrata* were exposed to 'T. granifera water' than to 'B. glabrata water', they were similar to numbers in the control group exposed to spring water. There was thus little evidence from this limited trial that *T. granifera* suppressed egg laying of *B. glabrata* by chemical means. Embryo development was normal in each group (M. A. Prentice, unpublished data).

Helisoma duryi

Earlier work in Puerto Rico (Ferguson 1977), Egypt (Abdallah & Nasr, 1973) and Tanzania (Rasmussen, 1974) suggested that *H. duryi* may control snail intermediate hosts of schistosomiasis. More recently it was shown that *H. duryi* caused a marked inhibition of growth and reproduction of *Biomphalaria camerunensis* and *Biomphalaria alexandrina*, possibly by food competition and mechanical interference with their eggs (Madsen & Frandsen, 1979; Madsen, 1979).

Table 12.2. *Number of egg masses and eggs (in parentheses) laid by 5 × 3 B. glabrata exposed to water from a T. granifera colony, a B. glabrata colony and a spring*

	Day number								
	2	3	4	5	6	7	8	9	Total
15 *B. glabrata* exposed to *T. granifera* water	1 (11)	5 (55)	—	2 (15)	—	7 (63)	2 (20)	1 (10)	18 (174)
15 *B. glabrata* exposed to *B. glabrata* water	—	6 (74)	—	7 (59)	—	8 (75)	—	7 (74)	28 (282)
15 *B. glabrata* exposed to spring water	—	4 (36)	2 (7)	—	3 (20)	7 (53)	1 (6)	2 (16)	19 (138)

Semi-field investigations were made into the interaction between St Lucia *B. glabrata* and the Dominican strain of *H. duryi* in five simulated banana drains dug 1.2 m long by 0.5 m wide. They were lined with plastic sheeting and filled to a depth of 0.1 m with filtered river water. Twenty first-generation laboratory bred *B. glabrata* were placed in each of four 'drains', three of which also had 5, 10 or 20 *H. duryi* added; 20 *H. duryi* alone were added to the fifth 'drain'. Every two weeks the water was changed, the number of snails counted and their size recorded. The water level was maintained at the same depth by adding or removing water as necessary. Two experiments each lasting 70 weeks were carried out, one starting in February near the end of winter, the second starting in June in the middle of summer. Daily records were kept of temperature and rainfall (Christie *et al.*, 1981).

B. glabrata were gradually eliminated from the drains regardless of the initial number of *H. duryi* though this affected the rate at which control was effected. The other major factor was high temperature which affected the reproduction of *B. glabrata* adversely but had less effect on *H. duryi*. Complementary laboratory studies showed that the intrinsic rate of increase of *B. glabrata* is greater than that of *H. duryi* at or below 25 °C, but at higher temperatures it declines below that of *H. duryi*. As the temperature of the water increased, *B. glabrata* fecundity decreases, and as populations age and die without replacement, *H. duryi*, sharing the same niche, continue to breed with their young snails filling the gap left by mortality of the *B. glabrata*. In view of these findings it is likely that *H. duryi* will be of use as a biological control agent only in those geographical regions and microhabitats where temperatures are high enough and other environmental variables favourable enough to give this species a competitive advantage.

However, while *Helisoma* spp. and *Biomphalaria* spp. are basically pond dwellers, *B. glabrata* adapt to living in streams and rivers. On the other hand, a large population of *H. duryi* was found in a fish pond in Dominica but none occurred in the effluent stream (Prentice, unpublished). As *H. duryi* has a higher and less streamlined shell than *B. glabrata*, it may be unable to withstand running water.

Laboratory studies were made to investigate the dislodgement velocity of the two snails; two methods were used (Prentice & Barnish, unpublished). Snails were allowed to crawl onto a thin metal plate which could be whirled round in a 39 cm diameter circle 3 cm below the surface of water in a flat tray. The speed of rotation could be gradually increased, and the velocity of the plate measured the instant at which snails were dislodged. Eight *H. duryi* ranging from 7 to 12 mm in diameter were dislodged at velocities of 60 cm/sec or less, while similar sized *B. glabrata* withstood velocities of between 70 and 110 cm/sec.

In a further experiment 25 snails of each species were individually subjected to increasing water velocity in a 15 mm diameter clear plastic tube. Velocity at the centre of the tube was measured by a micro-pitot tube 1.5 mm in diameter. The geometric mean of velocity that dislodged *B. glabrata* was 137 cm/sec compared with 79 cm/sec for *H. duryi*. Both methods used thus support the hypothesis that *B. glabrata* would have a selective advantage over *H. duryi* in a stream habitat.

However, *H. duryi* were released into three different areas in St Lucia where they would not be affected by stream flow (M. A. Prentice & G. Barnish, unpublished). A spring-fed pool and dasheen marsh–pool complex at Monier seemed ideal habitats, particularly as *B. glabrata* had been under pressure during a series of molluscicide trials. In December 1977 a total of 1200 *H. duryi* were introduced, in groups of 400, into the main watercress bed, a dasheen/marsh pool and the spring-fed pool, but within a week only six could be recovered from all sites and none were found in subsequent monthly searches.

A further 1000 *H. duryi* were introduced into a marsh/stream complex near Soufriere. Recovery rates gradually declined and the habitat temporarily dried. Although *B. glabrata* were rapidly re-established, when the rains came *H. duryi* were never found.

A final release of 2000 *H. duryi* was made in a high level pond in the Canaries valley, but again recoveries dropped quickly and the snail failed to establish itself.

The reason for these failures is unknown, but it is apparent that the snail has no chance of being a biological control agent in St Lucia.

Pomacea glauca

In Brazil, laboratory tests indicated that *Pomacea australis* were able to eliminate *Biomphalaria* (Paulinyi & Paulini, 1972), and there was evidence from some sites in St Lucia that *B. glabrata* population were depressed by *P. glauca* although the two snails were often found together in banana drains in Cul de Sac valley.

To investigate any suppressive effect, 400 *P. glauca* were introduced into the headwaters of a marsh/stream complex at Rock, on the western edge of Marquis valley, where *B. glabrata* were known to have been for at least five years. An isolated tributary, supporting colonies of *B. glabrata*, which joined the main stream below a series of small waterfalls, served as a control. The numbers of *B. glabrata* and *P. glauca* were assessed at monthly intervals by quantitative searches over a period of 39 months. Although the number of *P. glauca* increased, they had no discernible effect on *B. glabrata* (M. A. Prentice, unpublished data).

Laboratory studies
Predation of B. glabrata *by freshwater shrimps*

Freshwater shrimps are common in St Lucia and 13 species have been identified (Barnish, 1984). As a shrimp was observed eating a snail under natural conditions (Sturrock, 1974c) and predation of mature *B. glabrata* by shrimps had been observed during an unrelated laboratory study, their potential as biological control agents was investigated (Barnish & Prentice, 1982).

The snail-eating ability of four of the most common species of shrimp, *Macrobrachium faustinum*, *M. crenulatum*, *M. heterochirus* and *Atya innocous*, was investigated. Single specimens of each species were placed in 3 l aquaria and starved for 24 hours when 10 live *B. glabrata* were added. All three *Macrobrachium* had eaten within 24 hours but the atyid did not begin eating for 62 hours.

The individual daily consumption by six *M. faustinum* and six *M. crenulatum* of *B. glabrata* (8 mm diameter) was studied. Over a 14-day period

Fig.12.3. Shells of *B. glabrata* eaten by shrimps. The shell on the left has been opened opposite the retracted foot. (From Barnish & Prentice, 1982.)

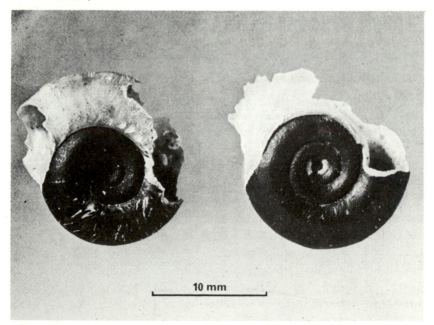

10 mm

the number of snails eaten by individual shrimps varied considerably, ranging from 3 to 74 and from 6 to 109 for *M. faustinum* and *M. crenulatum* respectively. Daily consumption likewise varied for individual shrimps and ranged from zero to 20 (the maximum number offered in a day) for one *M. crenulatum*. A single specimen of the largest shrimp in St Lucia, *M. carcinus*, was observed to consume 37 snails in 14 days. When *M. faustinum* was offered a choice of *B. glabrata* or the thinner-shelled *Physa marmorata*, daily observations showed that *Biomphalaria* were eaten before *Physa*.

Shrimps were observed to hold the snail with their maxillipeds and turn them until the shell opening faced the mandibles, which then broke the shell until the body of the snail was reached (Fig. 12.3). After regular feeding on *B. glabrata*, one *Macrobrachium* would come to the surface and take a hand-offered snail from above the water surface.

B. glabrata were the only food offered in these experiments, but in a limited trial to test food preference three newly caught shrimps appeared to prefer *B. glabrata* when offered them with crushed mouse pellets and boiled dasheen leaves. On examining the stomach contents of 31 *M. faustinum* from the field, remains of snails were found in five.

Although it is apparent that shrimps consume snails in natural conditions and may form part of the complex of factors that restrain *B. glabrata* populations, they are unlikely to be effective control agents since they form a common human food in St Lucia.

Predation of cercariae by Poecilia (L.) reticulata.

Although Prentice was able to detect carcariae 500 m from the point of release in a stream in St Lucia (see Chapter 13), it is apparent that their numbers declined. Apart from losses due to penetration of abnormal 'hosts' (Warren & Peters, 1967), fatigue and other causes, the predatory habits of fish such as guppies has been documented (reviewed by Jordan *et al.*, 1980a).

Predation by *P. reticulata* was investigated in still and moving water (M. A. Prentice & G. Barnish, unpublished). Four beakers, of 1000 ml capacity, were half filled with cercariae in the range of 100–500/100 ml, and number estimated by filtration and staining of two aliquots of 50 ml taken while the suspension was magnetically stirred. Two beakers were surrounded by white and black material respectively, and two (one a control with no fish) left with the natural laboratory surround. Five *P. reticulata* were introduced into each beaker and the reduction in numbers of cercariae determined at the end of a 4-hour period.

The control beaker showed only a reduction of cercariae of 11.2% while the others showed cercarial losses of between 92.4% and 99.3%. In a similar experiment, the effect of muddy water was investigated. In the control beaker (with fish in clear water) there was a 98.3% reduction in cercarial numbers compared with 94.3% and 67% reductions with turbidities of 200 and 500 JTUs (Jackson Turbidity Units) respectively. In a further beaker with a 500 JTU turbidity but no fish, cercarial numbers were reduced by 29.9% in the 4-hour observation period. It is apparent that muddy water caused a loss of cercariae but the predatory power of guppies was also reduced. Whether this was due to inability of fish to see cercariae or inhibition of feeding was not investigated.

A comparison was made of cercarial loss in a 3 l aquarium and an equal volume of water moving at 7.5 cm/sec in a trough built of rectangular section plastic gutter pipes (Fig. 12.4). The current was maintained by means of a paddle-wheel belt driven by a variable speed motor. Water velocity was measured by timing floating particles as they passed markers in the rear chamber. Turbulence at the paddle and the 180° turn at each end of the trough caused uniform distribution of particles after about 5 minutes.

Numbers of cercariae were estimated by taking ten 50 ml samples, and placing them in a beaker that was magnetically stirred (to minimise clumping). Three 50 ml aliquots were drawn from the edge of the bulked sample, filtered and stained, the balance of 350 ml cercarial suspension being returned to the experimental vessel.

The loss of cercariae without added fish was found to be high in the trough, 50% compared with 11.2% in the aquarium. Turbulence due to

Fig.12.4. Trough for investigating cercarial loss in moving water.

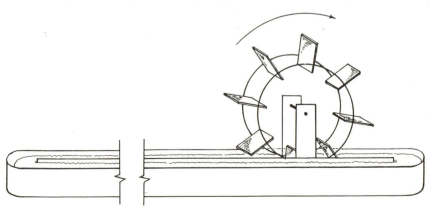

Table 12.3. *Per cent reduction in the number of cercariae by various species of shrimp over a period of four hours*

No shrimps (control)	Atya	Micratya	Micratya	Macro-brachium	Macro-brachium
14.7	35.0	8.13	80.9	21.1	31.5

Fig.12.5. Arrangement for generating water movement by air jet.

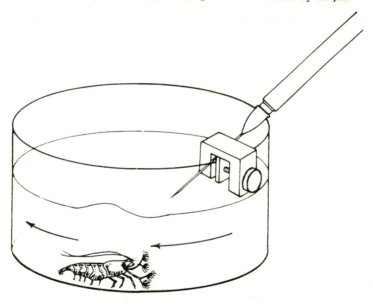

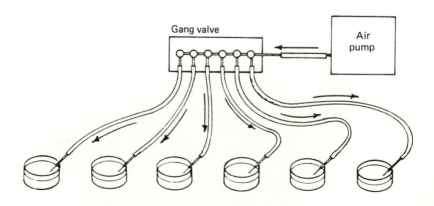

paddle action may have accounted for this as, in another experiment, losses were much less in water stirred by an air jet. When fish were added cercarial loss was 75.4% compared with 82.7% in still water; allowing for the 50% loss without fish being present it is apparent that guppies were much less effective in moving water.

Predation of cercariae by shrimps

Shrimps of the genera *Atya* and *Micratya* (and others) are found in many streams in St Lucia (Barnish, 1984). They have chelipeds modified into brushes, or fans, which can be used either to sweep small particles of food from the substrate or as passive filters to remove particles from flowing water.

An attempt was made to investigate the ability of shrimps to feed on cercariae in moving water in the trough, but they were either damaged by the paddle or, if protected from it, they crowded against the screen and failed to feed. After some trials it was found that they could be induced to extend their fans in a current generated by blowing air across the surface of the water close to the edge of a circular crystallising dish (Fig. 12.5). Initially a comparison was made between *Micratya*, *Atya* and *Macrobrachium*. Each shrimp was supplied with approximately 1500 cercariae and allowed to feed for four hours. Results are shown in Table 12.3.

The reduction due to *Macrobrachium*, which does not possess fans and is not a filter feeder, is interesting and possibly due to cercariae being damaged in their passage through the gill chambers.

The experiment was repeated with 5 individual *Micratya* after adjusting water velocity to the preferred rate. One shrimp did not feed, and the cercarial loss was only 7.3% (control loss 5.7%); the loss with the remaining 4 varied only between 96.7 and 98.9%.

The experiment was carried out under identical conditions with individual *P. reticulata* substituted for the shrimp. In three successful experiments the number of cercariae were reduced between 59 and 89%.

Under these conditions the shrimps were not significantly more efficient than the guppies. It is interesting to note, however, that the guppies were much more capable of feeding in the whirlpool in the crystallising dishes than they were in the more linear current in the trough. In nature fish are free to choose their own feeding groups and will choose conditions where the velocity is most suitable.

13

Epidemiology

Epidemiology of schistosomiasis encompasses the definitive human host, the intermediate snail host, all stages of the life cycle of the parasite, its relationship with the two hosts, and the development of schistosomal disease.

In addition to the various control programmes described in Part I, different aspects of epidemiology were investigated. These investigations included levels of contamination of the environment with *S. mansoni* ova, hatchability of eggs, dispersion of miracidia, intermediate host/parasite relationships, shedding and dispersion of cercariae, water contact studies, infection of man and development of disease. These studies are described below.

S. mansoni in St Lucia and other endemic areas

The importance of intensity of infection in the development of hepatosplenomegaly was first demonstrated in Brazil (Kloetzel, 1962) and, in spite of different quantitative techniques, there appeared to be a similar relationship between intensity of infection and prevalence in children in Uganda, Tanzania, Brazil and St Lucia (Jordan, 1967). With the wide acceptance of the Kato technique for quantitative and qualitative surveys, results from different endemic areas should now be more generally comparable, but the methods of giving quantitative results vary with either the arithmetic or geometric mean of egg output being reported.

Although the Kato quantitative technique was not used routinely in the St Lucia project, it was used in one village survey and the prevalence and arithmetic mean of *S. mansoni* egg output compared with findings of Siongok *et al.* (1976) in a Kenya village (Bartholomew, Peters & Jordan, 1981). Comparable results from other Kenyan villages are also available (A. E. Butterworth, personal communication; Smith, Warren & Mahmoud,

1979) and shown in Fig. 13.1. Comparable results of Kato examinations in terms of geometric means are also available from Kenya (Butterworth, *loc. cit*; Smith *et al.*, *loc. cit.*), Egypt (El Alamy & Cline, 1977) and Ethiopia (Hiatt, 1976), and are shown.

Apart from one village in Ethiopia where a very low prevalence was found (10.7%), the results confirm the close relationship between prevalence and intensities of infection in different endemic areas, and show that in St Lucia schistosomiasis is of moderate intensity but comparable to other areas relative to overall prevalence.

Infection of the snail intermediate host

Environmental contamination

In the course of the St Lucia project 48 villages were found with overall prevalence rates greater than 10%. They were grouped according to prevalence being low (10–29%), moderate (30–49%), or high (50% or more) at surveys before control; 11 700 persons were examined with between 3600 and 4200 in each group. Age specific prevalence and intensities of infection (arithmetic and geometric means of those infected) in the three village groupings are shown in Fig. 13.2.

The level of environmental contamination with *S. mansoni* eggs in the three village groups was investigated using the arithmetic mean of egg output for different age groups to give a more realistic figure of the actual number of *S. mansoni* eggs likely to be contaminating the environment. The population structure as found in surveys was used. The sum of the product of prevalence, arithmetic mean of egg output and the proportion of each

Fig.13.1. Relationship between overall prevalence and intensity of *S. mansoni* infection, as determined by the Kato technique, in different endemic areas. ([1] Siongok *et al.*, 1976; [2] A. E. Butterworth, personal communication; [3] Smith, *et al.*, 1981; [4] Hiatt, 1976; [5] Abdel-Wahab *et al.*, 1980.) (△ geometric mean, ▲ arithmetic mean).

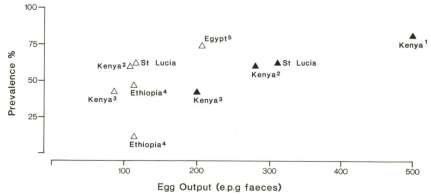

Fig.13.2. Age prevalence and intensity of infection in areas of differing endemicity.

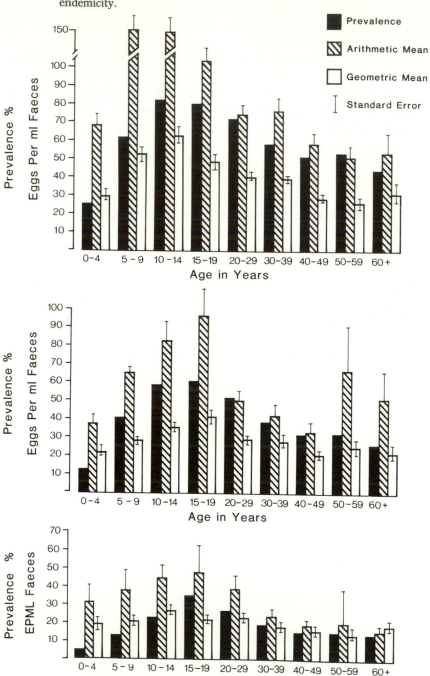

age group in the total population represents the egg-load in 1 ml of stool of a standard 100 persons (i.e. as represented by the age structure of the population). The total egg output per day from a village of 1000 persons with an average faecal output of 125 g per day (mean faecal output of patients in hospital) was calculated. In the villages of low endemicity (mean prevalence 18%) the daily *S. mansoni* egg excretion was calculated to be just over three quarters of a million (762 500), in villages of moderate endemicity (mean prevalence 38%) over 3 million (3 151 250), and in highly endemic villages (mean prevalence 58%) over $7\frac{1}{2}$ million (7 666 250). As these calculations are based on results of stool examination techniques less sensitive than those recently developed they represent the minimum levels of contamination. The increase in the level of contamination from nearly $\frac{3}{4}$ million eggs per day in the areas of low endemicity to nearly $7\frac{1}{2}$ million in areas of high endemicity – although prevalence increased only threefold (from 18 to 58%) – emphasises the importance of the increase of intensity of infection as prevalence increases.

Daily egg output by age group is shown in Fig. 13.3. On the basis of these calculations, as endemicity increases, the 5–14-year age groups play an increasing role as the major contributor to the total contamination of the environment (Fig. 13.4). In low, medium and highly endemic areas they may be responsible for 36, 46 and 55% of contamination, proportions which are increased to 44, 50 and 60% when the hatchability of eggs

Fig.13.3. Potential daily *S. mansoni* egg output by age in villages of 1000 population in areas of differing endemicity.

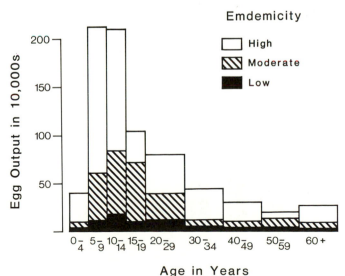

Emdemicity

☐ High

▨ Moderate

■ Low

excreted by this age group of the community is considered (Upatham, Sturrock & Cook, 1976) (see below).

The contribution to the total level of contamination of individuals with different levels of egg output is relevant in control schemes if chemotherapy is targeted towards high egg excretors. Fig. 13.5 was designed to show the expected reduction in contamination resulting from the treatment of individuals with different levels of egg excretion. The upper part shows the frequency distribution of the egg output in the low, moderate and high endemicity areas: the lower graph shows the contribution to the total contamination of different levels of egg output. It has been suggested that for disease control treatment should be targeted to persons excreting more than 400 e.p.g of faeces (Warren & Mahmoud, 1976) which reduced contamination in Kenya by 80% (Mahmoud *et al.*, 1983). From the upper graph, however (Fig. 13.5), it is seen that in the high transmission areas only about 5% of counts were greater than 400 e.p.ml and accounted for about 40% of contamination. The difference between the Kenyan (80%) and St Lucian (40%) figures is due to the use of the Kato quantitative technique in Kenya compared with the Bell technique in St Lucia (Chapter 3), with lower intensities of infection the lower the proportional reduction in contamination from treating persons with a given level of intensity.

A 50% reduction of contamination would be effected by treatment of individuals with counts above 300 e.p.ml, 140 e.p.ml and 75 e.p.ml in the high to low endemic areas, equivalent to treating the 8%, 13% and 16% of the infected population. However, in the high prevalence group of villages a reduction of 50% in contamination will still leave nearly 4

Fig.13.4. Relative IPC (%) by age in areas of differing endemicity.

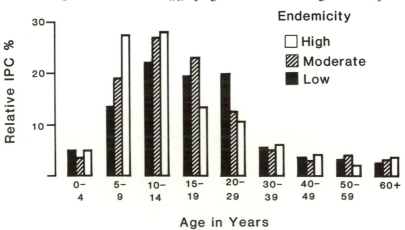

million eggs contaminating the environment each day. To reach the daily level of contamination in the low prevalence areas (*circa* 90% reduction in contamination), all persons with counts above 45 e.p.ml would need treatment, or over 40% of all infected.

Contamination of water

The transfer of *S. mansoni* eggs to a water environment is probably the least understood part of the life cycle of the parasite. There is ample evidence from the field that faecal contamination of river banks occurs (apparently more frequently once the river is not used as a main domestic

Fig.13.5. Frequency distribution of *S. mansoni* egg output in areas of differing endemicity and contribution to contamination of different levels of egg excretion.

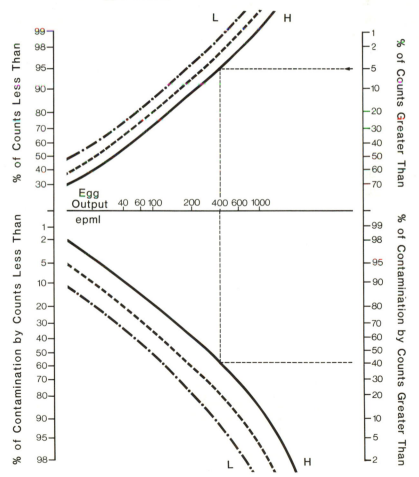

water supply – Chapter 7) and excreta are seen on rocks above the water surface in streams. However, in both situations the faecal material is exposed to the hot sun (in the dry season) so that eggs may be destroyed. In the rainy season when snail populations may be low faecal matter is washed into the river or, if on rocks, is submerged by rising water levels. In these situations it is paradoxical that in St Lucia the main transmission season is when there is least rain but with greater snail population, and it is evident that sufficient faecal matter is washed in – or is deposited directly into the water – to continue transmission. While in the wet season greater quantities of faecal matter are washed in, not only are snail populations lower than in the dry season but the greater volume of water present and the velocity of flow reduce the chance of effective miracidia–snail contact and the perpetuation of the life cycle.

Infected *B. glabrata* were found in a small pool formed by a leaking roadside standpipe. Direct defaecation at the site seems unlikely, but *S. mansoni* eggs may have been introduced from the rinsing of faecal contaminated hands. This may also be a source of infection in other habitats, and Husting (1970) has referred to contamination from adhering perianal faecal material while bathing. The role of this source of eggs and from faecal soiled clothing has not been investigated.

Hatching of S. mansoni *eggs*

Epidemiologically, any variation with age of the hatchability of excreted *S. mansoni* eggs may be important in transmission and, in control through chemotherapy, any differential rate may indicate those groups to which special attention should be paid. A study of the hatchability of *S. mansoni* eggs excreted by persons having different intensities of infection, age and sex was therefore carried out (Upatham, Sturrock & Cook, 1976). Considerable variation was found among eggs in consecutive stools from the same individual but overall higher rates were associated with younger subjects and those with high egg loads. The hatching rate of eggs in persons to the age of 19 was found to be 0.4222, among persons 20–39 years of age 0.3254, and older persons 0.2536.

Duration of hatching

Although there have been several laboratory studies of the hatching of miracidia, little was known about the rapidity or duration of hatching when infected faeces were deposited in natural water. A series of experiments was designed to investigate these aspects of the parasite's life cycle, using large tanks, 120 cm in diameter holding 178 l of water, and caged snails located at the periphery. Adequate aliquots of hard and soft stools to provide 1400 miracidia (from infected St Lucian children) were introduced at the centre of the tanks. Caged snails were removed after exposure to miracidia for varying lengths of time, and maintained in aquaria for 12–14 days before being examined for sporocysts.

Hatching times were found to vary with consistency of stool, starting within 24 and 32 hours for soft and hard stools respectively and extending to 48 and 128 hours. The finding that hatching of eggs from hard stools may go on for at least 5 days may lead to wider dispersion of infection, especially in flowing water (Upatham, 1972a).

Further experiments were made in the field. Relays of caged snails were located in a banana drain and a stream and exposed to calculated numbers of miracidia expected to hatch from hard, soft and mushy stools. It was again found that duration of hatching varied with consistency of stool. In static water it started after about 12 hours and extended to 72 hours for hard stools, and to 48 hours for soft and mushy stools. In running water similar results were obtained except that in mushy stools hatching took place between 12 and 24 hours. Although hatchability of eggs in the stools was high, less than 1 % of miracidia successfully infected snails (Upatham, 1972b). This could have been due to the distance between point of release of stool and the cages, 30.2 cm in the standing-water habitat but 152 cm in flowing-water, although it was shown in other experiments that miracidia could locate snails up to 914 cm and 9754 cm in standing and flowing-water habitats (Upatham, 1973a).

It was thought possible to estimate the number of miracidia penetrating *B. glabrata* from the number of daughter sporocysts found on dissection (Upatham, 1973a), but this could not be confirmed in a later study (Christie & Prentice, 1978). Although the maximum number of sporocysts found did relate to increasing miracidial challenge, the range for each showed too much overlap for accurately assessing the intensity of the miracidial inoculation.

Miracidial dispersion and survival

The development of the sentinel snail technique enabled studies to be carried out in semi-natural and field conditions on the dispersion and survival of miracidia. Chernin & Dunavan (1962) had shown that in a Petri dish miracidia tended to concentrate at its margin and this was found to be so in large outdoor tanks and in a natural pond (Upatham, 1972c). It was also shown that similar infection rates in sentinel snails were obtained in cages located at the surface and on the bottom of the pond. Miracidia located caged snails at a depth of 122 cm and moved horizontally 107 cm but a distance of 914 cm was recorded after experiments in banana drains (Upatham, 1972*d*).

The interference by other aquatic snails, tadpoles and guppies on the capacity of miracidia to infect *B. glabrata* was investigated. *Physa* and *Drepanotrema* were found to reduce the infection rate in *B. glabrata* more than guppies and tadpoles (Upatham, 1972*e*). It was found also that the degree of the reduction in the infection rate of *B. glabrata* was directly proportional to the logarithm of the decoy surface area and inversely proportional to the logarithm of the miracidial concentration (Upatham & Sturrock, 1973).

The infection rate in snails was also affected by salinity, pH, turbidity and volume. As the sodium chloride concentration increased from 0.5 p.p.m. to 4200 p.p.m. the infection rate decreased from 79% to 2%. Highest infection rates were obtained at pH 7–9, low rates were obtained at pH 5 and 10, but no infections were obtained at pH 4. Although *B. glabrata* tolerated all pH levels, miracidial activity was of short duration in water with a low pH, 1–2 minutes in pH 4, peaked at 5–6 hours in pH 7–9 and decreased to 2 hours in pH 10 (Upatham, 1972*f*). As turbidity increased to 100 p.p.m. the infection rate decreased sharply but more slowly as turbidity increased to 500 p.p.m. Snails appeared unaffected by turbidity in the one hour of exposure. While extreme conditions in the laboratory affected infection, they are unlikely to affect infection rates severely in natural snail habitats under normal circumstances.

The effect of temperature was investigated: no infections were found in *B. glabrata* exposed at temperatures lower than 16 °C when 14% became infected. A peak infection rate of 71% was obtained at 34 °C but at 40 °C it dropped to 10% when there was a high mortality of snails and miracidia. As the annual range of temperature in St Lucia is from 22–30 °C natural infections are generally unlikely to be affected by temperature, although this may occur in a few small foci in very hot weather in the summer months (Upatham, 1973*b*).

The parasitised snail

Laboratory studies were carried out to investigate different aspects of the snail/parasite relationship (Sturrock & Sturrock, 1970*a*).

Age of the snail and infection

Snails at 2, 6, 12, 24 and 44 weeks after hatching were individually exposed to five miracidia. The pre-patent period varied between 21 and 35 days, but was not related to the snails' age: snails aged 2 weeks at the time of the infection showed a 100% infection rate, the oldest snails

(44 weeks at exposure) a 93% rate; other rates varied from 70% to 83% but there was no direct relationship with age and no indication of resistance to infection with increased age.

Mortality was greater in all groups compared with uninfected controls and there was evidence that it occurred earlier in the snails that were older at the time of exposure. Bleeding that was observed in some snails during or after exposure, particularly in the younger snails, was not associated with death.

Except in the youngest group the rate of growth of snails temporarily increased after infection but eventually uninfected controls were larger than those infected at 6 and 12 weeks. The stunting of growth was associated with deformity of the shell aperture, due to a reversal from ventral to dorsal of the deflection found in uninfected snails. The distortion occurred at the time of cercarial shedding and increased in size linearly as the infection progressed. Using data from the laboratory findings, it was possible to estimate that naturally infected field B. glabrata, showing the deformity, had been shedding cercariae for an average of less than three weeks (Sturrock & Sturrock, 1971).

Compared with uninfected snails, egg production was severely reduced and many snails were sterilised by the infection, though some later resumed limited egg production and simultaneously produced cercariae as well; no self cures were observed. The average total output of cercariae per infected snail was estimated at nearly 250 000. The high infection rates, high cercarial outputs and long life-span of the infected snails suggest a well adapted relationship between the St Lucian strains of B. glabrata and S. mansoni.

Miracidial load and cercarial infection rates

Groups of snails were exposed to 1, 2, 4 and 8 miracidia; except for a 53% infection rate with 2 miracidia a rate of 80% was obtained with 1 and 4 miracidia, the highest rate, 95%, being obtained with 8 miracidia. The mean daily cercarial output of infected snails showed a similar pattern to the infection rate – the highest output being 2872 cercariae from the 8 miracidia infections, 2643 with 1 miracidia but 1115 and 1476 with 2 and 4 miracidia respectively.

Survival of cercariae

The dispersion and survival of cercariae are important factors in the epidemiology of schistosomiasis and investigations were made in static and flowing habitats; cercariae were detected by Sandt's technique (Sandt, 1973b) and sentinel mice exposure.

As indicated in Chapter 1, the first recorded patient in St Lucia acquired his infection while washing under a waterfall after bathing in the sulphurous waters at the Sulphur Springs. The infectivity of cercariae surviving the 6 m drop was investigated by releasing 32 000 cercariae during a 2-hour period at the top of the falls and assessing infection in groups of caged mice floated in the pool at the bottom and in a further pool 50 m downstream. On dissection seven weeks after exposure only 1 of 18 mice in the waterfall pool was infected, suggesting considerable loss of infectivity. However, the result indicates that tourists and others in the population may be exposed to infection while bathing in pools below the many waterfalls in St Lucia (Upatham, 1973c). None of 19 mice in the more distant pool was infected, although in other experiments it was shown that cercariae retained their infectivity to mice for at least 97 m downstream in water with a medium velocity of about 40 cm/sec, and were detected by cercariometry as far as 195 m. In fast flowing water (velocity 74 cm/sec) they were detected, and they infected mice at 12 m below the point of entry. It was calculated that between 0.100% and 0.18% of cercariae infected mice (Upatham, 1974a).

Although static water habitats in St Lucia (marshes and banana drains) probably play little role in transmission owing to limited human water contact and cercarial immobility, in theory, where such habitats border streams, cercariae may drain into the running water; this would extend their dispersion and increase the risk of persons being infected, particularly

Fig.13.6. Sketch map of streams used for cercariometry. *a*: Ti Bourg; *b*: Talvern; *c*: Ravine Saut.

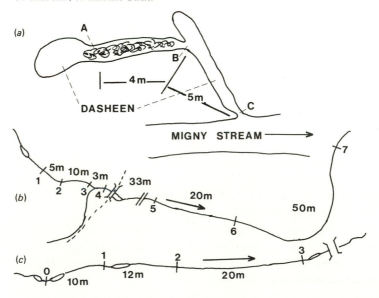

if the water enters a slow flowing pool (Upatham, 1974*b*). Local conditions may, however, reduce the number of cercariae available for infection and attenuation of cercarial density was investigated in two field locations where naturally infected snails were found and in another where laboratory infected snails were introduced (M. A. Prentice, unpublished).

At Ti Bourg (see Chapter 6), infected snails were found in a seepage pool and dasheen marsh feeding a watercress bed before flowing into the main Migny stream in the Fond St Jacques area (Fig. 13.6*a*). Discharge was 0.2 l/s at B and 0.4 l/s at C. Water samples were collected for cercariometry at sites A, B and C. Results from three days of sampling are shown in Table 13.1 (*a*).

At Talvern in Marquis valley (see Chapter 5), snails were found infected in a small stream with a discharge of 0.4 l/s (Fig. 13.6*b*). Preliminary sampling showed that cercarial density was highest at station 1. Samples were taken at seven stations as shown. The section between 1 and 3 was overgrown with *Comelina* spp. to such an extent that the water surface was

Table 13.1. *Cercariae counts/litre of water on 9 cm diameter glass filter pads strained with Lugol's iodine*

Station	No. of samples	Sample volume	Distance below prev. station (m)	cerc./l	Attenuation relative to station A (%)	Attenuation between stations (%)
(a) Ti Bourg watercress/dasheen gutter, March 1978. Discharge 0.2–0.4 l/s						
A	9	180	—	0.52	—	—
B	4	74	4	0.0	100	100
C	10	200	5	0.005	99	—
(b) Talvern, June 1978. Discharge, station 1–3 0.27 l/s; 3–7 0.4 l/s						
1	5	42	—	12.07	—	—
2	5	53	5	3.43	71.5	71.5
3	5	67	10	0.16	98.7	95.3
4	5	85	3	0.06	99.5	62.5
5	5	100	33	0.00	100	100
6	5	62	20	0.03	99.8	—
7	5	100	50	0.01	99.9	66.6
(c) Ravine Saut, June 1978. Discharge 1.1 l/s						
0	8	160	—	1.29	—	—
1	8	160	10	0	100	100
2	8	160	12	0	100	—
3	8	160	20	0	100	—

Prentice, unpublished data.

invisible; from station 3 onwards the stream was open with rocky shallow sections interspersed with pools. Attenuation of cercarial numbers was greatest in the overgrown section and thereafter declined more slowly. The cercariae collected at stations 6 and 7 were present in the 12.00 and 13.00 hours samples, i.e. 1–2 hours after peak shedding (Table 13.1(*b*)).

Ravine Saut, a remote ravine high in the hills above Anse La Raye, was chosen for the experimental release of cercariae from laboratory infected snails. The stream flowed rapidly in a narrow gravel and rock channel but was interrupted by two pools each of approximately 500 l volume. The discharge was 1.1 l/s and the mean velocity over a 40 m stretch was 1.3 m/min, as determined by a marker dye. The layout of the stream is shown in Fig. 13.6*c*. A drip feed of niclosamide maintained a concentration of 2 mg/l below site 3 throughout the experimental period to kill cercariae and prevent their further dispersion (Table 13.1(*c*)).

The very high levels of attenuation found in these experiments even in unobstructed streams as at Ti Bourg and Ravine Saut, suggest that infected snails in marshes and banana drains contribute little to transmission.

It was apparent that in seepages and small streams where the wetted perimeter is large in proportion to the volume of water, considerable loss of cercariae occurs. However, in experiments in a section of the Cul de Sac river without turbulence or tributaries, with a clean, sandy bottom and no vegetation, cercariae were shown to travel at least 500 m. Collecting stations at 100 m intervals were marked off over a distance of 500 m and pooled cercariae from about 500 infected snails were dripped into the river from a constant flow device. Approximately 40 l samples of water were collected at each station and passed through fibre-glass filters, stained with iodine and the cercariae counted. (A niclosamide drip was maintained for an hour below the last sample site to kill cercariae, and men stationed at intervals along the experimental stretch warned the population not to enter the river.)

The time of collecting water samples was based on a preliminary timing of a dye marker passing the collecting stations, water samples being collected 20 minutes after the calculated time of arrival of the first cercariae. Results of three replicates are shown in Table 13.2.

A similar trial was made in a much smaller stream (discharge *circa* 50 l/sec). Cercariae were detected 500 m from point of discharge, by which time there had been a loss of approximately 90% of cercariae. Although this loss is not unlike that from the Cul de Sac river, a greater per cent loss might have been expected owing to the high wetted perimeter/volume ratio. It seems likely that this was compensated for by a lower loss from exhaustion of cercariae in the slowly moving water compared with that in Cul de Sac river with a higher rate of discharge. Although it is apparent that cercariae can travel a considerable distance, their infectivity was not established, and it has been shown recently that mortality among schistosomula may be high within 24 hours of penetration, possibly due to exhaustion of energy reserves (Lawson & Wilson, 1983). In this respect it is of interest that in Cul de Sac valley and on the northern side of Richefond valley higher rates of prevalence and intensity of infection were found in settlements at the head of the rivers than in villages lower downstream, suggesting that although cercariae may be carried downstream, even if they penetrate the human host they do not develop to adult worms.

Exposure to infection – water contact activities

Although the lifecycle of *S. mansoni* was finally understood in 1915 it is only within the last few years that studies have been made to investigate the water contact patterns of communities to provide detailed and quantitative data on the exposure to infection of different sections of the population. Data from the 1975 water contact study on the northern side of Richefond valley (Chapter 7) have been analysed in an attempt to define the relative risks of different domestic contacts and to investigate evidence for the development of immunity.

Methods used have been described in Chapter 3. Observations were made in 1975, 1976 and 1977 at seven main contact points used by the population of Derniere Riviere, Belmont and Morne Panache II. Results

Table 13.2. *Number of* S. mansoni *cercariae (and cerc./l) recovered from 40 l samples of water collected at 100 m intervals from point of cercarial release in Cul de Sac river*

Approx. no. cercariae released	Stream discharge (l/s)	Theoretical cerc./l	Distance below release (m)				
			100	200	300	400	500
			Number and (cerc./l)				
170000	265	0.36	14 (0.3)	7 (0.16)	7 (0.16)	1 (0.02)	0
Sample fault	329	?	5 (0.11)	7 (0.15)	9 (0.2)	9 (0.2)	10 (0.2)
110000	178	0.34	3 (0.08)	1 (0.03)	1 (0.03)	0	1 (0.02)

Prentice, unpublished data.

Table 13.3. Analysis by age and activity of 1473 water contacts among 362 females (computer analysis)

Age group	Total			Activities					
	Contacts	Persons	Contacts/person	Washing	Bathing	Playing	Collecting water	Fording	Other
0–4	88	32	2.75	n.o.[a]	23 (19)	57 (24)	n.o.	7 (7)	1 (1)
5–9	261	76	3.43	43 (16)[b]	41 (31)	110 (53)	2 (2)	58 (27)	7 (6)
10–14	337	81	4.16	143 (41)	52 (37)	57 (38)	1 (1)	77 (42)	7 (4)
15–19	256	49	5.22	161 (33)	32 (24)	18 (12)	n.o.	45 (18)	n.o.
20–29	170	45	3.78	117 (31)	20 (16)	9 (9)	1 (1)	23 (15)	n.o.
30–39	162	31	5.23	132 (27)	11 (10)	7 (5)	n.o.	10 (7)	2 (1)
40–49	127	29	4.38	96 (23)	10 (8)	7 (7)	1 (1)	13 (10)	n.o.
50–59	56	13	4.30	39 (8)	1 (1)	9 (6)	3 (1)	4 (4)	n.o.
60+	16	6	2.67	14 (4)	n.o.	2 (2)	n.o.	n.o.	n.o.
Total	1473	362	4.07	745 (183)	190 (146)	276 (156)	8 (6)	237 (130)	17 (12)
% of contacts				51	13	19	<1	16	1
% of individuals				51	40	43	2	4	3

[a] Not observed.
[b] No. in brackets refers to no. of individuals.

from 1975 only, obtained before the introduction of laundry and shower units, are analysed. At the 1975 stool survey 817 women and 750 men were recorded as living in the area; 362 women (44% of the women) and 186 or 25% of men were observed at the contact points. The analysis is restricted to the females.

Number of contacts

Water contact activities were classified as washing (mainly clothes), bathing, playing, fording, collecting water and 'other'. While play by children is obvious, amongst adults this was usually casual contact for no obvious reason. 'Other' contacts involved such activities as fishing, washing cars or animals, collecting river sand, or washing boots. Collecting water was infrequently observed as the area was served by a community standpipe water supply.

Observations were made at a different site on each of the seven days in the seven months period of study. Results therefore represent 49 site observation days out of the total of 1392 in the period of study, 7×28 (days) $\times 7$ (sites). The actual number of contacts over the period was, therefore, many times that recorded. A breakdown of the observed 1473 female water contact activities is shown in Table 13.3.

The greatest proportion of contacts was for washing (51%) and 51% of females observed were engaged in the activity. Playing, fording and bathing contributed 19, 16 and 13% of contacts, with 40% and 43% respectively of women being observed to bath or play. The mean number of contacts per person increased to 5.23 in the 30–39-year age group but

Fig.13.7. Changes in pattern of water contact with age among females.

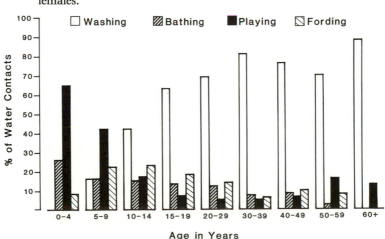

Age in Years

remained high, falling only in those over the age of 60 years. The pattern of contact, however, changed with increasing age (Fig. 13.7).

As a per cent of the total contacts, washing increased with age, while playing and bathing contacts declined rapidly from peaks in the 0–4-year age group to the 15–19-year age group. Fording activities were greatest in the 5–14-year age group and were seen mainly by children going to school.

Apart from the frequency of water contact the risk of acquiring *S. mansoni* probably varies with the water contact activity. The duration of exposure and the degree of body exposed during contact appear important factors that may affect it. In addition, owing to the diurnal shedding of cercariae by infected snails, the time of day of water contact may be relevant, particularly in flowing water habitats where carcariae do not remain at the contact point as they might in a static water site. These factors and combinations of them were investigated in relation to infection in the human population in an attempt to define those most important in acquiring the infection.

Duration of contact

The overall mean duration per contact gradually increased to the 30–49-year age group, and then declined (Table 13.4). For washing the mean time of contact increased to the age of 40–49 and was the most prolonged activity with a mean of 16 minutes per contact: the mean

Table 13.4. *Mean duration per contact by age and activity (computer analysis)*

| Age group | Mean duration of all contacts | Mean duration for activity | | | | | |
		Washing	Bathing	Playing	Collecting water	Fording	Other
0–4	6.7	n.o.[a]	4.7	8.4	0.3	n.o.	6.0
5–9	6.0	10.7	7.0	6.6	1.3	0.3	11.3
10–14	8.6	14.3	8.1	5.5	0.2	0.3	16.0
15–19	11.2	16.1	6.7	3.3	n.o.	0.2	n.o.
20–29	12.5	16.5	6.2	6.3	2.5	0.4	n.o.
30–39	14.7	17.2	5.5	0.8	n.o.	0.4	24.0
40–49	14.6	18.5	6.3	2.0	1.0	0.3	n.o.
50–59	12.0	16.3	5.0	2.6	0.8	0.3	n.o.
60+	12.6	14.4	n.o.	0.6			
Mean	10.3	16.0	6.7	6.1	1.1	0.3	14.4

[a] Not observed.

Table 13.5. *Mean contact time of individuals observed in various activities (computer analysis)*

	Washing		Bathing		Playing		Collecting water		Fording		Other	
	No. observed	Mean time	No. observed	Mean time	No. observed	Mean time	No. observed	Mean time	No. observed	Mean time	No. observed	Mean time
0–4	—	—	19	5.74	24	19.85	—	—	7	0.25	1	6.00
5–9	16	28.75	31	9.22	53	13.71	2	1.33	27	0.65	6	13.17
10–14	41	49.86	37	11.36	38	8.22	1	0.17	42	0.45	4	28.00
15–19	33	78.68	24	8.87	12	4.87	1	—	18	0.41	—	—
20–29	31	62.30	16	7.75	9	6.24	1	2.50	15	0.61	—	—
30–39	27	84.08	10	6.03	5	1.10	—	—	7	0.52	1	48.00
40–49	23	77.00	8	7.88	7	1.95	1	1.00	10	0.39	—	—
50–59	8	79.63	1	5.00	6	3.90	1	2.37	4	0.34	—	—
60+	4	50.25	—	—	2	0.63	—	—	—	—	—	—
	183	65.09	146	8.77	156	10.73	1	1.45	130	0.49	12	20.42

contact for the few 'other' activities observed was 14.4 minutes, bathing 6.7 minutes (peaking in the 10–14-year age group), playing 6.1 minutes, (decreasing from the longest in the 0–4-year age group), but collecting water, 1.1 minutes, and fording, less than a minute, were of minimal duration in all age groups.

The mean total contact time for washing by individual women increased to a peak of 84 minutes in the 30–39-year age group (Table 13.5) and for bathing it increased in children to 11.36 minutes among the 10–14-year-old girls followed by a steady decline. The greatest total contact time for individuals at play was nearly 20 minutes in the youngest age group, and although 'other contacts' were infrequently seen they had a similar mean of total duration.

Extent of body exposed

The proportion of the body exposed to contact with water varies with activity and, for the same activity, the actual surface area of the body exposed, in terms of m², will vary with age. Tables of mean height and weights by sex and age were derived from measurements of nearly 3000 patients attending the schistosomiasis clinic and were used to calculate the surface area of the body. The proportion of the total surface area exposed was derived from surgical charts used in the management of burn victims (see Chapter 3), so that the actual area of skin in contact with water could be calculated for different activities (Table 13.6).

The effect of surface area exposed is most clearly seen in respect of bathing, which involves virtually complete submersion. Among the

Table 13.6. *Mean area of skin in m² exposed to water contact by age and activity* (*computer analysis*)

| Age group | Mean of all contacts | Activity | | | | | |
		Bathing	Washing	Playing	Collecting water	Fording	Other
0–4	0.199	0.494	n.o.	0.094	n.o.	0.101	0.120
5–9	0.217	0.707	0.148	0.118	0.107	0.128	0.095
14–14	0.323	1.042	0.221	0.201	0.064	0.138	0.129
15–19	0.375	1.346	0.268	0.207	n.o.	0.136	n.o.
20–29	0.401	1.391	0.291	0.213	0.300	0.177	n.o.
30–39	0.366	1.404	0.309	0.178	n.o.	0.150	0.207
40–49	0.334	1.399	0.258	0.204	0.302	0.148	n.o.
50–59	0.210	1.390	0.204	0.182	0.100	0.110	n.o.
60+	0.232	n.o.	0.231	0.238	n.o.	n.o.	n.o.

[a] Not observed.

0–4-year-olds this involves only 0.494 m² of surface area compared with 1.404 m² for the 30–39-year age group who would, therefore, presumably be exposed to nearly three times the risk of infection of the child for the same activity.

Time of exposure

The shedding of cercariae has been shown to start a few hours after daybreak and to increase during the morning, after which it declines (Webbe & Jordan, 1966.) From these findings a risk time factor $r(t)$, was calculated with a maximum value of 100 at midday. The particular value for a given time of day was given by the function:

$$r(t) = \frac{C}{2\pi\sigma^2} \exp\left(-\frac{1}{2\sigma^2}(t-\tau)^2\right)$$

where $\tau = 12$ $\sigma^2 = 4$ $C = 501.326$.

This is a normal density function with mean at midday, a variance of 4 hours and adjusted by C to have a maximum of 100. No specific units can be ascribed to this measure of exposure as the $r(t)$ factor is an arbitrary function.

The number of contacts observed at different times is shown in Table 13.7. More contacts occurred between 11 a.m. and midday, when the risk of infection is greatest, than in any other period of the day.

Table 13.7. *Number of observed water contacts in relation to time of day (computer analysis)*

Time activity started		Total contacts	Activity				
			Washing	Bathing	Playing	Fording	Other
a.m.	6–7	4	1	n.o.[a]	1	2	n.o.
	7–8	86	52	4	7	23	n.o.
	8–9	137	72	4	24	35	2
	9–10	225	117	19	39	48	2
	10–11	223	150	16	34	18	5
	11–12	246	122	29	63	30	2
p.m.	12–1	191	98	42	34	14	2
	1–2	144	73	33	21	9	4
	2–3	136	46	37	36	16	n.o.
	3–4	61	11	6	12	30	n.o.
	4–5	203	3	n.o.	5	12	n.o.
	Total	1473	745	190	276	237	17

[a] Not observed.

The risk of infection

At the end of the 1975 water contact study 260 of the women who had been observed in contact with water provided a stool sample for examination. The level of infection (IPC – prevalence multiplied by geometric mean of egg output) among different age groups was compared with different factors generally thought to be involved in individuals becoming infected. The following indices of risk were considered: (a) the number of contacts, (b) the duration of contact in minutes, (c) duration and exposure (mins/m² exposed), and (d) duration and exposure adjusted by the *rt* factor. Results are shown in Fig. 13.8.

The IPC increased in parallel with all indices of risk to the age of 15–19 years, but in spite of higher levels of risk (except for the mean number of contacts) in the 20–29-year age group, there was no change in the level of infection, and this fell markedly in the 30–39-year age group although risk factors were at their peak. The lowest level of infection in the 60 + age group was associated with risk factors similar to those of the 15–19 age group.

The declining prevalence and intensity of infection usually found in the early years of adulthood in most endemic areas have been considered, amongst other causes, to be an indication of developing immunity to re-infection, but changing patterns of water activity with age (Fig. 13.5) could not exclude reduced exposure to cercarial infested water accounting for the declines (Warren, 1973). However, results of the St Lucia study suggest that although major changes in water contact do occur with age, when duration of exposure, surface area of skin exposed and the risk time factor are considered, an overall reduction in risk of infection is only apparent in the 40–49-year age group. The results suggest therefore that in the group of women studied, immunity to re-infection was apparent in the 20–29-year age group. While the risk factors considered in this study would appear to warrant consideration, other investigations suggest their role is not fully understood. Prentice (1983*b*) found that cercarial densities in natural waters did not correlate with worm loads in sentinel mice exposed in natural habitats; low cercarial densities were associated with a disproportionately large number of adult worms recovered compared with exposure to high cercarial densities. This supports laboratory experiments where a 50% reduction in worm load in mice was obtained when cercarial concentration was reduced by a factor of 80 (Warren & Peters, 1967). The results suggest that low cercarial densities that may be present in the early morning are disproportionately more dangerous than high concentrations at midday. In further animal studies it was shown that although cercarial penetration may appear to be rapid, maturation of

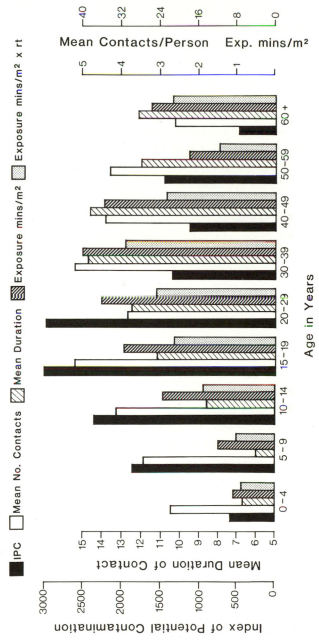

Fig.13.8. Index of potential contamination by age and corresponding indices of the risk of infection during water contact.

cercariae to adult worms requires more prolonged exposure and cercariae that have not penetrated completely while exposed die as the skin dries (Warren & Peters, 1967); there may therefore be very little risk of infection from fording or collecting water.

In studies with mice and *S. mansoni*. cercariae, Stirewalt (1953) found a local inhibition of penetration by cercariae when a second exposure followed the first by an interval of up to one day and, from direct observation of cercariae penetrating human skin, entry points were, without exception, wrinkles (Stirewalt, 1956). If this applies under natural conditions the wrinkled skin of the elderly may be more attractive to cercariae than the unblemished skin of a baby! While these investigations into the process of infection refer mainly to mice, it is not known whether findings apply also to the human host and how they could affect infection and indices of risk.

Infection of the individual
Intensity of first infection

Data from cross-sectional epidemiological surveys indicate that intensity of infection increases with age to a peak in the second decade of life, and that the frequency distribution of excreted *S. mansoni* eggs is log normal. There is, however, no information on the intensity of first infections ('quantitative incidence'), and nothing to indicate whether it varies yearly with the level of transmission or age, or how the egg distribution pattern is attained. Do children when first infected all have a similar, low level of egg excretion which gradually builds up in some individuals with greater exposure, or is the distribution of eggs log normal following first exposure? Futhermore, how does quantitative incidence compare with the intensity of infection of similar aged children known previously to have been infected?

Data from the annual stool surveys carried out in the Richefond valley high transmission comparison area (Chapter 4) enabled some of these questions to be answered. Analyses were made of results of stool examinations from children who had two stools negative for *S. mansoni* at consecutive annual surveys, followed, the third year, by a positive stool for which a quantitative result was obtained. The only exception to this was if no specimen had been examined when the child was in its first year of life, it being assumed it would have been uninfected. Table 13.8 illustrates the method of selecting cases and gives examples of equivocal results which were rejected.

Quantitative incidence data were available from 249 individuals age 1–12 years for six 2-year periods between 1969 and 1975; results are shown in Table 13.9 and compared with the corresponding incidence of new infections (Table 4.9).

It is apparent that quantitative incidence varied from year to year depending on the transmission pattern and was highest in infections acquired between 1971 and 1972, corresponding to the peak transmission year in the area.

Table 13.8. *Method of determining intensity of infection at the first year of known infection.*

Numbers under the columns 'Year of survey' indicates S. mansoni *eggs/ml faeces*

Age at 1968	Year of survey							Age at first infection
	1968	1969	1970	1971	1972	1973	1974	
Acceptable cases								
0	n.s.[a]	—[b]	20					2
0	n.s.	—	—	40				3
2	n.s.	—	n.s.	—	—	70		7
4	—	n.s.	—	—	300			8
7	—	—	10					9
−1	n.b.[c]	—	n.s.	—	—	50		4
−4	n.b.	n.b.	n.b.	n.b.	n.s.	—	60	2
Rejected cases								
4	—	—	+[d]	20				6
6	—	n.s.	—	50				Unknown
8	—	—	—	n.s.	20			Unknown

[a] No specimen.
[b] Stool negative for *S. mansoni* ova.
[c] Not born at time of survey.
[d] Stool *S. mansoni* positive on qualitative examination for ova but insufficient stool for quantitative examination.

Table 13.9. *Quantitative incidence data from 249 1–12-year-old children by year and comparable per cent incidence of new infections*

Transmission period	No. new infections	Mean log egg output	SD	GM	% inc.
1969–70	37	1.1502	0.2850	14.13	21.8
1970–71	43	1.2792	0.4046	19.02	21.0
1971–72	87	1.3971	0.4234	24.95	39.4
1972–73	34	1.3601	0.4238	22.92	28.2
1973–74	28	1.2995	0.4036	19.93	28.3
1974–75	20	1.1729	0.2488	14.89	18.5

New infections in 1972 provided the greatest number of cases – 87 – for further analysis and the frequency distribution of egg output of new infections was investigated. From Fig. 13.9 it is apparent that the egg output follows the typical log normal distribution found in endemic areas. It is of interest that water contact studies carried out later (1975–77) showed a similar distribution of the duration of water contacts among children in the same area.

Data from these 87 children who acquired their infection between 1971 and 1972 were analysed by age group – 1–4, 5–8 and 9–12 years (Table 13.10). The 1–4-year age group had the lowest intensity of infection,

Table 13.10. *Intensity of infection in 1972 in those newly infected and those known to be previously infected*

Age in 1972	New infections				Old infections			
	No. of children	GM	Mean log	SD	No. of children	GM	Mean log	SD
1–4	16	18.40	1.2648	0.3783	25	21.31	1.3286	0.4245
5–8	50	25.67	1.4094	0.4107	95	33.73	1.5280	0.4597
9–12	21	29.42	1.4686	0.4803	144	39.27	1.5940	0.4826

Fig.13.9. Frequency distribution of *S. mansoni* egg output in newly acquired infection in children (quantitative incidence) and duration of observed water contact in children to the age of 12 years.

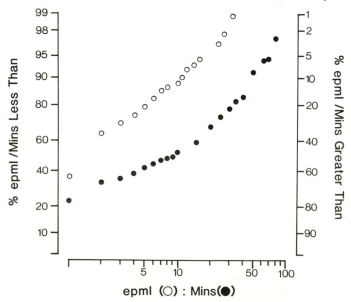

epml (O) : Mins(●)

geometric mean 18.4 e.p.ml, which was significantly different from the 29.4 e.p.ml of the 9–12-year group. These findings were compared with similar data from 264 children who were known to have been infected in 1971 and for whom quantitative data were available for 1972: they lived in the same villages as the 87 in the above study and were thus exposed to a similar high level of transmission.

The intensity of infection increased with age among children in both groups and was consistently lower in those recently infected, though the difference between the two groups was not significant ($Z = 1.94$). However, in view of the level of infection in the new cases, those previously infected might have been expected to have considerably higher levels of infection.

Increasing intensity of infection

Among children with old infections quantitative data for 1971 and 1972 were available from 110 aged between 7 and 16 years; changes in intensity of infection in three age groups are shown in Table 13.11.

The per cent increase in egg output in 1972 decreased with increasing age, in spite of increasing indices of risk, supporting the concept of developing immunity among the children.

Schistosomal morbidity

The majority of *S. mansoni* infections are asymptomatic with only a few persons developing hepatosplenomegaly – the most frequent serious sequelae of the infection. However, as this may be caused by conditions other than *S. mansoni* it was necessary to confirm this parasite as the most common cause of it in St Lucia.

Table 13.11. *Comparison of change in egg output between 1971 and 1972 in three age groups of cohort of 110 children*

	Age group		
	7–10	11–13	14–16
Number in cohort	32	38	40
Geometric mean 1971	21.8	28.1	45.7
Geometric mean 1972	55.5	45.4	54.1
% increase	148	62	19
No. counts increasing	18[a]	23	22
No. counts decreasing	7[a]	11	16
No change	7	4	12

[a] Difference significant at 5% level.

Owing to limited investigational facilities in the island five children excreting *S. mansoni* eggs and with hepatosplenomegaly were admitted to Queen Elizabeth Hospital, Barbados for full investigation to exclude other aetiologies. Two children were found to have portal hypertension with oesophageal varices, but no cause other than schistosomiasis could be found to account for the organomegaly, suggesting a schistomal origin in at least the majority of cases in children in St Lucia.

Intensity of infection and hepatosplenic disease

In the 1960s there appeared to be no explanation for the variation in the prevalence of hepatosplenomegaly in different areas where *S. mansoni* is endemic, and there was speculation that pre-disposition to disease may be genetically influenced, affected by diet, co-existing disease or differences in the pathogenicity of parasites from different regions. It was not until faecal egg counts were used in Brazil as a measure of the intensity of infection that a relationship with splenomegaly was shown (Kloetzel, 1962).

Cheever (1968) confirmed that egg output is a reliable measure of the adult worm burden with the faecal egg output being generally proportional to the number of worm pairs recovered by post-mortem perfusion of the mesenteric veins. His studies also suggested that heavy infection was a prerequisite for the development of Symmers' clay-pipe stem fibrosis of the liver – the hallmark of schistosomal liver disease. However, some heavy infections were noted without accompanying Symmers' fibrosis which was also associated in some cases with light infections. In these, past heavy infections could not be excluded as a cause of the fibrosis.

Confirmation of the relationship between intensity of infection and hepatosplenomegaly in St Lucia came from a study of 138 school children, with quantitative egg excretion data and a comparable uninfected control group (Cook, Baker, Warren & Jordan, 1974). The uninfected group of 23 children, and groups of children having three levels of intensity of infection, were investigated – light infections, 10–75 e.p.ml (57); moderate, 100–300 e.p.ml (32); and heavy, 400 or more e.p.ml of faeces (26). All subjects had stable egg excretion levels over the previous 2–4 years; medical histories were taken and clinical examinations were made 'blind'.

Although symptoms referable to the gastro-intestinal tract are frequently attributed to *S. mansoni*, in this carefully controlled study there was no difference between the three groups in respect of the frequency of complaints of weakness, abdominal pain, cramp, aches, epigastric pain, diarrhoea or blood in stools. Anthropometric measurements of height, weight, arm circumference and skinfold thickness were similar in all groups, and the only difference found on examination was the frequency of liver enlargement, to more than 2.5 cm below the costal margin, which increased from 8.7% in the uninfected group 12.3% in the lightly infected, and 25.9% in the combined heavy/moderate group; this was significantly different at the 5% level, compared with the combined light and uninfected groups. In addition, the extent of enlargement was related to intensity of infection (Fig. 13.10). Five children had splenomegaly – all were in the heavy/moderate groups.

Liver enlargement and nutritional status

Although in the above study there was no difference in anthropological measurements in the groups, in a further study at a school in Richefond valley, among children with hepatomegaly there was evidence that anthropological measurements may be affected in the long term.

In April 1967 811 children aged 5–15 years were examined: 428 were boys, 383 were girls. Livers were palpable in 22.9% and 18.0% of males and females respectively, and spleens in 1.4 and 4.4%. The frequency of palpable livers increased to 30% at the age of 9 and 10, then declined to 7% at 15 years. Two of 105 8–year-old children had hepatosplenomegaly but the rate increased to 5% in the children aged 14 and 15 years.

Fig.13.10. Correlation of mean liver size below the costal margin in mid-sternal and mid-clavicular lines, with intensity of schistosomiasis mansoni. (From Cook *et al.*, 1974.)

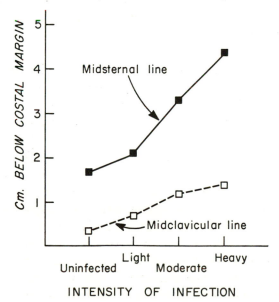

For further study, 108 children with palpable livers were formed into a 'clinical group' and matched, as nearly as possible, for age, sex and village of residence with children whose livers were not palpable – forming a 'non-clinical group'. The children were weighed and measured and over the next 18 months three stool examinations were made and two further physical examinations were carried out. By November 1968 it was apparent that some palpable livers had regressed and in other children the liver became palpable. There were thus four groups – group 1 (44 children), liver never palpable; group 2 (20), liver normal in April 1967, palpable November 1968; group 3 (50), liver enlarged throughout period; and group 4 (36), liver enlarged April 1967 and not palpable by November 1968. Groups 1 and 2 formed the original non-clinical group (64 children), groups 3 and 4 the clinical group (86 of the original 108 children).

The children were examined by Dr Robert Cook of the Caribbean Food and Nutrition Institute. Examinations included a physical, height, weight, arm circumference (AC), triceps skinfold thickness (from these measurements the calculated mid-arm muscle circumference – CMAMC – was derived), and a haemoglobin estimation.

For each group the per cent of standard weight and height for age at April 1967 and November 1968 were calculated, as well as the per cent standard AC, CMAMC and haemoglobin at the November examination. The composition of the groups and parasitological data are shown in Table 13.12; other results are summarised in Table 13.13. The following comparisons are made:

Groups 1 and 2 *versus* groups 3 and 4 (the original non-clinical and clinical groups);

Findings did not differ significantly except for the mean haemoglobin which was higher in the non-clinical group, 11.8g, than in the clinical group, 11.3 g (significant at 5% level).

Group 1 *versus* group 3 (liver never palpable and persistently palpable):

Data from these groups suggest there was a significant difference in anthropological measurements and haemoglobin between those with a persistently palpable liver and those whose livers were never felt. In April 1967 and November 1968 the mean per cent of standard weight for age was greater in those whose liver never enlarged. The mean height for age in April 1967 and mean haemoglobin in November 1968 were also greater in the group with non-palpable livers.

Group 4 *versus* group 3 (liver regressing and persistently palpable):

At the beginning of the study height and weight measurements were significantly better amongst those whose livers were to regress compared with those with persistent liver enlargement, and at the end of the study

Table 13.12. *Hepatomegaly: sex and age structure and parasitological findings in four study groups*

Group	No.	Sex		Age in months		S. mansoni egg output					
		M	F	Mean	SD	% +ve	Mean log	SD	GM	AM[d]	SD
(1) Liver never palpable	44[a]	17	27	112.5	21.9	83.7	1.1855	0.8693	15.33	58.05	84.69
(2) Normal 1967, palpable 1968	20[b]	9	11	119.5	26.1	94.7	1.4206	0.7580	26.34	74.50	120.80
(1)+(2)	64	26	38	114.7	23.3	87.1	1.2513	0.8437	17.84	62.65	95.99
(3) Liver always palpable	50[c]	20	30	118.0	23.0	95.8	1.4977	0.8247	31.36	122.64	280.66
(4) Enlarged 1967, normal 1968	36	14	22	112.6	20.0	86.1	1.1808	0.8592	15.16	55.44	77.20
(3)+(4)	86	34	52	115.7	21.9	89.5	1.3582	0.8541	22.81	93.31	218.86

[a] Stools from 43 examined.
[b] Stools from 19 examined.
[c] Stools from 48 examined.
[d] Arithmetic mean of e.p.ml.

Table 13.13. *Hepatomegaly: indices of nutritional status April 1967 and November 1968*

| Group | N | % of standard wt for age | | | | % of standard ht for age | | | | November 1968 | | | | | |
| | | April 1967 | | Nov 1968 | | April 1967 | | Nov. 1968 | | % standard AC for age | | % standard CMAMC for age | | Haemoglobin g/100 ml | |
		Mean	SD	Mean	SD	Mean	SD	Mean	SD	Mean	SD	Mean	SD	Mean	SD
(1)	44	85.7[a,g]	11.5	83.2[b]	12.3	94.8[c]	4.6	93.7[d]	4.4	87.9	6.9	91.3	7.2	11.8[e]	1.5
(2)	20	84.0	7.2	82.7	6.7	93.5	4.0	93.3	3.4	87.7	4.7	91.4	5.3	11.9	1.5
(1)+(2)	64	85.2	10.4	83.1	10.8	94.4	4.4	93.7	4.0	87.8	6.3	91.3	6.6	11.8[f]	1.5
(3)	50	80.4[a,g]	10.6	77.6[b,h]	10.1	92.2[c,j]	4.2	91.4[d,k]	4.2	85.1[m]	6.4	88.7[n]	6.8	11.0[e]	1.6
(4)	36	88.5[g]	13.2	86.1[h]	13.5	95.0[j]	5.5	93.5[k]	5.4	90.2[m]	6.9	93.5[n]	7.0	11.6	1.3
(3)+(4)	86	83.4	12.4	81.1	12.3	93.3	5.0	92.3	4.8	87.3	7.0	90.7	7.2	11.3[f]	1.5
All	150	84.4		82.0		93.8		92.9		87.5		91.0		11.5	

Differences between means which are statistically significant are indicated by pairs of letters:

a–a: t = 2.33	e–e: t = 2.40	j–j: t = 2.70
b–b: t = 2.44	f–f: t = 2.26	k–k: t = 2.05
c–c: t = 2.86	g–g: t = 3.15	m–m: t = 3.51
d–d: t = 2.58	h–h: t = 3.33	n–n: t = 3.20

all anthropological measurements (height, weight, AC and CMAMC) were significantly better in the children whose livers became normal, suggesting that regression of the liver is more likely in the better nourished child.

Group 1 *versus* group 2 (liver never palpable and becoming palpable):

No significant differences were noted between those never found with enlarged liver and those whose livers enlarged over the period of the study.

Overall, these results suggest that the nutritional status influences the development of hepatomegaly – those never developing a palpable liver being better nourished than those with persistent liver enlargement – and, where enlargement did occur, in the better nourished, regression was more likely. Although these results could indicate that the nutritional status influences the development of hepatomegaly, those with persistent liver enlargement had a higher mean intensity of *S. mansoni* infection than persons with no liver enlargement, and than persons with regressing livers, which could have affected the anthropological findings.

The socio-economic circumstances at the homes of affected children were investigated in an attempt to establish whether anthropological findings could be due to a lower food intake. In the homes of children with persistent liver enlargement the mean size of families was found to be higher, 7.8 persons per household, than in other groups (range 7.1–7.6) but the mean expenditure per head *per annum* on food and on animal protein was higher (ECC $130.38 and $51.47 respectively) than in other groups (range $83.9–117.5 and $35.8–47.3). In view of this it seems likely that the lower anthropological measurements in those with persistent hepatomegaly were not primarily due to nutritional factors but may have been caused by the parasitic infection.

Further examinations of the children were made but the number of children available gradually decreased. One hundred and seven were available at a final examination in 1971. Over the years, only one child in the 'non-clinical' group developed hepatosplenomegaly compared with 11 of those in the clinical group, possibly indicating that the condition is more likely to develop if hepatomegaly occurs at an early age. Based on the three stool examinations between April 1967 and November 1968, the geometric mean of egg output of those who developed splenomegaly was 79 e.p.ml (arithmetic mean 130 e.p.ml) compared with 23 e.p.ml (arithmetic mean 74 e.p.ml) of those who were found to have splenomegaly at the first examination, suggesting that as the spleen enlarges intensity of infection falls.

It was encouraging to find that at a survey of the school in 1981 among 115 10–14-year-old children living in the villages supplied with water ten years previously, no case of hepatosplenomegaly was detected.

Racial predisposition to hepatosplenic schistosomiasis

Although epidemiological, clinical and autopsy evidence relates severity of disease to intensity of infection (Kloetzel, 1962; Cheever, 1968; Cook *et al.*, 1974), it is not unknown for severe disease to develop in persons with light infections; previous heavy infections cannot be excluded, but there is evidence that some persons are predisposed to develop hepatosplenic complications – those with blood group A (Khattab, El-Gengehy & Sharaf, 1968; Camus, Bina, Carlier & Santoro, 1977; Pereira *et al.*, 1979) – and there is evidence from Egypt that organomegaly may be related to histocompatibility lymphocyte-A A1 and B5 (Salam, Ishaac & Mahmoud, 1979).

On the other hand, some patients appear to tolerate heavy infections and show no sign of hepatosplenomegaly. The condition appears to be rare in Africans south of the Sahara (Billinghurst, 1965; Gelfand, 1966), though severe disease is reported from the West Nile region of Uganda where extremely high levels of egg output are common (Ongom, Ower, Grundy & Bradley, 1972). In Egypt, the Sudan and Brazil such cases are common, suggesting some races, and particularly Negroes, may be less susceptible than others to late stage disease (Bina, Tavares-Neto, Prata & Azevedo, 1978). However, few comparable studies on quantitative aspects of infection, nutritional status, natural heterologous immunity and zooprophylaxis (Nelson, 1974) have been made. Further, it has been postulated that as schistosomes spread from their original home in the Great Lake Region of Africa (Nelson, Teesdale & Highton, 1962), differences in the ancestral experience that various races have had with the infection may be affecting their immunological response now, and may account for differences in pathology (Foster, 1973).

Although the population of St Lucia is predominantly Negro of African origin, as indicated in Chapter 2, East Indians were brought to the island at the time of emancipation and now make up about 5 % of the population. These two ethnic groups, with those of mixed Negro/East Indian ancestry, make up 99 % of the population; other racial and ethnic groups, – Caucasian, Syrian and Amerindian – are miniscule in comparison.

In spite of East Indians forming such a small proportion of the community there was subjective evidence that they were presenting with hepatosplenomegaly more frequently than Negroes, thus prompting more detailed investigations (R. W. Goodgame, unpublished data).

At the time of a retrospective study, 203 patients with hepatosplenic disease had been seen and documented. These came from more than 3000 patients attending the clinic as referrals from all over the island, and from amongst more than 5000 infected persons examined during extensive field campaigns when chemotherapy was offered in rural areas. An analysis was made of the racial distribution among the hepatosplenic patients and the general population. Race was assessed by asking patients the race of their parents; if these were different they were classified as of 'mixed' origin. Racial data were unobtainable in 16 of the 203 patients.

Table 13.14 shows the racial distribution of the total population of the island and of 187 with organomegaly – a disproportionately high number were of East Indian background.

The race of all the 8000 persons examined was not recorded, but assuming the racial distribution was the same as in the general population, the difference in the racial distribution of the hepatosplenic patients is highly significant at the 0.01% level.

Splenic enlargement in the East Indians tended to be greater than in the other groups and a history of haematemesis was more frequently obtained (Table 13.15).

A more detailed community study was made of the comparison settlements in Richefond north where longitudinal parasitological studies had been carried out. After the 1977 survey, all persons who had been found infected were offered treatment; of 959 persons 93% accepted therapy and were examined, their racial origin determined and the presence of

Table 13.14. *Hepatosplenic patients: radical distribution compared with distribution in population*

	Negro		East Indian		Mixed	
	Number	%	Number	%	Number	%
Island population[a]	90154	91.1	3253	3.3	5503	5.6
Hepatosplenic patients[b]	137	73.2	31	16.6	19	10.2

[a] Excludes small number of Caucasians, Syrians and other races.
[b] 187 patients from approximately 8000 patients examined.

Table 13.15. *Hepatosplenomegaly: mean spleen size and frequency of haematemesis among patients of different racial groups*

	Negro	East Indian	Mixed
Number of patients	137	31	19
Mean spleen size (cm)	3.2	5.5	3.5
No. with haematemesis	7 (5.1%)	4 (12.9%)	2 (10.5%)

hepatosplenomegaly noted and related to the level of *S. mansoni* infection in the different racial groups. Results are shown in Table 13.16.

The racial distribution of the population in the community was similar to that of the whole island except that more had a mixed racial background, reflecting the greater number of East Indians in the villages and the frequent intermarriage with Negroes. There was no difference in the composition of the racial groups presenting for treatment, and no difference in age of patients. As hepatosplenomegaly takes some years to develop, the overall intensity of infection was calculated for the three racial groups based on results of surveys in 1968, 1970 and 1972 (i.e. between 5 and 9 years before the physical examinations in 1977). Intensity of infection was lowest amongst the East Indians, but the difference was not statistically significant.

Hepatosplenomegaly was found in 33 of the 896 examined (3.7%), but the distribution within the racial groups varied considerably, with a disproportional number, 6 of the 33 cases (18.2%), being found in East Indians, giving a hepatosplenic rate in this ethnic group of 14.3% compared with 4.1% and 3.0% in those of mixed blood and Negroes respectively; the difference between East Indian and the other groups combined being significant at the 1% level.

This is the first report of increased susceptibility of East Indians to disease, but anecdotal reports from East and South Africa suggest that compared to Negroes, Caucasians are predisposed to hepatosplenic schisto-

Table 13.16. *Hepatosplenomegaly: details of Negro, East Indian and 'mixed' households examined in community study*

	Negro	East Indian	Mixed
Population (% of total)	1776 (84.8)	101 (4.8)	218 (10.4)
No. ever known infected	1072	66	127
% known infected	60.4	65.4	58.3
Intensity of infection			
GM e.p.ml faeces	36	33	39
Mean log (SD)	1.5519 (0.4943)	1.5225 (0.4798)	1.5896 (0.5655)
No. examined	757	42	97
% examined	70.6	63.6	76.4
% < 20 years of age	57	60	61
Hepatosplenomegaly	23	6	4
% of total	69.7	18.2	12.1
Hepatosplenic rate			
(in persons examined)	3.0%	14.3%	4.1%

somiasis. Comparable findings were reported from autopsy studies in Puerto Rico (Cheever & Andrade, 1967; Tsutsumi, 1972), and in a similar, well controlled study in Brazil (Bina *et al.*, 1978) there was a significant deficiency of black individuals with hepatosplenic and pulmonary complications compared with whites and mulattoes. Further, in a longitudinal study, although white, mulatto and black youngsters were equally infected in terms of quantitative egg output, and at the commencement of the study 25% of whites, 1% of mulattoes and 0% of blacks had hepatosplenomegaly, six years later the respective figures were 36%, 27% and 0%. Other workers in Brazil report a similar predisposition of whites to severe disease (Prata & Schroeder, 1967; Numesmaia, Azevedo, Arandas & Widmer, 1975).

With increasing numbers of whites visiting areas where *S. mansoni* is endemic, these reports are of more than academic interest. Although tourists might acquire only light infections they may be at a greater risk of developing severe disease than dark skinned visitors or nationals. Case reports from Australia and Canada of hepatosplenic schistosomiasis diagnosed in two Poles 16 and 20 years after exposure of *S. mansoni* infection in Tanganyika illustrate the chronicity of the condition and the longevity of the worms – both patients were still excreting *S. mansoni* ova (Chartes, Jackson & Vivian, 1969; Little, 1972). The past intensity of infection is of course unknown.

Other genetic and immunologic studies are needed to try to identify host factors which either reduce or enhance the risk of developing the severe forms of schistosomiasis. Other studies of the host response in different racial groups in endemic areas might be profitable.

Hepatosplenomegaly in the community

Community based physical examinations were not made but during the course of the chemotherapy campaigns in the different valleys large numbers of infected persons in the community had abdominal examinations when the finding of hepatosplenomegaly was noted. To obtain more complete data on the prevalence of this condition the Research Ward and clinic records were re-examined to identify the home location of other patients with organomegaly to provide a profile of its distribution in the island and to relate findings to the prevalence and intensity of *S. mansoni* infection in different areas prior to control. Parasitological data from 5–14-year-old children from the first surveys made were used in this analysis, and spleen findings related to infected persons of all ages. Results are shown in Table 13.17.

Except for the quantitative result from Cul de Sac, both the prevalence and geometric mean of egg output correlate closely with the spleen rate (correlation with prevalence, $r = 0.960$; with geometric mean excluding Cul de Sac, $r = 0.935$). The regression for splenomegaly and geometric mean of egg output was calculated to be 0.104 GM -0.799.

(The data from Cul de Sac was collected in 1967 – the first survey of the project. The high geometric mean is likely to have been due to inexperienced microscopists and to quality control not, at the time, being in operation.)

It was calculated that hepatosplenomegaly would probably occur only rarely if intensity of infection in 5–14-year-old children was below about 10 e.p.g (Kato technique) equivalent to a prevalence of about 30%.

Hepatosplenic schistosomiasis in St Lucia and other endemic areas

Data from community based studies are available from a number of areas, but a direct comparison with the St Lucian hepatosplenomegaly data can be made with only one study from Brazil (Lehman *et al.*, 1976) where the geometric mean of egg output (determined by the Bell technique) among 5–14-year-old children was 187 e.p.g. Extrapolating from the St Lucia data this egg load would be associated with an 18.6% spleen rate – a rate of 19.1% was actually found!

Although results from other areas are not strictly comparable with the St Lucian and Brazilian findings, it can be shown that results from a study in Kenya (Siongok *et al.*, 1976) are similar. In the 5–14-year age range the arithmetic mean of egg output is shown to be approximately 800 e.p.g. Allowing for the difference between Kato and Bell results (Chapter 3), this would mean about 100 e.p.g by the Bell technique, or about 40 e.p.g geometric mean. (Data show that the arithmetic mean in high prevalence areas is about 2.7 times greater than the geometric mean). An e.p.g of 40 would

Table 13.17. *Prevalence and intensity of* S. mansoni *among children aged 5–14 and per cent of infected persons with splenomegaly in different valleys*

	Population	Prev. (%)	GM	Population examined	% with splenomegaly
Richefond South	2000	64	55	846	5.4
Richefond North	3000	61	51	896	3.7
Calypso South	2500	53	33	879	3.4
Cul de Sac	5000	49	94	989	2.9
Banse	1000	40	24	374	1.6
Marquis	3000	32	20	1250	1.0

be associated with a spleen rate of 3.5%. In the small Kenya community of 416 people, 12 were found to have splenic enlargement out of 343 infected, or 3.5%. Results from a study in Ethiopia, however, show that no cases of splenomegaly were found among nearly 300 children, although the geometric mean of their egg count was a high 259 e.p.g by Kato (Hiatt & Gebre-Medhin, 1977). If this is equivalent to about 30 e.p.g by the Bell technique, between 2 and 3% would be expected to have splenomegaly.

In St Lucia liver enlargement greater than 2.5 cm was found in 8.7% of uninfected persons and increased with intensity of infection to 25.9% among those excreting more than 400 *S. mansoni* e.p.ml (Cook *et al*; 1974). In Marquis valley 26% of 5–14-year-old infected children had palpable livers, but less than 10% of adults being treated in the first campaign had hepatomegaly. Although in Brazil liver enlargement increased with intensity of infection, it was found, overall, in 68% of those infected; this may have been related to heavy intensities of infection but it was found in 61% and 48% of uninfected children and adults respectively.

Hepatomegaly was also common in the Ethiopian children studied. In the uninfected, 28% had left lobe liver enlargement greater than 2 cm, as did 41% with egg excretion levels greater than 500 e.p.g. Data from the Machakos area of Kenya are similar, though results are given for the examination of all age groups. Amongst the uninfected 21% had palpable livers, and overall 44% of those infected had enlargement greater than 3 cm.

In relation to the intensity of infection in St Lucia, hepatosplenomegaly was found to occur as frequently as in Brazil and more frequently than in Kenya and Ethiopia. Liver enlargement in St Lucia did not appear to be as common as in Brazil or Africa, where it was frequently found in the uninfected. Whatever the aetiology of this hepatomegaly, it does not appear to predispose to schistosomal hepatosplenomegaly in Africa.

Longevity of adult worms

Although there are reports in the literature of emigrés found infected with *S. mansoni* many years after leaving endemic areas (Chartes *et al.*, 1969; Little, 1972), these tend to establish extreme limits of longevity of 20 to 30 years rather than the mean or average life-span. Attempts have been made to calculate this indirectly from schistosome egg excretion data obtained during different epidemiological investigations (Hairston, 1965; Warren *et al.*, 1974). Using decreasing egg count data from individuals in Grande Ravine (Richefond south) and Cul de Sac valley after the introduction of control measures, in hosts 10 years of age and older a mean life span of 3.3 years for adult worms was calculated. Results for younger persons were inconclusive, but it was suspected that the mean life-spans are greater (Goddard & Jordan, 1980).

These results are not unlike those obtained by other workers and provide evidence that the worm's life-span is much less than the extremes recorded in the literature. Nevertheless, with an exponential survival and mean life-span of 3.3 years some individuals will harbour a few worms that survive 20 to 30 years.

14

Immunological studies

Dr Daniel G Colley

Significant strides have been made in the last two decades in the understanding of the immunology of schistosomiasis (Smithers & Terry, 1976; Phillips & Colley, 1978). In experimental systems there is now a good conception of the basis of egg-focused pathogenesis (Warren, 1972) and its immunoregulation (Colley, 1981; Damian, 1984), and insights into the development of fibrosis are being made (Wyler, 1983). Also, while a vaccine practical for use in man has not yet been developed, experimental systems studying both concomitant and artificially produced immunity to challenge infection now allow studies regarding protective immune mechanisms (James, Sher, Lazdins & Meltzer, 1982; Sher, Heiny, James & Asofsky, 1982; Damian, 1984). Concurrent investigations in antigen purification, immunodiagnostic developments, monoclonal antibody production and molecular genetics related to schistosomes now contribute to the hope of future gains that will aid in diagnosis, evaluation, and immunisation related to this infection (Colley, 1983; Hillyer, 1979; Cordingley, Taylor, Dunne & Butterworth, 1984). Studies of the human immune responses during schistosomiasis, and following curative chemotherapy, have begun to define the range of host responses that develop, and their regulation during the establishment and maintenance of chronic conditions (Colley, 1981; Ottesen, 1982).

Studies on the immunology of schistosomiasis that were conducted at the Research and Control Department span a period of more than 14 years and are the collaborative efforts of multiple investigators. Consequently, they reflect the varied interests of these researchers, and the rapidly changing developments that have occurred during this period in the field of immunology. The three major areas of investigation represented in these studies are immune protection, immunodiagnosis and immune responses and their regulation that occur during schistosomiasis. This chapter is intended to review the Research and Control studies that are related to each of these areas, and discuss them in relationship to the work of other groups that have investigated similar aspects of the overall subject of the immunology of schistosome infections.

Immune protection

A variety of experimental animal models have provided evidence that the mammalian host is capable of mounting significant, partially protective immune responses against challenge infections by schistosome cercariae (Smithers & Terry, 1976; Phillips & Colley, 1978; Dean, 1983; Damian, 1984). However, although epidemiologic data, such as age-prevalence curves, suggest that schistosome-infected human patients also develop similar immunity, direct evidence in support of this conclusion is not available (Warren, 1973). Three early studies at Research and Control attempted to provide such definitive evidence. In the first (Warren, Cook & Jordan, 1972), a gamma globulin fraction was obtained from the plasma of 45 adult *S. mansoni* infected patients. This preparation was termed 'anti-*S. mansoni* gamma globulin', or 'immune' gamma globulin. A similar preparation was obtained from plasma from uninfected subjects (control gamma globulin). Six pairs of children, between the ages of 3 and 7 years, were matched in regard to their age, sex and faecal output of *S. mansoni* eggs. One of each of the pair then received three consecutive daily doses of either 'immune' or 'control' gamma globulin, totalling 100 mg protein/kg body weight. Prior to, and two weeks following these transfers, the patients were studied by immediate and delayed intradermal tests against *S. mansoni* adult worm antigens. Anti-cercarial circulating antibody titres were determined in the sera of the children by immunofluoresence, before and one week after the transfers. Faecal egg counts were obtained frequently from these patients, and all recipients were treated with hycanthone, between two and three weeks after the gamma globulin transfers.

This study thus sought to evaluate the effect of passive gamma globulin administration on already established *S. mansoni* infections in children. It was seen that those pair members that received the 'immune' globulin increased their immediate anti-adult worm skin test reactivity, and to some degree their anti-cercarial fluorescent antibody titres. As expected, transfer of control or 'immune' globulin did not alter delayed skin test reactivity. Neither did it have any effect on faecal egg output. It seems clear that the transfer of what amounts to additional anti-schistosomal serum globulins to young patients with existing infections and normal immune reactivities had no demonstrable adverse effect on the fecundity of their adult schistosome populations.

A transfer study was also done to evaluate the prophylactic capacity of similar control and 'immune' gamma globulin preparations (Cook, Warren & Jordan, 1972). Recipients were uninfected, but naturally exposed children followed over a year. In this case, 50 young children (mean age of 2 years) were matched by age and placed randomly into two groups. At the beginning of the study, all were stool negative for *S. mansoni*, but both groups were infected to similar extents with intestinal helminths (hookworm, *Ascaris* and *Trichuris*). Initially, and at three month intervals thereafter, each child received a total dose of 108 mg gamma globulin per kg body weight. Stools were collected in hospital at given intervals. At one year after the beginning of the study it was observed that 10 children in each of the groups of 25 had become stool positive for *S. mansoni* eggs, giving an equal incidence of 40%. The mean output of eggs/ml of faeces from those children that became infected did not differ significantly between the control or 'immune' globulin groups. This study indicated that protective immunity, if it existed in the infected donor patients, was not transferable by humoral components using this protocol, in this setting.

Considering the possibility that protective immunity might depend, either in part or entirely, on cell-mediated immune mechanisms, a study was also done to assess the effect of transfer factor from sensitised donors on early infections in children (Warren, Cook, David & Jordan, 1975).

Dialysed transfer factor was carefully prepared from the leucocytes of chronic, non-hepatosplenic schistosomiasis patients who exhibited large intradermal delayed skin reactions to adult worm extracts. it was administered to six children with mild *S. mansoni* infections and six uninfected parallel subjects. Unfortunately, only one child in each group exhibited evidence (by delayed skin tests) that the transfer had been effective. Three of the treated and one of the control group demonstrated positive reactivity of their peripheral blood mononuclear cells (PBMN) in *in vitro* cultures stimulated with *S. mansoni* adult worm antigens. There was no observable effect of treatment with transfer factor on the faecal egg output of any of the infected transfer recipients. In the light of the difficulty in demonstrating positive transfers, it remains unclear whether augmented cell-mediated reactivity against schistosomes would affect the fecundity of established adult worms.

In sum, these transfer studies provided no evidence that protective immunity against schistosomes develops in infected patients. While lacking such direct evidence, several *in vitro* schistosomular-killing assays have been developed using human antibodies and/or peripheral blood cells as possible candidate correlates of resistance in this infection (Phillips & Colley, 1978; Colley, 1981). One of these, an eosinophil-mediated, antibody-dependent system, was evaluated using plasma from St Lucian patients in relation to the duration and intensity of their infections (Sher *et al.*, 1977). Quantitatively, the cytotoxicity-mediating antibody activity correlated significantly with the intensity of *S. mansoni* infection (faecal egg count). It was also directly correlative with the PBMN blastogenic responsiveness of the patients' cells to crude saline antigenic preparations obtained from *S. mansoni* eggs (SEA), adult worms (SWAP), and cercariae (CAP). There was no correlation observed between the duration of known *S. mansoni* infection and the levels of this antibody in patient's plasma. Because the epidemiological evidence for immunity indicates that it might develop slowly, and be expressed in relationship to the duration of infection, this last observation could be interpreted as indicating a lack of correlation between this *in vitro* assay and protection. It remains conjectural as to how any of the schistosomulae-killing assays relate to the state of immunity of the donor patient. Such studies have, however, begun to contribute considerably to an insight into new potential effector mechanisms available to the host in response to multicellular parasites (Butterworth *et al.*, 1982; Capron, Dessaint, Haque & Capron, 1982; Ellner & Mahmoud, 1982).

Immunodiagnosis

The immunodiagnosis of schistosomiasis has been evaluated by a wide variety of methodologies ranging from antibody detection (including different isotypes and specificities) (Kagan & Pellegrino, 1961; Nash, 1982), antigen demonstration (Carlier, Nzeyimana, Bout & Capron, 1980; Carlier *et al.*, 1975), and immediate, Arthus-type and cell-mediated intradermal skin tests (Warren *et al.*, 1973a; Moriearty & Lewert, 1974; Camus *et al.*, 1977). Studies at Research and Control contributed to several different aspects of the development and evaluation of immunodiagnostic procedures.

In an experimental animal study it was demonstrated that it was theoretically possible that the occasional, apparently false, positive reactions obtained using the anti-cercarial fluorescent antibody assay might be attributable to single sex infections (Sturrock & Woodstock, 1973). Groups of mice infected with cercariae of either one or both sexes were seen to develop anti-cercarial antibodies detectable by indirect immunofluorescence at equivalent rates, and to similar degrees. It was postulated that single sex infections in humans, that would be undiagnosed by faecal examination, could account for positive immunofluorescent assays using the sera of stool negative persons for endemic areas.

In an extensive serological study using the sera from almost 200 St Lucians and 200 St Vincentians (a topographically similar island 30 kilometres from St Lucia that has never been known to have schistosomiasis), Warren *et al.* (1973*b*) compared three assay systems (complement fixation, cholesterol–lecithin flocculation and immunofluorescence). The complement fixation assay used an adult worm antigenic extract, and the other two systems detected anti-cercarial antibodies. The complement fixation and cholesterol–lecithin flocculation assays were proved to be very insensitive, producing many false negatives with the St Lucian sera, and the former also gave unacceptable false positives with some of the St Vincentian sera. The anti-cercarial immunofluoresence test was superior to the other two assays in overall sensitivity and specificity.

Continued progress toward more sensitive and specific serological diagnostic systems was evaluated in subsequent studies of an enzyme linked immunosorbent assay (ELISA) (McLaren, Long, Goodgame & Lillywhite, 1979) and a comparison between an ELISA and a radioimmunoassay (RIA) (Long *et al.*, 1981). Using a soluble egg antigenic preparation and detecting IgG antibodies of this specificity in a peroxidase or phosphatase ELISA, it was seen that 82–99.5% sensitivity was obtained. The degree of sensitivity was directly related to the intensity of the infection as measured by the e.p.ml of stool. Furthermore, the specificity, as determined using St Vincentian control sera, was 100%. Upon repeated stool examinations of a group of apparent false positives in the St Lucian population, at least half of them proved to be infected, with very low levels of e.p.g. Another aspect of this study demonstrated that finger-prick blood samples harvested and stored on filter papers were perfectly adequate for later elution and ELISA evaluation (Long, Lawrence & Augustine, 1981). The ease, safety and decreased expense of this method of serum sampling makes it a logical choice for field epidemiological or survey work.

In a further evaluation and comparison of diagnostic assays, the ELISA, while very sensitive, was somewhat less so than an RIA using the purified SEA fraction termed MSA_1. Also, in comparison with the RIA, the ELISA was somewhat less specific. Two serological and two parasitological diagnostic assays were done on each patient, and then were analysed by the Armitage's 'J' index. The Kato thick smear faecal assay was seen to be the best (most reliable) indicator of the presence or absence of infection. Next, in order of reliability, came the RIA, the ELISA and the Bell filtration faecal examination. This study was performed using a community of 516 untreated persons and was based on a combination of parasitological and serological data, rather than any one pre-selected standard test. The results indicate the feasibility of the ELISA system, and suggest that in combination with more purified antigens this might provide a useful adjunct to stool examinations for monitoring *S. mansoni* infections (see also Chapter 3).

Studies of the intradermal reactivity of schistosomiasis patients to schistosomal antigens indicated that the immediate (IgE-mediated) response is highly sensitive (90–95%) in detecting current or past infections (Warren *et al.*, 1973*b*; Moriearty & Lewert, 1974). However, this is primarily only true in adult patient populations, being far less sensitive in children. Also, some antigens, such as an *S. mansoni* cercarial preparation, may give large numbers of false positive reactions in control populations. It was also seen that the *S. mansoni* infected patients on St Lucia responded generally very well to antigenic materials prepared from *S. japonicum* and *S. haematobium* eggs. Delayed reactions were again less reliable in younger patients. They were also less sensitive, although apparently more specific, than immediate reactions (Warren *et al.*, 1973*a,b*). There was no observable differences in the ability of adult worm antigenic preparations from four different geographic strains of *S. mansoni* to elicit positive responses. The sensitivity of the delayed reactions was not appreciably enhanced by adjusting the antigen concentration used. However, upon a repeat skin test one month after the initial testing, delayed but not immediate reactions were observed to be significantly increased.

To evaluate further the possible reasons for the lack of sensitivity of immediate and delayed schistosomal skin tests in children, anthropometric, parasitological and intradermal tests were performed in 97 5–11-year-old St Lucian children (McKay, Warren, Cook & Jordan, 1973). While marginal malnutrition was observed in this population, its presence or absence did not correlate with intradermal reactivity. It was, however, seen that there was a striking correlation between skin reactivity and the intensity of infection. Thus, for both immediate and delayed reactions to adult worm antigens, the likelihood of obtaining a positive skin test was directly related to the number of eggs per ml of faeces.

Immune responses and immunoregulation

Until the recent development of field-applicable relatively non-toxic drugs for the treatment of schistosomiasis, it was not possible to consider altering a patient's infection status for experimental purposes. Even now, with acceptable chemotherapy, the community considerations and logistics of doing so may not coincide in a reasonable manner. Therefore insight into the immune mechanisms that occur during various stages and conditions of this chronic infection has been sought by experiments involving study of the reactivity of patient materials, usually peripheral blood samples, rather than direct experimentation with the patient–host. Several groups of investigators have now persued basic immunological questions related to human schistosomiasis in this manner (Colley, 1981;

Ottesen, 1982). Through such studies it has become obvious that the uncomplicated, asymptomatic, chronic condition (intestinal schistosomiasis) and the severe, hepatosplenic state, are both complex conditions that heavily involve multiple responses and regulatory mechanisms to a wide variety of schistosomal immunogens.

In a study of general immunological parameters, Kellermeyer *et al.*, (1973) carefully documented concentrations of serum immunoglobulin isotopes in three age groups of St Lucians and St Vincentians. The St Lucian 5–9-year age group had higher levels of IgG and IgM than their St Vincentian counterpart groups, but did not differ in their IgA, IgD or IgE levels. Only the IgG and IgA levels of the St Lucian 10–14-year age group were significantly higher than the St Vincentian 10–14-year olds. The adult St Lucian group also demonstrated elevated IgG concentrations, and had a greater than five-fold higher level of IgE than the parallel St Vincentian group. The two island 10–14-year groups were also compared with an age-matched control black population from Cleveland, Ohio. In these comparisons both island groups had elevated IgM, IgD and IgE levels, while only the St Lucian group had higher levels of IgG and IgA than the Cleveland control group. Between the schistosome endemic island of St Lucia and the comparable, but non-endemic island of St Vincent, it would seem that the endemicity is consistently, at all age groups, associated with elevated IgG levels. In the younger age group higher concentrations of IgM paralleled schistosome infection, while in the adult group chronic schistosomiasis appeared to be related to very elevated levels of IgE.

Two studies were performed at Research and Control to compare directly the immunological capacities of groups of matched pairs of intestinal and hepatosplenic schistosomal patients. In the first, (Cook, Woodstock & Jordan, 1972), seven pairs of patients (one pair partner having intestinal and the other hepatosplenic disease) matched for age, sex and faecal egg counts were seen to be comparable in their IgM and IgA serum concentrations, their anti-cercarial fluorescent antibody titres, and their skin test reactivities (both immediate and delayed) to an adult worm extract. Their abilities to develop a cell-mediated immune response to the contact sensitiser dinitrochlorobenzene were also equal. The only significant difference in any of the parameters compared, and it was minimally so, was that the intestinal partners of each pair generally had higher total serum concentrations of IgG.

In a later study (Goodgame *et al.*, 1978), 24 similarly matched pairs were examined in regard to several other humoral immune capacities. The assays evaluated the patients' sera for anti-MSA$_1$ RIA activity, anti-egg and anti-worm extract ELISAs for total and IgM antibodies, and their abilities to suppress schistosome antigen-induced PBMN blastogenesis in *in vitro* culture (Colley, Hieny, Bartholomew & Cook, 1977b). No difference was found, using any of these criteria, between the patients with intestinal or hepatosplenic disease.

These studies did not find any obvious serological difference between patients presenting with these differing clinical conditions. However, subsequent studies in other endemic areas have demonstrated certain abnormalities, primarily in cell-mediated reactivities, as assessed by PBMN and spleen cell responses. In Egypt, splenic adherent cells (Reiner *et al.*, 1979) and non-adherent T-lymphocytes (Ellner *et al.*, 1980) obtained from surgically removed spleens from hepatosplenic patients have been observed to non-specifically suppress mitogen- and schistosomal antigen-induced blastogenesis. In Brazil (Colley *et al.*, 1983), phenotyping of PBMN from hepatosplenic patients demonstrated a decreased T4 + :T84 + ratio that was due to a decreased number of cells of the T4 + (mainly 'helper') phenotype. This lower ratio correlated with less responsiveness to the worm extract SWAP in blastogenesis assays. Parallel examinations of PBMN from intestinal patients did not reveal any alterations in lymphocyte phenotypes. Even within the hepatosplenic population, however, considerable hetero-geneity of SWAP-induced responsiveness exists and in some cases correlates with the intensity of infection (Ellner *et al.*, 1981).

In the 1970s, the Research and Control Department was a unique environment for cellular immunologists interested in human schistosomi-asis. The relative contiguous nature of the experimental laboratory bench and the schistosomal patient population in an endemic, well documented field setting provided the opportunity to ask a variety of questions related to the basic immune response capabilities of patients. The work was based on *in vitro* studies of patients' PBMN responses when exposed to the three crude, saline soluble, antigenic preparations mentioned previously, (SEA, SWAP or CAP), or the unrelated antigenic material *Candida albicans* extract, or the mitogen phytohaemaglutinin P (PHA). Optimal antigen concentra-tions and the general culture conditions were established and standardised (Colley *et al.*, 1977a). Normal human serum was used as the medium supplement, and good general cellular responsiveness was observed with patients' PBMN. It was seen that when a chronic patient's mean intensity of infection (individual means of the study population were from 40–210 e.p.ml of faeces for the previous three years) was compared with his or her PBMN reactivity to SEA, SWAP or CAP, there was no relationship between the two parameters. It must, however, be made clear that the levels of intensity observed in the St Lucian patient population studied were low to moderate in comparison with some later studies that observed an inverse relationship in these parameters (Ellner *et al.*, 1981). Perhaps the major surprise in the early St Lucia standardisation data concerned patient PBMN responsiveness to the schistosomal extracts in relationship to the known longevity of their schistosome infections. In most chronic patients it was observed that the SEA response was minimal, but that in earlier infections SEA responses were often quite high. These observations thus resembled the condition described in *S. mansoni* infected mice, termed modulation, wherein responsiveness to eggs or SEA waxes early in infection, attaining a peak at about 8 weeks, and wanes to a minimal level that is then maintained throughout chronic infections (Andrade & Warren, 1964; Domingo & Warren, 1968; Colley, 1975). In contrast to SEA, patient PBMN responses to SWAP, and to some degree CAP appeared to increase during early infections and attain even higher levels at later times. These data are in general agreement with those of others (Ottesen, 1979; Rocklin *et al.*, 1980).

As described above, PBMN from chronic patients generally respond much better to SWAP and CAP than to SEA. In addition, it soon became apparent that if the cultures were supplemented with serum from the patient (autologous) or from other chronic patients (heterologous), the responses to all three of these schistosomal preparations were considerably reduced when compared with parallel cultures in medium supplemented with serum from uninfected individuals. This particular form of serosup-

Fig.14.1. Individual patient (infected with *S. mansoni* for more than 8 years) lymphocyte transformation capabilities in homologous-normal (striped bars), or autologous (open bars) serum-supplemented media. Data presented as counts per minute and the per cent change and direction of change caused in autologous serum supplemented medium *vs.* homologous-normal serum is indicated for each condition. (From Colley *et al.*, 1977a.)

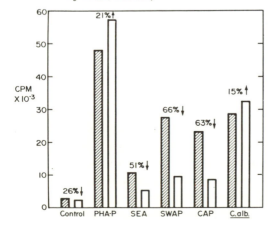

pression did not affect either PHA responsiveness or that to the unrelated antigenic preparation from *C. albicans* (Colley *et al.*, 1977*b*; Ottesen & Poindexter, 1980) (Fig. 14.1). This regulatory phenomenon develops during the early months and years of infection and is maintained throughout chronicity. Approximately 75% of all chronic patients clearly express this regulation, which, in retrospective analysis, requires the presence of undetermined factors in the serum and the co-existence of appropriate (suppressible) cells in the PBMN population (Todd, Goodgame & Colley, 1980). This observation allowed the categorisation of patients based on the presence or absence of these components (suppressive serum and suppressible cells, 75% having both), but the categories thus established do not yet relate to any given clinical conditions. The mechanisms underlying serosuppression are still unclear. They have been attributed in part to antibody and antigen/antibody complexes in the patients' sera (Rocklin *et al.*, 1980). In some situations (Cottrell, Humber & Sturrock, 1980), especially in hepatosplenic disease (Kamel & Higashi, 1982), non-specific suppression of some responses can also be mediated by patient sera.

Studies regarding cellular suppressor mechanisms in cultured PBMN from chronically infected patients demonstrated that 88% (15 of 17) of such individuals on St Lucia had cells (presumably T-lymphocytes) that could be stimulated by concanavalin A to express suppressor activity against autologous PBMN responding in a separate culture to PHA (Colley, Lewis & Goodgame, 1978). When the schistosomal antigenic preparations, SEA and SWAP, were substituted for concanavalin A in the stimulation culture, the percentage of patients that developed PHA response-suppressive activity was 36% (8 of 22) and 39% (9 of 23), respectively. The generation of non-specific suppressor cells by specific schistosomal antigenic materials indicates the potential, at least in some patients, to mount powerful immunoregulatory responses upon stimulation. The ability of a given patient to do so was not correlated with clinical condition, but was possibly associated with the duration of infection, in that it increased in the second decade of life. These antigen-induced suppressor cells appeared to be better induced in the presence of suppressive serum. Also seen clearly in this study, and another (Colley, Todd, Lewis & Goodgame, 1979), was the observation that in the St Lucian patient population the PHA responsiveness was entirely normal (Fig. 14.2). Subsequently, it has been shown that antigen-specific suppression can be induced by SEA, or a protein fraction of SEA, acting on T-lymphocytes (Rocklin, Tracy & El Kholy, 1981). In this study, a partially purified glycoprotein fraction of SEA was also capable of inducing a non-specific suppressor mechanism.

The SEA or CAP induction of non-specific suppressor activity, as expressed in PHA cultures, was seen using the PBMN from a variety of subjects on St Lucia (Colley *et al.*, 1979). In these studies the antigenic materials were added to cultures of PBMN exposed simultaneously to concentration curves of PHA (Fig. 14.3). Although the SEA or CAP were not toxic to the cultures, they could, at appropriate concentrations, suppress PHA responsiveness of PBMN from early, chronic treated or schistosome-normal individuals. Therefore, in addition to the early studies of antigen-specific stimulation of suppressors (Colley *et al.*, 1978), these investigations demonstrate a further ability of some schistosomal preparations to cause non-specific suppression by unsensitized PBMN. This activity required T-lymphocyte involvement and affected the early portion of the PHA response. It required rather high concentrations of SEA or CAP, but it might be possible that such amounts of these materials accumulate locally in the microenvironments surrounding impacted eggs or penetrating cercariae.

Another schistosome antigen-specific immunoregulatory mechanism that occurs in the PBMN of a majority of schistosome patients is mediated by cells that are adherent to either plastic (Todd, Goodgame, Colley & Lewis, 1979) or nylon wool (Ottesen, 1979). St Lucian studies of this mode of regulation demonstrated that greater than 80% of chronic patients express

Fig.14.2. Incorporation of ^{3}H-TdR in response to optimum concentrations of PHA by peripheral blood mononuclear cells from either uninfected subjects (Controls) or chronically infected patients (< 4 yr) (Chronics) in either (*a*) tube cultures (10, 16), or (*b*) microtitre well cultures. Data given as mean ±SEM c.p.m. Each mean was derived from the number of subjects depicted in parentheses below each bar. (From Colley *et al.*, 1979.)

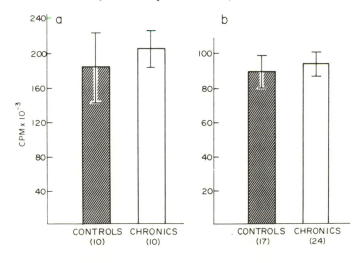

this suppression, but it was not found in transiently infected or treated patients, or in uninfected control subjects Table 14.1). With chronic patients' PBMN, removal of adherent cells (likely to be monocytes) greatly augmented the response of the remaining cells to either SWAP or CAP, but not to SEA, PHA or *C. albicans* extract. These augmented responses were not just increases in tritiated thymidine uptake, but actually represented greater blastogenesis of the lymphoid population, as observed morpholog-

Fig.14.3. Incorporation of ³H-TdR, in response to PHA concentration gradient, of two individual patient's cells (A: chronic infection; B: early infection) in the presence of PHA alone (○——○), or PHA and 50 µg/ml SEA (■---■). (From Colley *et al.*, 1979.)

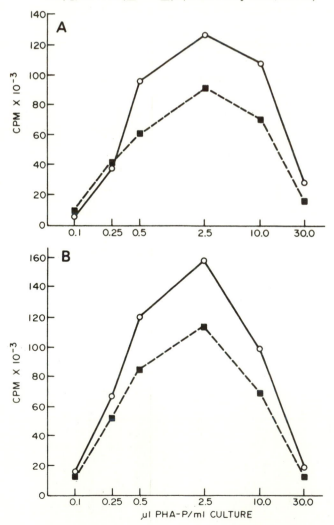

Table 14.1. *Effect of adherent/phagocytic cell removal on antigen-induced responsiveness of lymphocyte cultures*

Patient groups	Cell populations	Antigens			
		SWAP	CAP	SEA	C. albicans
Chronic infections (24)[a]	Unseparated	21208±3160[b]	14324±2320	10642±3405	18720±3065[c]
	NA/NP[d]	37632±5740**	29940±4350**	9234±3437	18752±4420
Treated patient (3)	Unseparated	18835±6966	15096±5910	36181±20418	5700±395
	NA/NP	29256±13593	17363±7892	27661±14973	4884±1713
Transient infections (3)	Unseparated	8164±3265	7792±1704	9544±2408	17681±9065
	NA/NP	4521±2274	4042±878	3843±1512*	6778±1324
Uninfected controls (4)	Unseparated	3981±1624	4079±1957	3448±1008.	12357±5400
	NA/NP	920±366	2009±903	568±241	4734±1517

[a] Numbers in parentheses indicate number of subjects contributing to each mean.
[b] Mean c.p.m. ^{3}H-TdR incorporation ± SEM. Group data were analysed by individual paired Student's *t*-tests. Means noted by asterisks indicate significant differences between NA/NP and unseparated response (*, $P < 0.05$; **, $P < 0.2$).
[c] Only 18 patients tested.
[d] NA: None adherent; NP: none phagocytic.
From Todd *et al.*, 1979.

ically. Furthermore, in Ottesen's parallel study of this regulatory phenomenon the re-addition of esterase-positive, phagocytic, mononuclear cells (monocytes/macrophages) reasserted control over antigen-induced responses of the non-adherent, responsive cell populations (Ottesen, 1979). Subsequent studies of the possible mechanistic basis of adherent cell (macrophage/monocyte) mediated suppression have investigated the potential role of prostaglandins (Barsoum *et al.*, 1983). It appears that some 30% of those patients examined for PBMN reactivity in the presence *versus* absence of indomethacin (a prostaglandin synthetase inhibitor) demonstrated elevated PBMN responses. In a very limited portion of this study, it seemed that in one of 4 patients the reversal of regulation by indomethacin was lost if adherent cells were first removed. It would seem that in some patients the adherent suppressor cell activity might be explained by a prostaglandin-mediated regulation. However, in the majority of the cases this mechanism is not sufficient to account for the suppression, nor does it explain the antigen-specificity of the regulation. Although their actual mode of suppression remains largely unknown, adherent suppressor cells remain one of the most universally observed regulatory phenomena when studying the PBMN of chronic intestinal patients (Todd *et al.*, 1979; Ottesen, 1979).

In an interesting study of the basic immunology of endemic schistosomiasis, Lees & Jordan (1968) performed serological analyses by anti-adult slide flocculation on the cord sera from 100 St Lucian infants and their mothers. A subgroup of 19 pairs was also examined by anti-cercarial immunofluoresence. Thirty-three of the 100 pairs of sera were positive. Twenty-nine seropositive mothers had seronegative infants, but no seronegative mothers had seropositive infants. Thirty-one seropositive infants were tested monthly for antibodies. At from 1 to 6 months after birth the positive:total ratios were 31:31, 31:31, 15:31, 7:31, 2:31 and 0:31 respectively. These data clearly indicate the transplacental transfer of maternal antibody to a relatively high percentage of their children. Furthermore, the decay rates of that maternal antibody demonstrate a period during which the child loses maternal 'coverage', but has not yet been stimulated to develop its own humoral responsiveness. This could have consequences in regard to early cercarial exposures and protection, but this is clearly conjectural. Perhaps even more importantly (but even more speculative), it is possible that such *in utero* exposure to maternal idiotypes of schistosome specificity (Wikler, Demeur, Dewasme & Urbaine, 1980; Kresina & Nasinoff, 1983) might well influence the subsequent anti-schistosomal repertoire expressed by the child upon subsequent exposure at challenge and during the development of chronic infection. The

St Lucian study and several others (Carlier *et al.*, 1975; Sontoro *et al.*, 1977; Hillyer, Menedwy-Corrada, Lluberes & Hernandez-Morales, 1970) clearly demonstrate the occurrence of transplacental and breast milk transfer of antigens and antibodies related to schistosomes, from mother to child, and that sensitisation of the child can arise from such exposure (Camus *et al.*, 1976; Tachon & Borojevic, 1978). However, the potentially central nature of such influences on their later immune response capabilities of endemic populations has not been adequately pursued.

The immunological studies of schistosomiasis performed on St Lucia have addressed a wide variety of questions relevant to the areas of protection, immunodiagnosis and immune responsiveness and its regulation. The question of human resistance to invading schistosomes remains a focus of current interest, and it may well be that the advent of field-applicable, acceptable chemotherapy will soon allow more direct approaches to this important point. Once defined, the question of the mechanisms responsible for human resistance and their potential manipulation in regard to vaccine development remains for the future. Immunodiagnostic tools are continuing to be developed in regard to both the technology and the purification of the antigens that are available (Colley, 1983). It can be envisioned that the development and use of the molecular genetics of schistosomes, now underway in at least a dozen laboratories, will contribute considerably to the production of diagnostically useful antigens. The broad patterns of immune responses and immunoregulatory mechanisms that have emerged from basic studies of human responses during schistosomiasis indicate that the majority of chronic, intestinal patients respond and immunoregulate their responses very effectively. Such interactions are presumably essential for the development and maintenance of the generally balanced host-parasite relationship characteristic of a successful chronic parasitic infection. The challenge of defining, understanding and hopefully manipulating the more aberrant situations that occur in hepatosplenic patients remains ahead.

Appendices

APPENDIX 1

Sedimentation concentration stool examination technique

(1) Add an estimated 5 g of stool to 100 ml formal glycerol solution*
    in a urine sedimentation glass and emulsify with a glass rod.
(2) Sieve through copper-wire gauze (mesh 15/cm) into a second
    sedimentation glass.
(3) Add formal glycerol to about 3 cm below top and allow to
    sediment for a minimum of 20 minutes at room temperature.
(4) Pour off supernatant to leave approximately 25–30 ml of fluid
    containing sedimented deposit.
(5) Re-suspend in formal glycerol and sediment for 20 minutes.
(6) Gently pour off supernatant to leave approximately 15–20 ml of
    suspended deposit.
(7) Use a straw (cheap, disposable and hygienic) to transfer about
    0.1 ml of deposit to each of 3 microscope slides and cover each
    with a plastic coverslip 20 mm × 50 mm.
(8) Examine all 3 slides and record all helminth eggs observed.

* Formal glycerol solution: 5 ml formaldehyde; 10 ml glycerol; 985 ml water.

APPENDIX 2

Balanced incomplete block design for studying water contact at 15 major sites in Richefond valley (south)

		Sun.	Mon.	Tues.	Wed.	Thurs.	Fri.	Sat.
Month	1	L	I	C	M	H	J	A
	2	K	H	B	L	G	I	O
	3	O	L	F	A	K	M	D
	4	G	D	M	H	C	E	K
	5	C	O	I	D	N	A	G
	6	F	C	L	G	B	D	J
	7	E	B	K	F	A	C	I
	8	N	K	E	O	J	L	C
	9	H	E	N	I	D	F	L
	10	A	M	G	B	L	N	E
	11	M	J	D	N	I	K	B
	12	J	G	A	K	F	H	N
	13	B	N	H	C	M	O	F
	14	I	F	O	J	E	G	M
	15	D	A	J	E	O	B	H

APPENDIX 3

Snails identified in various collections from different parts of the island

In 1966 and 1967 qualitative snail surveys were made in the Cul de Sac, Richefond, Roseau and Marquis valleys. Specimens were preserved and sent to various authorities for identification, including Dr E. Malek, Dr Mandahl-Barth, Dr W. J. Clench and Dr L. Paraense.

Aquatic snails

Operculates:

Potamopyrgus coronatus (Pfeiffer)
Pomacea glaucus (Linn.)
Neritina virginea Linn.
Neritina punctulata Lam.
Neritilia succinea (Recluz)

Pulmonates:

Biomphalaria glabrata (Say)
Drepanotrama surinamensis (Clessin)
Lymnaea cubensis (Pfeiffer)
Physa marmorata Guilding
Ferrissea radiata Guilding

Bivalves:

Psidium punctiferum (Guppy)

Terrestrial snails

Pulmonates:

Succinea approximans Shuttleworth
Pleurodonte orbiculata Férrussac
Bulimulus pilosus (Guppy)

Bulimulus exilis (Gmélin)
Diaphora bicolor (Hutton)
Subulina octona (Brugière)
Brachypodella tatei (Crosse & Bland)
Omalonyx unguis (Férrussac)
Veronicella occidentalis (Guilding)

In 1976, in order to confirm that there had been no introduction of other *Biomphalaria* spp., specimens from River Doree (Saltibus), Ravine Beranger (Banse), Sallée River (Desruisseau) and from Cul de Sac and Canaries valleys and Fond St Jacques were sent to Dr L. Paraense. All specimens were identified as *B. glabrata*.

APPENDIX 4

Post-mortem results of St Lucian wild animal helminth survey

Host species	No. exam.	Parasites found	Location in host	No. infected
Mongoose (*Herpestes auropunctatus*)	26	**Nematoda:**		
		Capillaria spp.	Stomach	10
		Spirurid	Stomach	1
		Unidentified	Kidney	6
Brown rat (*Rattus rattus*)	24	**Cestoda:**		
		Taenia taeniaformis	Liver	3 +
		Hymenolepis diminuata	Small intestine	1
		Nematoda:		
		Aspicularis tetraptera	Large intestine	4
		Nippostrongylus braziliensis	Small intestine	4
		Ascarid	Stomach	4 +
House mouse (*Mus musculis*)	3	**Nematoda:**		
		A. tetraptera	Large intestine	—
		N. braziliensis	Small intestine	—
		Capillaria hepatica	Liver	—
Opossum (Manicou) (*Didelphis marsupialis insularis*)	1	**Nematoda:**		
		Spirurid	Stomach	1
		Oxyurid	Large intestine	1
		Unknown	Mesenteric blood vessels	1
Domestic cat (*Felis domesticus*)	1	**Cestoda:**		
		T. taeniaformis	Intestine	1
		Nematoda:		
		Ancylostoma caninum	Intestine	1
		Toxacara cati	Intestine	1
		Trematoda:		
		Platynosomum fastosum	Bile duct	1

Host species	No. exam.	Parasites found	Location in host	No. infected
Little blue heron (*Florida caerula*)	8	**Nematoda:**		
		Tetrameres spp.	Proventriculus	2
		Unidentified	Proventriculus	1
		Trematoda:		
		Ribieroia marini	Proventriculus	3
		Clinostomum spp.	Mouth	1
		Amphistome	Bursa	2
		Echinostome	Intestine	5
		Holostome	Intestine	1
		Strigeid	Intestine	2
Green heron (*Butorides viricens*)	6	**Cestoda:**		
		Unidentified 1	Intestine	4
		Unidentified 2	Intestine	1
		Nematoda:		
		Contracaecum spp.	Proventriculus	2
		Spirurid	Proventriculus	1
		Trematoda:		
		Amphimerus anatus	Bile duct	1
		Distome	Bursa	1
		Echinostome	Intestine	5
		Holostome	Intestine	3
		Strigeid	Intestine	3
Lesser Antilles Grackle (*Quiscalus lugubris*)	6	**Acanthocephala:**		
		Unidentified	Intestine	—
		Cestoda:		
		Unindentified	Intestine	—
		Nematoda:		
		Unidentified 1	Orbit	—
		Unidentified 2	Kidney	—
		Unidentified 3	Proventriculus	—
		Trematoda:		
		Unidentified 1	Kidney	—
		Unidentified 2	Bursa	—
Least sandpiper (*Calidus manutilla*)	2	**Cestoda:**		
		Unidentified	Intestine	—
Lesser Yellow Legs (*Totanus flavipes*)	1	**Cestoda:**		
		Unidentified	—	—
		Trematoda:		
		Unidentified	—	—

Host species	No. exam.	Parasites found	Location in host	No. infected
Semipalmated sandpiper (*Ereunetes pusillus*)	1	**Cestoda:** Unidentified	—	—
		Trematoda: Unidentified	—	—
Sandwich Tern (*Thalasseus sandvicensis*)	1	**Nematoda:** Unidentified 1	Lung	—
		Unidentified 2	Stomach	—
		Trematoda: Unidentified 1	Intestine	—
		Unidentified 2	Intestine	—
		Unidentified 3	Lung	—
Common Ground Dove (*Columbigallina passerina*)	1	Nil		

APPENDIX 5

Identification of freshwater fish killed by molluscicide

Order	Family	Genus and species	Common name English	Patois
Anguilliformes	Anguillidae	*Anguilla rostrata*	Eel	Zanji blanc
Atheriniformes	Poeciliidae	*Poecilia coucana*	Guppy	Badenmowo
		P. reticulata	Guppy	Badenmowo
Perciformes	Carangidae	?		Cavawy
	Cichlidae	*Tilapia mossambica*	Tilapia	Acansin
	Eliotridae	*Dormitator maculatus*	—	Jamawe
		Gobiomorus dormitor	—	Zadomé
		Eliotris pisonis	—	Toma
	Gobiesocidae	?	Clingfish	Téta
	Gobiidae	*Awaous tajasica*	Goby	Loash
		Evorthodus lyricus	Goby	Loash
		Gobionellus sp.	Goby	Si si sals
		Sycidium spp.	Goby	Si si sals
	Mugilidae	*Agonostomus monticola*	Mullet	Millet, Como
		Mugil spp.	Mullet	'Blanche'
Synbranchiformes	Synbranchidae	*Synbranchus marmoratus*	Brown eel	Zanji noire
Syngnathiformes	Syngnathidae	*Syngnathus* sp.	Pipefish	Soufflet

APPENDIX 6

Details of design of latrines used in the Calypso north area

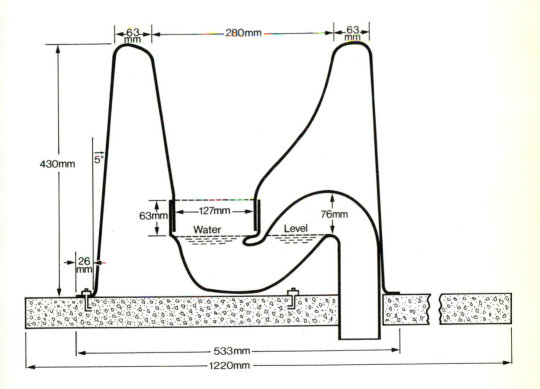

APPENDIX 7

Manufacture of molluscicidal granules

Gelatine granules GB/H 33% active ingredient

Materials:	Gelatin	120 g
	'Bayluscide'	120 g
	Water	1 litre

Method: Dissolve the gelatin in warm water. Cool to 25 °C (to thicken the gelatin and discourage settling), stir in 'Bayluscide' wettable powder and pour on to a plastic sheet. Allow to air dry to hardness, break into pieces and immerse in 5% formalin for one hour. Re-dry, and when brittle grind into granules in a hand-operated coffee mill; sieve for size. Any powder can be used again.

Sand Granules SG 5% active ingredient

Materials:	Sieved sand (1–2 mm diameter particles)	1000 g
	'Bayluscide'	75 g
	5% solution of PVA adhesive	100 ml

(e.g. Evostik Resin 'W', Weldbond or Elmers Glue-all)

Method: Mix the 'Bayluscide' and adhesive solution into a paste. Add sand and continue mixing until all grains are wetted and a uniform colour. Spread on a plastic sheet to dry in the shade. Break up any accretions and sieve.

From Prentice & Barnish, 1980.

REFERENCES

Abdallah, A. (1973). A resumé of some pilot control projects carried out in Egypt in the past 20 years. *Journal of the Egyptian Public Health Association*, **48**, 290–307.

Abdallah, A. & Nasr, T. (1973). *Helisoma H. duryi* as a means of biological control of schistosomiasis vector snails. *Journal of the Egyptian Medical Association*, **56**, 514–20.

Abdel-Wahab, M. F., Strickland, G. T., El-Sahly, A., Ahmed, L., Zakaria, S., El Kady, N. & Mahmoud, S. (1980). Schistosomiasis mansoni in an Egyptian village in the Nile Delta. *American Journal of Tropical Medicine and Hygiene*, **29**, 868–74.

Adams, R. & Rogers, E. F. (1939). The structure of monocrotaline, alkaloid in *Crotalaria spectabilis* and *Crotalaria retusa*. *Journal of the American Chemical Society*, **63**, 2815–9.

Alves, W. (1946). The public health cure of bilharziasis with one-day course of antimony. *South African Medical Journal*, **20**, 146–7.

Amin, M. A., Fenwick, A., Teesdale, C. H., McLaren, M., Marshall, T. F. & Vaughan, J. P. (1982). The assessment of a large scale snail control programme over a three-year period in the Gezira irrigated area of the Sudan. *Annals of Tropical Medicine and Parasitology*, **76**, 415–24.

Andrade, Z. A., Santos, H. A., Borojevic, R. & Grimaud, J. A. (1974). Lesoes hepáticas produzidas por hycanthone (Etrenol). *Revista do Instituto de Medicina Tropical de São Paulo*, **16**, 160–70.

Andrade, Z. A. & Warren, K. S. (1964). Mild prolonged schistosomiasis in mice. Alterations in host response with time and the development of portal fibrosis. *Transactions of the Royal Society of Tropical Medicine and Hygiene*, **58**, 53–7.

Anon. (1918). *Report of Medical and Sanitary Department of St Kitts, 1918*.

Anon. (1967). *Annual Report to the Pan American Health Organisation of the Schistosomiasis Snail Identification Centre for the Americas*.

Anon. (1976). *A National Food and Nutrition Survey of St Lucia, 1974*. Kingston 7, Jamaica: Caribbean Food and Nutrition Institute.

Anon. (1982a). Ministry of Health St Lucia. *Report to Caribbean Health Ministers' Conference*, Belize.

Anon. (1982b). *World Development Report 1982*. Published for the World Bank. Oxford University Press.

Barbosa, F. S. & Costa, D. P. P. (1981). A long term schistosomiasis control project with molluscicide in a rural area of Brazil. *Annals of Tropical Medicine and Parasitology*, **75**, 41–52.

Barbosa, F. S., Pinto, R., & Souza, O. A. (1971). Control of schistosomiasis mansoni in a small north east Brazilian community. *Transactions of the Royal Society of Tropical Medicine and Hygiene*, **65**, 206–13.

Barlow, C. H. (1937). The value of canal clearance in the control of schistosomiasis in Egypt. *American Journal of Hygiene*, **27**, 327–48.

Barnish, G. (1982). Evaluation of chemotherapy in the control of *Schistosoma mansoni* in Marquis valley, Saint Lucia. II. Biological results. *American Journal of Tropical Medicine and Hygiene*, **31**, 111–15.

Barnish, G. (1984). The freshwater shrimps of Saint Lucia, West Indies (Decapoda: Natantia) *Crustaceana* **47**, 314–20.

Barnish, G., Christie, J. D. & Prentice, M. A. (1980). *Schistosoma mansoni* control in Cul de Sac Valley, Saint Lucia. I. A two-year focal surveillance–mollusciciding programme for the control of *Biomphalaria glabrata*. *Transactions of the Royal Society of Tropical Medicine and Hygiene*, **74**, 488–92.

Barnish, G., Jordan, P., Bartholomew, R. K. & Grist, E. (1982). Routine focal mollusciciding after chemotherapy to control *Schistosoma mansoni* in Cul de Sac valley, Saint Lucia. *Transactions of the Royal Society of Tropical Medicine and Hygiene*, **76**, 602–9.

Barnish, G. & Prentice, M. A. (1981). Lack of resistance of the snail *Biomphalaria glabrata* after nine years of exposure to Bayluscide. *Transactions of the Royal Society of Tropical Medicine and Hygiene*, **75**, 106–7.

Barnish, G. & Prentice, M. A. (1982). Predation of the snail *Biomphalaria glabrata* by freshwater shrimps in St Lucia, West Indies. *Annals of Tropical Medicine and Parasitology*, **76**, 117–20.

Barnish, G., Prentice, M. A. & Harris, S. (1980). *Fasciola hepatica* in St Lucia, West Indies. *British Veterinary Journal*, **136**, 299–300.

Barnish, G. & Sturrock, R. F. (1973). Aerial application of a molluscicide to a marsh. *Transactions of the Royal Society of Tropical Medicine and Hygiene*, **67**, 610.

Barsoum, I. S., Todd, C. W., Habib, M., El Alamy, M. A. & Colley, D. G. (1983). The effects of indomethacin on *in vitro* peripheral blood mononuclear cell reactivity in human schistosomiasis. *Parasite Immunology*, **5**, 441–7.

Bartholomew, R. K. & Goddard, M. (1978). Quality control in laboratory investigations on *Schistosoma mansoni* on St Lucia, West Indies: a staff assessment scheme. *Bulletin of the World Health Organisation*, **56**, 309–12.

Bartholomew, R. K. & Jordan, P. (1978). Quality control in laboratory investigations on *Schistosoma mansoni* in St Lucia, West Indies. Maintenance of artificial prevalence as a laboratory guide. *Bulletin of the World Health Organisation*, **56**, 655–6.

Bartholomew, R. K., Peters, P. A. S., & Jordan, P. (1981). Schistosomiasis in St Lucia and Kenyan communities – a comparative study using the Kato stool examination technique. *Annals of Tropical Medicine and Parasitology*, **75**, 401–5.

Basch, P. & Sturrock, R. F. (1969). Life history of *Ribeiroia marini* (Faust & Hoffman, 1934) comb. N (Trematoda: Cathaemasiidae). *Journal of Parasitology*, **55**, 1180–4.

Bell, D. R. (1963). A new method of counting *S. mansoni* eggs in faeces with special reference to therapeutic trials. *Bulletin of the World Health Organisation*, **29**, 525–30.

Berg, C. O. (1964). Snail control in trematode diseases: the possible value of sciomyzid larvae, snail killing Diptera. *Advances in Parasitology*, **2**, 259–309.

Billinghurst, J. R. (1965). The clinical features of infection with *Schistosoma mansoni* in Uganda. *East Africa Medical Journal*, **42**, 620–8.

Bina, J. C., Tavares-Neto, J., Prata, A. & Azevedo, E. S. (1978). Greater resistance of development of severe schistosomiasis in Brazilian negroes. *Human Biology*, **50**, 41–9.

Branch, S. (1922). Letter from Director of hookworm campaign to Acting Colonial Secretary, St Lucia. Rockefeller Foundation Archives.

Breen, H. H. (1844). *St Lucia: Historical, statistical and descriptive*. Republished 1970. London: Frank Cass.

Bundy, D. A. P. (1984). Caribbean schistosomiasis. *Parasitology* **89**, 377–406.

Butterworth, A. E., Taylor, D. W., Veith, M. C., Vadas, M. A., Dessein, A., Sturrock, R. F. & Wells, E. (1982). Studies on the mechanisms of immunity in human schistosomiasis. *Immunological Review*, **61**, 5–39.

Calderbank, A. & Tomlinson, T. E. (1968). The fate of paraquat in soils. *Outlook on Agriculture*, **5**, 252–7.

Cameron, T. W. M. (1928). A new definitive host of *Schistosoma mansoni*. *Journal of Helminthology*, **6**, 219–22.

Camus, D., Bina, J. C., Carlier, Y. & Santoro, R. (1977). ABO blood groups and clinical forms of schistosomiasis mansoni. *Transactions of the Royal Society of Tropical Medicine and Hygiene*, **61**, 626.

Camus, D., Carlier, Y., Bina, J. C., Borojecvic, R., Prata, A. & Capron, A. (1976). Sensitization of *Schistosoma mansoni* antigen in uninfected children born to infected mothers. *Journal of Infectious Diseases*, **134**, 405–8.

Camus, D., Carlier, Y., Capron, M., Bina, J. C., Figueredo, J. F. M., Prata, A. & Capron, A. (1977). Immunological studies in human schistosomiasis. III. Immunoglobulin levels, antibodies, and delayed hypersensitivity. *American Journal of Tropical Medicine and Hygiene*, **26**, 482–90.

Capron, A., Dessaint, J. P., Haque, A. & Capron, M. (1982). Antibody-dependent cell-mediated cytotoxicity against parasites. *Progress in Allergy*, **31**, 234–67.

Carlier, Y., Bout, D., Bina, J. C., Camus, D., Figueredo, J. F. M. & Capron, A. (1975). Immunological studies in human schistosomiasis. I. Parasitic antigen in urine. *American Journal of Tropical Medicine and Hygiene*, **24**, 949–54.

Carlier, Y., Nzeyimana, H., Bout, D. & Capron, A. (1980). Evaluation of circulating antigens by a sandwich radioimmunoassay, and of antibodies and immune complexes, in *Schistosoma mansoni*-infected African parturients and their newborn children. *American Journal of Tropical Medicine and Hygiene*, **29**, 74–81.

Chaia, G., Chaia, A. B. Q., McAullife, J., Katz, N. & Gasper, D. (1968). Coprological diagnosis of Schistosomiasis. II. Comparative study of quantitative methods. *Revista do Instituto do Medicina Tropical de São Paulo*, **10**, 349–53.

Chartes, A. D., Jackson, J. G. & Vivian, A. B. (1969). A case of severe schistosomiasis (*Schistosoma mansoni*) in Western Australia. *Medical Journal of Australia*, **2**, 299–302.

Cheever, A. W. (1968). A quantitative post-mortem study of schistosomiasis mansoni in man. *American Journal of Tropical Medicine and Hygiene*, **17**, 38–60.

Cheever, A. W. & Andrade, A. Z. (1967). Pathological lesions associated with *Schistosoma mansoni* infection in man. *Transactions of the Royal Society of Tropical Medicine and Hygiene*, **61**, 626–39.

Chernin, E. & Dunavan, C. A. (1962). The influence of host parasite dispersion upon the capacity of *S. mansoni* miracidia to infect *A. glabratus*. *American Journal of Tropical Medicine and Hygiene*, **11**, 455–71.

Christie, J. D., Edward, J., Goolaman, K., James, B. O., Simon, J., Dugat, P. S. & Treinen, R. (1981). Interactions between St Lucian *Biomphalaria glabrata* and *Helisoma duryi*, a possible competitor snail, in a semi-natural habitat. *Acta Tropica*, **38**, 395–417.

Christie, J. D. & Prentice, M. A. (1978). The relationship between numbers of *Schistosoma mansoni* daughter sporocysts and miracidia. *Annals of Tropical Medicine and Parasitology*, **72**, 197–8.

Christie, J. D., Prentice, M. A., Upatham, E. S. & Barnish, G. (1978). Laboratory and field trials of a slow-release copper molluscicide in St Lucia. *American Journal of Tropical Medicine and Hygiene*, **27**, 616–22.

Christie, J. D. & Upatham, E. S. (1977). Control of *Schistosoma mansoni* transmission by chemotherapy in St Lucia. II. Biological results. *American Journal of Tropical Medicine and Hygiene*, **26**, 894–8.

Christopherson, J. B. (1918). The successful use of antimony in bilharziasis administered as intravenous injections of antimonium tartaratium, tartar emetic. *Lancet*, **2**, 325–7.

Chu, K. Y., Vanderburg, J. A. & Klumpp, R. K. (1981). Transmission dynamics of miracidia of *Schistosoma haematobium* in the Volta Lake. *Bulletin of the World Health Organisation*, **59**, 555–60.

Clarke, V. de V., Blair, D. M. & Weber, M. C. (1969). Field trial of hycanthone (Etrenol Winthrop) in the treatment of urinary and intestinal bilharziasis. *Central African Journal of Medicine*, **15**, 1–6.

Clarke, V. de V., Shiff, C. J. & Blair, D. M. (1961). The control of snail hosts of bilharziasis and fascioliasis in Southern Rhodesia. *Bulletin of the World Health Organisation*, **25**, 549–58.

Coats, G. E., Funderbury, H. H., Lawrence, J. M. & Davis, D. E. (1966). Factors affecting persistence and inactivation of diquat and paraquat. *Weed Research*, **6**, 58–66.

Colley, D. G. (1975). Immune responses to a soluble schistosomal egg antigen preparation during chronic primary infection with *Schistosoma mansoni*. *Journal of Immunology*, **115**, 150–6.

Colley, D. G. (1981). Immune response and immunoregulation in experimental and clinical schistosomiasis. In *Parasitic Diseases. The Immunology*, ed. J. M. Mansfield, pp. 1–83. New York: Marcel Dekker.

Colley, D. G. (1983). Schistosome antigen laboratory workshop: A summary of a meeting sponsored by the Edna McConnell Clark Foundation. *Journal of Parasitology*, **69**, 45–8.

Colley, D. G., Cook, J. A., Freeman, G. L., Bartholomew, R. K. & Jordan, P. (1977*a*). Immune responses during human schistosomiasis mansoni. I. *In vitro* lymphocyte blastogenic responses to heterogeneous antigenic preparations from schistosome eggs, worms and cercariae. *International Archives of Allergy and Applied Immunology*, **53**, 420–33.

Colley, D. G., Hieny, S. E., Bartholomew, R. K. & Cook, J. A. (1977*b*). Immune responses during human schistosomiasis mansoni. III. Regulatory effect of patient sera on human lymphocyte blastogenic responses to schistosome antigen preparations. *American Journal of Tropical Medicine and Hygiene*, **26**, 917–25.

Colley, D. G., Katz, N., Rocha, R. S., Abrantes, W., da Silva, A. L. & Gazzinelli, G. (1983). Immune reponses during human schistosomiasis mansoni. IX. T-lymphocyte subset analysis by monoclonal antibodies in hepatosplenic disease. *Scandinavian Journal of Immunology*, **17**, 297–302.

Colley, D. G., Lewis, F. A. & Goodgame, R. W. (1978). Immune responses during human schistosomiasis mansoni. IV. Induction of suppressor cell activity by schistosome antigen preparations and concanavalin A. *Journal of Immunology*, **120**, 1225–32.

Colley, D. G., Todd, C. W., Lewis, F. A. & Goodgame, R. W. (1979). Immune responses during human schistosomiasis mansoni. VI. *In vitro* non-specific suppression of phytohemagglutinin responsiveness induced by exposure to certain schistosomal preparations. *Journal of Immunology*, **122**, 1447–53.

Cook, J. A., Baker, S. T., Warren, K. S. & Jordan, P. (1974). A controlled study of morbidity of schistosmiasis mansoni in St Lucian children, based on quantitative egg excretion. *American Journal of Tropical Medicine and Hygiene*, **23**, 625–33.

Cook, J. A. & Jordan, P. (1971). Clinical trial of hycanthone in schistosomiasis mansoni in St Lucia. *American Journal of Tropical Medicine and Hygiene*, **20**, 84–8.

Cook, J. A. & Jordan, P. (1976). Absence of liver toxicity in 2723 patients treated with hycanthone in St Lucia. *Annals of Tropical Medicine and Parasitology*, **70**, 109–11.

Cook, J. A., Jordan, P. & Armitage, P. (1976). Hycanthone dose-response in treatment of schistosomiasis mansoni in St Lucia. *American Journal of Tropical Medicine and Hygiene*, **25**, 602–7.

Cook, J. A., Jordan, P. & Bartholomew, R. K. (1977). Control of *Schistosoma mansoni* transmission by chemotherapy in St Lucia. I. Results in man. *American Journal of Tropical Medicine and Hygiene*, **26**, 887–93.

Cook, J. A., Jordan, P., Woodstock, L. & Pilgrim, V. (1977). A controlled trial of hycanthone and placebo in schistosomiasis mansoni in St Lucia. *Annals of Tropical Medicine and Parasitology*, **71**, 197–203.

Cook, J. A., Sturrock, R. F. & Barnish, G. (1972). An allergic reaction of a new formulation of the molluscicide clonitralide (Bayluscide). *Transactions of the Royal Society of Tropical Medicine and Hygiene*, **66**, 954–5.

Cook, J. A., Warren, K. S. & Jordan, P. (1972). Passive transfer of immunity in human schistosomiasis mansoni: Attempt to prevent infection by repeated injections of hyperimmune antischistosome gamma globulin. *Transactions of the Royal Society of Tropical Medicine and Hygiene*, **66**, 777–80.

Cook, J. A., Woodstock, L. & Jordan, P. (1972). Immunological studies in *Schistosoma mansoni* infection in St Lucia. *Annals of Tropical Medicine and Parasitology*, **66**, 369–73.

Cook, J. A., Woodstock, L. & Jordan, P. (1974). Two-year follow-up of hycanthone-treated schistosomiasis mansoni patients in St Lucia. *American Journal of Tropical Medicine and Hygiene*, **23**, 910–14.

Cordingley, J. S., Taylor, D. W., Dunne, D. W. & Butterworth, A. E. (1984). Clone banks of cDNA from the parasite *Schistosoma mansoni*: Isolation of clones containing a potentially immunodiagnostic antigen gene. *Genealogy*, **26**, 25–39.

Cottrell, B. J., Humber, D. & Sturrock, R. F. (1980). An immunosuppressive factor in the serum of schistosomiasis patients. *Transactions of the Royal Society of Tropical Medicine and Hygiene*, **74**, 415–16.

Cram, E. B. & Files, V. S. (1946). Laboratory studies on the snail host of *Schistosoma mansoni*. *American Journal of Tropical Medicine*, **26**, 715–20.

Crossland, N. O. (1962). A mud-sampling technique for the study of the ecology of aquatic snails, and its use in the evaluation of the efficacy of molluscicides in field trials. *Bulletin of the World Health Organisation*, **27**, 125–33.

Crossland, N. O. (1967). Field trials to evaluate the effectiveness of the mulluscicide N-tritylmorpholine in irrigation systems. *Bulletin of the World Health Organisation*, **37**, 23–42.

Cumper G. E. (1984). *Determinants of Health Levels in Developing Countries*. New York: Research Studies Press Ltd. John Wiley & Sons Inc.

Dalton, P. (1976). A socio-ecological approach to the control of *Schistosoma mansoni* in St Lucia. *Bulletin of the World Health Organisation*, **54**, 587–95.

Damian, R. T. (1984). Immunity in schistosomiasis: A holistic view. *Contemporary Topics in Immunobiology*, **12**, 359–420.

Davis, A. (1961). Suppressive management of schistosomiasis with antimony dimercaptosuccinate. *Annals of Tropical Medicine and Parasitology*, **55**, 256–61.

Davis, A. (1963). An attempted suppression of endemic urinary bilharziasis with thioxanthones. *East African Medical Journal*, **40**, 628–34.

Davis, A., Biles, J. E., Ulrick, A. M. & Dixon, H. (1981). Tolerance and efficiency of parziquantel in phase IIA and IIB therapaeutic trials. *Arzneimittel Forschung/Drug Research*, **31**, 568–74.

Dean, D. A. (1983). A review, *Schistosoma* and related genera: Acquired resistance to schistome infection in mice. *Experimental Parasitology*, **55**, 1–104.

Diem, K. & Lentner, C. (eds.) (1970). In *Scientific Tables*, 7th edn, p. 537. Basle, Switzerland: J. R. Geigy, S. A.

Domingo, E. O. & Warren, K. S. (1968). Endogenous desensitization. Changing host granulomatous response to schistosome eggs at different stages of infection with *Schistosoma mansoni*. *American Journal of Pathology*, **52**, 369–79.

Duncan, J. (1980). The toxicology of molluscicides. The organotins. *Pharmacology and Therapeutics*, **10**, 407–29.

Economist, The (1980). *The World in Figures*. p. 144. London: Macmillan Press.

El Alamy, M. A. & Cline, B. L. (1977). Prevalence and intensity of *Schistosoma haematobium* and *S. mansoni* infection in Qalyub, Egypt. *American Journal of Tropical Medicine and Hygiene*, **26**, 470–2.

Ellner, J. J. & Mahmoud, A. A. F. (1982). Phagocytes and worms: David and Goliath revisited. *Review of Infectious Diseases*, **4**, 698–714.

Ellner, J. J., Olds, G. R., Kamel, R., Osman, G. S., El Kholy, A. & Mahmoud, A.A.F. (1980). Suppressor splenic T-lymphocytes in human hepatosplenic schistosomiasis mansoni. *Journal of Immunology* **125**, 308–12.

Ellner, J. J., Olds, G. R., Osman, G. S., El Kholy, A. & Mahmoud, A. A. F. (1981). Dichotomies in the reactivity to worm antigen in human schistosomiasis mansoni. *Journal of Immunology*, **126**, 309–12.

Etges, F. J. & Maldonado, J. F. (1969). The present status of bilharziasis in the Dominican Republic. *Malacologia*, **9**, 40–1.

Evans, A. S., Cook, J. A., Kapikian, A. Z., Nankervis, G., Smith, A. L. & West, B., (1979). A serological survey of St Lucia. *International Journal of Epidemiology*, **8**, 327–32.

Eyakuze, V. M. (1974). Experience with niridazole and niclosamide in a *Schistosoma haematobium* pilot project. *East African Journal of Medical Research*, **3**, 203–7.

Faria, H. F. (1972). Control of schistosomiasis in Venezuela. In *Proceedings of a symposium on the future of Schistosomiasis Control*, ed. Max J. Miller, pp. 100–3. Tulane University Press.

Farooq, M., Hairston, N. G. & Samaan, S. A. (1966*a*). The effect of area–wide snail control on the endemicity of bilharziasis in Egypt. *Bulletin of the World Health Organisation*, **35**, 369–75.

Farooq, M. & Mallah, M. G. (1966). The behavioural pattern of social and religious water-contact activities in the Egypt-49 bilharziasis project area. *Bulletin of the World Health Organisation*, **35**, 377–87.

Farooq, M., Nielson, J., Samaan, S. A., Mallah, M. B. & Allam, A. (1966*b*). The epidemiology of *Schistosoma haematobium* and *S. mansoni* infections. 3. Prevalence of bilharziasis in relation to certain environmental conditions. *Bulletin of the World Health Organisation*, **35**, 319–30.

Farooq, M. & Samaan, S. A. (1967). The relative potential of different age groups in the transmission of schistosomiasis in the Egypt-49 project area. *Annals of Tropical Medicine and Parasitology*, **61**, 315–20.

Ferguson, F. F. (1977). *The Role of Biological Agents in the Control of Schistosome-bearing Snails*. CDC Atlanta: US Department of Health, Education and Welfare Public Health Services.

Ferguson, F. F. & Buckmire, K. W. (1974). Notes on the freshwater molluscs of Grenada, British West Indies. *Caribbean Journal of Science*, **14**, 147–8.

Ferguson, F. F., Palmer, J. R. & Jobin, W. (1968). Control of schistosomiasis on Vieques Island, Puerto Rico. *American Journal of Tropical Medicine and Hygiene*, **17**, 858–63.

Ferguson, F. F., Richards, C. S., Sebastian, S. S. & Buchanan, I. C. (1960). Natural abatement of *schistosomiasis mansoni* in St Kitts, British West Indies. *Public Health*, **74**, 261–5.

Ferguson, F. F. & Ruiz-Tibén, E. (1971). Review of biological control method for schistosome-bearing snails. *Ethiopian Medical Journal*, **9**, 95–103.

Foster, A. (1973). Oxamniquine symposium: Summary of round table discussion. *Revista do Instituto de Medicina Tropical de São Paulo*, **15**, 83–6 (Suppl. 1).

Friedheim, E. A. H. & De Jongh, R. T. (1959). The effect of a single dose of TWSb in urinary bilharziasis; suggestions for a suppressive management of bilharziasis. *Annals of Tropical Medicine and Parasitology*, **53**, 316–24.

Galgey, O. (1899). *Filaria demarquaii* in St Lucia, West Indies. *British Medical Journal*, **1**, 145–6.

Gelfand, M. (1966). The general or constitutional symptoms in *S. mansoni* infestation: a clinical comparison in two racial groups. *Journal of Tropical Medicine and Hygiene*, **69**, 230–1.

Goddard, M. J. & Jordan, P. (1980). On the longevity of *Schistosoma mansoni* in man on St Lucia, West Indies. *Transactions of the Royal Society of Tropical Medicine and Hygiene*, **74**, 185–91.

Golvan, Y. J., Houin, R., Combes, C., Deniau, M. & Lancastre, F. (1977). Natural transmission of *Schistosoma mansoni* infection in Guadeloupe, French Antilles. Preliminary note. *Annales de Parasitologie Humaine et Comparée*, **52**, 259–75.

Gönnert, R. & Schraufstatter, E. (1959). A new molluscicide: Molluscicide Bayer 73. In *Proceedings of the sixth International Congress on Tropical Medicine and Malaria, Lisbon 1958*, vol. 2, p. 197. Abstracts of the papers. Libson: Institute de Medicina Tropical.

Gönnert, R. & Strufe, R. (1961). The stability of the molluscicide Bayluscide. *Zeitschrift für Tropenmedischen und Parasitologie*, **12**, 220–34.

Gonzales-Martinez, J. (1904). Referring to a study of *Bilharzia haematobium* and bilharziasis in Puerto Rico. *Revista do Medicina Tropical*, **5**, 193–4.

Goodgame, R. W., Colley, D. G., Graper, C. C., Lewis, F. A., McLaren, M. L. & Pelley, R. P. (1978). Humoral immune responses in human hepatosplenic schistosomiasis mansoni. *American Journal of Tropical Medicine and Hygiene*, **27**, 1174–80.

Greany, W. H. (1952). Schistosomiasis in the Gezira irrigated area of the Anglo-Egyptian Sudan. 1. Public health and field Aspects. *Annals of Tropical Medicine and Parasitology*, **46**, 250–67.

Guerra, F. (1966). Influence of disease on race, logistics and colonisation in Antilles. *Journal of Tropical Medicine and Hygiene*, **69**, 23–35.

Haddock, K. C. (1981). Control of schistosomiasis: the Puerto Rican experience. *Social Science and Medicine*, **15D**, 501–14.

Hairston, N. G. (1965). An analysis of age prevalence data by catalytic models. *Bulletin of the World Health Organisation*, **33**, 163–75.

Harley, J. (1986). On the endemic haematuria of the Cape of Good Hope. *Medico-Chirological Transactions*, **47**, 55–72.

Harrison, A. D. & Rankin, J. J. (1978). Hydrobiological studies of Eastern Lesser Antillean Islands. III. St Vincent: Freshwater Mollusca – their distribution, population dynamics and biology. *Archiv fur Hydrobiologie*, **54**, 123–88.

Hartman, P. E., Berger, H. & Hartman, Z. (1973). Comparison of hycanthone (Etrenol), some hycanthone analogs, myxin, and 4-nitroquinoline-L-oxide as frameshift mutagens. *Journal of Pharmacology and Experimental Therapeutics*, **186**, 390–8.

Hartman, P. E., Levine, K., Hartman, Z. & Berger, H. (1971). Hycanthone: a frameshift mutagen. *Science*, **172**, 1058–60.

Henry, F. (1981). Environmental sanitation, infection and nutritional status of infants in rural St Lucia, West Indies. *Transactions of the Royal Society of Tropical Medicine and Hygiene*, **75**, 507–13.

Hetrick, F. M. & Kos, W. L. (1973). Transformation of Rauscher virus infected cell cultures after treatment with hycanthone and lucanthone. *Journal of Pharmacology and Experimental Therapeutics*, **186**, 425–9.

Hiatt, R. A. (1976). Morbidity from *Schistosoma mansoni* infections: an epidemiological study based on quantitative analysis of egg excretion in two highland Ethiopian villages. *American Journal of Tropical Medicine and Hygiene*, **25**, 808–17.

Hiatt, R. & Gebre-Medhin, M. (1977). Morbidity from *Schistosoma mansoni* infections: an epidemiological study based on quantitative analysis of egg excretion in Ethiopian children. *American Journal of Tropical Medicine and Hygiene*, **26**, 473–81.

Hillyer, G. V. (1979). Immunodiagnosis of infection with *Schistosoma mansoni*: comparison of ELISA, radioimmunoassay, and precipitation tests performed with antigens from eggs. *American Journal of Tropical Medicine and Hygiene*, **28**, 661–9.

Hillyer, G. V., Menedewy-Corrada, R., Lluberes, R. & Hernandes-Morales, F. (1970). Evidence of transplacental passage of specific antibody in schistosomiasis mansoni in man. *American Journal of Tropical Medicine and Hygiene*, **19**, 289–91.

Holcomb, R. C. (1907). West Indian bilharziosis. *Military Surgeon*, **20**, 450–67.

Hollister, A. C., Beck, D., Gittelsohn, A. M. & Hemphill, E. C. (1955). Influence of water availability on *Shigella* prevalence in children of farm labour families. *American Journal of Public Health*, **45**, 354–62.

Husting, E. L. (1970). Sociologic patterns and their influence on the transmission of bilharziasis. *Central African Journal of Medicine*, **16**, 5–10.

Iarotski, L. S. & Davis, A. (1981). The schistosomiasis problem in the world: results of a WHO questionnaire survey. *Bulletin of the World Health Organisation*, **59**, 115–27.

Jackson, J. A. J., Blair, W. E., Brinckman, F. E., & Iverson, W. P. (1982). Gas-chromatographic speciation of methylstannanes in the Chesapeake Bay using purge and trap sampling with a tin-selective detector. *Environmental Science and Technology*, **16**, 110–19.

James, S. L., Sher, A., Lazdins, J. K. & Meltzer, M. S. (1982). Macrophages as effector cells of protective immunity in murine schistosomiasis. II. Killing of newly transformed schistosomula *in vitro* by macrophages activated as a consequence of *Schistosoma mansoni* infection. *Journal of Immunology*, **128**, 1535–40.

Jelnes, J. E. (1977). Evidence of possible molluscicide resistance of *Schistosoma* intermediate host from Iran ? *Transactions of the Royal Society of Tropical Medicine and Hygiene*, **71**,451.

Jobin, W. R., Brown, R. A., Vélez, S. P. & Ferguson, F. F. (1977). Biological control of *Biomphalaria glabrata* in major reservoirs of Puerto Rico. *American Journal of Tropical Medicine and Hygiene*, **26**, 1018–24.

Jobin, W. R., Ferguson, F. F. & Palmer, J. R. (1970). Control of schistosomiasis in Guayama and Arroyo, Puerto Rico. *Bulletin of the World Health Organisation*, **42**, 151–6.

Jones, S. B. (1932). Intestinal bilharziasis in St Kitts, British West Indies. *Journal of Tropical Medicine and Hygiene*, **35**, 129–36.

Jordan, P. (1960). Cercarial action of soap. *East African Institute for Medical Research Report 1959–60*, p. 29. East Africa High Commission, Kenya.

Jordan, P. (1963). Some quantitative aspects of bilharzia with particular reference to suppressive therapy and mollusciciding in control of *S. haematobium* in Sukumaland, Tanganyika. *East African Medical Journal*, **40**, 250–60.

Jordan, P. (1966). Schistosomiasis in Tanzania: Long term results of TWSb and lucanthone hydrochloride combined in suppressive therapy in *Schistosoma haematobium*. *Transactions of the Royal Society of Tropical Medicine and Hygiene*, **60**, 83–8.

Jordan, P. (1967). Egg-output in bilharziasis in relation to epidemiology, pathology, treatment and control. In *Bilharzias*, ed. F. K. Mastafi, pp. 93–103. Berlin, New York: Springer-Verlag.

Jordan, P. (1969). Factors affecting results of chemotherapy in schistosomiasis. *Annals of the New York Academy of Science*, **160**, 602–11.

Jordan, P. (1977). Schistosomiasis – research to control. *American Journal of Tropical Medicine and Hygiene*, **26**, 877–86.

Jordan, P., Barnish, G., Bartholomew, R. K., Grist, E. & Christie, J. D. (1978). Evaluation of an experimental mollusciciding programme to control *Schistosoma mansoni* transmission in St Lucia. *Bulletin of the World Health Organisation*, **56**, 139–46.

Jordan, P., Bartholomew, R. K., Grist, E. & Auguste, E. (1982). Evaluation of chemotherapy in the control of *Schistosoma mansoni* in Marquis Valley, Saint Lucia. I. Results in humans. *American Journal of Tropical Medicine and Hygiene*, **31**, 103–10.

Jordan, P., Bartholomew, R. K. & Peters, P. A. S. (1981). A community study of *Schistosoma mansoni* egg excretion assessed by the Bell and modified Kato technique. *Annals of Tropical Medicine and Parasitology*, **75**, 35–40.

Jordan, P., Christie, J. D. & Unrau, G. O. (1980a). Schistosomiasis transmission with particular reference to possible ecological and biological methods of control. *Acta Tropica*, **37**, 95–138.

Jordan, P., Cook, J. A., Bartholomew, R. K., Grist, E. & Auguste, E. (1980b). *Schistosoma mansoni* control in Cul de Sac Valley, Saint Lucia. II. Chemotherapy as a supplement to a focal mollusciciding programme. *Transactions of the Royal Society of Tropical Medicine and Hygiene*, **74**, 493–500.

Jordan, P. & Randall, K. (1962). Schistosomiasis in Tanganyika: observations on suppressive management of *Schistosoma haematobium* with TWSb with particular reference to reduction in ova load. *Transactions of the Royal Society of Tropical Medicine and Hygiene*, **56**, 523–8.

Jordan, P. & Webbe, G. (1982). *Schistosomiasis – Epidemiology, Treatment and Control*. London: Heinemann Medical Books.

Jordan, P., Woodstock, L., Unrau, G. O. & Cook, J. A. (1975). Control of *Schistosoma mansoni* transmission by provision of domestic water supplies. *Bulletin of the World Health Organisation*, **52**, 9–20.

Jove, J. A. & Marszewski, P. (1961). Reduction of bilharziasis in the area of Tejerias in thirteen years of a public health campaign. *Revista Venezolana de Sanidad y Asistencia Social*, **26**, 615–26.

Kagan, I. G. & Pellegrino, J. (1961). A critical review of immunological methods for the diagnosis of bilharziasis. *Bulletin of the World Health Organisation*, **25**, 611–74.

Kamel, K. A. & Higashi, G. I. (1982). Suppression of mitogen–induced lymphocyte transformation by plasma from patients with hepatosplenic schistosomiasis mansoni; role of immune complexes. *Parasite Immunology*, **4**, 283–98.

Katz, N. (1971). Avaliação terapeutic da hycanthone em pacientes com periodo de infeção equistossomatica conhecido. *Revista da Sociedade Brasileira de Medicina Tropical*, **5**, 55–60.

Katz, N., Pellegrino, J., Ferreira, M. T., Oliveria, C. A. & Dias, C. B. (1968). Preliminary clinical trials with hycanthone, a new schistosomicidal agent. *American Journal of Tropical Medicine and Hygiene*, **17**, 743–6.

Katz, N., Pellegrino, J. & Oliveira, C. A. (1969). Further clinical trails with hycanthone, a new antischistosomal agent. *American Journal of Tropical Medicine and Hygiene*, **18**, 924–9.

Kellermeyer, R. W., Warren, K. S., Waldmann, T. S., Cook, J. A. & Jordan, P. (1973). Concentration of serum immunoglobulins in St Lucians with schistosomiasis mansoni compared with matched uninfected St Vincentians. *Journal of Infectious Diseases*, **127**, 557–62.

Khattab, M., El-Gengehy, M. T. & Sharaf, M., (1968). ABO blood groups in bilharzial hepatic fibrosis. *Journal of the Egyptian Medical Association*, **51**, 245–50.

Kikuth, W., Gönnert, R., Mauss, H. (1946). Therapeutic agent against intestinal bilharziasis. *Naturwissenschaften*, **33**, 253.

Kilgen, R. H. & Smitherman, R. O. (1971). Food habits of the white amur stocked in ponds alone and in combination with other species. *Progressive Fish-culturist*, **33**, 123–7.

Kloetzel, K. (1962). Splenomegaly in schistosomiasis mansoni. *American Journal of Tropical Medicine and Hygiene*, **11**, 472–6.

Knight, B. A. G. & Tomlinson, T. E. (1967). The interaction of paraquat (1:1'-dimethyl 4:4'-dipyridylium dichloride) with mineral soils. *Journal of Soil Science*, **2**, 233–43.

Kresina, T. F. & Nasinof, A. (1983). Passive transfer of the idiotypically suppressed state by serum from suppressed mice and transfer of suppression from mothers to offspring. *Journal of Experimental Medicine*, **157**, 15–23.

Lambert, C. R. (1964). Chemotherapy of experimental *Schistosoma mansoni* infections with a nitro-thiazole derivative CIBA 32 644-Ba. *Annals of Tropical Medicine and Parasitology*, **58**, 292–303.

Lavacuente, A., Brown, R. A. & Jobin, W. (1979). Comparison of four species of snails as potential decoys to intercept schistosome miracidia. *American Journal of Tropical Medicine and Hygiene*, **28**, 99–105.

Lawson, J. R. & Wilson, R. A. (1983). The relationship between the age of *Schistosoma mansoni* cercariae and their ability to penetrate and infect the mammalian host. *Parasitology*, **87**, 481–2.

Lees, R. E. M. (1966). Malnutrition: the infant at risk. *West Indian Medical Journal*, **15**, 211–16.

Lees, R. E. M. (1968). Suppressive treatment of Schistosomiasis mansoni with spaced doses of lucanthone hydrochloride. *Transactions of the Royal Society of Tropical Medicine and Hygiene*, **62**, 782–5.

Lees, R. E. M. (1973). A selective approach to yaws control. *Canadian Journal of Public Health*, **64**, suppl. 52–6.

Lees, R. E. M. & De Bruin, A. M. (1963). Review of yaws in St Lucia five years after an eradication campaign. *West Indian Medical Journal*, **12**, 98–102.

Lees, R. E. M. & Jordan, P. (1968). Transplacental transfer of antibodies to *Schistosoma mansoni* and their persistence in infants. *Transactions of the Royal Society of Tropical Medicine and Hygiene*, **62**, 630–1.

Lehman, J. S., Mott, K. E., Morrow, R. H., Muniz, T. M. & Boyer, M. H. (1976). The intensity and effects of infection with *Schistosoma mansoni* in a rural community in north east Brazil. *American Journal of Tropical Medicine and Hygiene*, **25**, 285–94.

Leiper, R. T. (1915). Report on the results of the bilharzia mission in Egypt 1915. *Journal of the Royal Army Medical Corps*, **25**, 1–55, 147–92, 253–67.

Lemma, A., Goll, P., Duncan, J. & Mazengia, B. (1978). control of schistosomiasis by the use of Endod in Adwa, Ethiopia: results of a 5-year study. *Proceedings of the International Conference on Schistosomiasis: Cairo, Egypt, October 18–25, 1975*. **1**. 415–36.

Letulle, M. (1904). A case of intestinal bilharziasis contracted in Martinique. *Revue de Médicine et d'Hygiène Tropicales*, **1**, 46–8.

Lie, K. J., Kwo, E. H. & Owyang, C. K. (1970). A field trial to test the possible control of *Schistosoma spindale* by means of interspecific trematode antagonism. *South East Asian Journal of Tropical Medicine and Public Health*, **1**, 19–28.

Lie, K. J., Kwo, E. H. & Owyang, C. K. (1971). Further field trial to control *Schistosoma spindale* by trematode antagonism. *South East Asian Journal of Tropical Medicine and Public Health*, **2**, 237–43.

Lim, H. K. & Heyneman, D. (1972). Intramolluscan inter-trematode antagonism: a review of factors influencing the host–parasite system and its possible role in biological control. *Advances in Parasitology*, **10**, 191–268.

Little, C. (1972). Schistosomiasis in a Canadian presenting with portal hypertension. *Canadian Medican Association Journal*, **106**, 905–6.

Long, E. G., Lawrence, M. C., & Augustine, T. (1981a). ELISA for *Schistosoma mansoni* infection: durability of blood spots on filter paper. *Transactions of the Royal Society of Tropical medicine and Hygiene*, **75**, 740–1.

Long, E. G., McLaren, M. L., Goddard, M. J., Bartholomew, R. K., Peters, P. & Goodgame, R. (1981b). Comparison of ELISA, radioimmunoassay and stool examination for *Schistosoma mansoni*. *Transactions of the Royal Society of Tropical Medicine and Hygiene*, **75**, 365–71.

Lyons, G. R. L. (1974). Schistosomiasis in north western Ghana. *Bulletin of the World Health Organisation*, **51**, 621–32.

McClelland, W. F. J. (1965). Exposure of laboratory bred snails in natural situations. *East African Institute for Medical Research Annual Report 1963–64*, pp. 18–20. East African High Commission, Nairobi, Kenya.

McCullough, F. (1973). WHO/Tanzania schistosomiasis pilot control and training project, Mwanza District, Tanzania. AFR/Schist/29.

Macdonald, G. (1965). The dynamics of helminth infections with special reference to schistosomes. *Transactions of the Royal Society of Tropical Medicine and Hygiene*, **59**, 489–506.

McKay, D. A., Warren, K. S., Cook, J. A. & Jordan, P. (1973). Immunologic diagnosis of schistosomiasis. III. The effects of nutritional status and infection intensity on intradermal test results in St Lucian children. *American Journal of Tropical Medicine and Hygiene*, **22**, 205–10.

McLaren, M. L., Long, E. G., Goodgame, R. W. & Lillywhite, J. E. (1979). Application of the enzyme linked immunosorbant assay (ELISA) for the serodiagnosis of *Schistosoma mansoni* infections in St Lucia. *Transactions of the Royal Society of Tropical Medicine and Hygiene*, **73**, 636–9.

McMahon, J. (1966). Suppressive therapy in *Schistosoma mansoni* infection; preliminary communication. *East African Medical Journal*, **43**, 409–11.

McMahon, J. E. (1981). Praziquantel: a new schistosomicide against *Schistosoma mansoni*. *Arzneimittel Forschung/Drug Research*, **31**, 592–4.

McMahon, J. P., Highton, R. B. & Marshall, T. F. de C. (1977). Studies on biological control of intermediate hosts of schistosomiasis in Western Kenya. *Environmental Conservation*, **4**, 285–9.

McMullen, D. B. (1952). Schistosomiasis and molluscicides. *American Journal of Tropical Medicine and Hygiene*, **1**, 671–9.

Madsen, H. (1979). Preliminary observations on the role of conditioning and mechanical interference with egg masses and juveniles in the competitive relationships between *Helisoma duryi* (Wetherby) and the intermediate host of *Schistosoma mansoni* Sambon: *Biomphalaria camerunensis* (Boettger). *Hydrobiologia*, **67**, 207–14.

Madsen, H. & Frandsen, F. (1979). Studies on the interspecific competition between *Helisoma duryi* (Wetherby) and *Biomphalaria camerunensis* (Boettger). Size-weight relationships and laboratory experiments. *Hydrobiologia*, **66**, 17–23.

Mahmoud, A. A. F., Siongok, T. Arap, Ouma, J., Houser, H. B. & Warren, K. S. (1983). Effect of targeted mass treatment on intensity of infection and morbidity in schistosomiasis mansoni. *Lancet*, **i**, 849–51.

Malek, E. (1975). *Biomphalaria havenensis* (Pfeifferi) from Grenada, West Indies. *The Nautilus*, **89**, 17–20.

Manson, P. (1902). Report on a case of bilharzia from West Indies. *Journal of Tropical Medicine*. **5**, 384–5.

Martin, L. K. & Beaver, P. C. (1968). Evaluation of Kato thick smear technique for quantitative diagnosis of helminth infections. *American Journal of Tropical Medicine and Hygiene*, **17**, 382–91.

Matthiessen, P. (1974). Some effects of bis(tri-*n*-butyltin) oxide on the tropical food fish, *Tilapia mossambica* Peters. In *Proceedings of the Controlled Release Pesticide Symposium, University of Akron, Ohio, September 16–18, 1974*, ed. N. F. Cardarelli, pp. 25.1–25.17. Akron: University of Akron:

Meyling, A. H. & Meyling, J. (1969). A modified method for the estimation of the molluscicide *n*-tritylmorpholine (Frescon) in field waters. *South African Chemical Processing*, **4**, 63–4.

Meyling, A. H. & Pitchford, J. (1966). Physico-chemical properties of substances used as molluscicides. Hydrolysis of N-tritylmorpholine (Shell WL 8008). *Bulletin of the World Health Organisation*, **35**, 733–6.

Mongeot, G. & Golvan, Y. J. (1977). Aspects de la bilharziose dans la mangrove douce et l'arriere mangrove de la Grande-Terre en Guadeloupe. *Annales de Parasitologie Humaine et Comparée*, **52**, 623–8.

Monroe, F. F. (1916). Report of a case of bilharzia. *Proceedings of the Medical Association of the Isthmian Canal Zone*, **9**, 77–9.

Moore, J. A. (1972). Teratogenicity of hycanthone in mice. *Nature*, **239**, 107–9.

Morgan, P. R. & Mara, D. D. (1982). Ventilated improved pit latrines: recent developments in Zimbabwe. *World Bank Technical Paper Number 3*.

Moriearty, P. L. & Lewert, R. M. (1974). Delayed hypersensitivity in Ugandan schistosomiasis. I. Sensitivity, specificity, and immunological features of intradermal responses. *American Journal of Tropical Medicine and Hygiene*, **23**, 169–78.

Morris, J. (1963). In *Pax Britannica: the Climax of an Empire*, p. 168, London: Faber & Faber.

Most, H. & Levine, D. (1963). Schistosomiasis in American tourists. *Journal of the American Medical Association*, **186**, 453–7.

Nash, T. E. (1982). Diagnostic serologic responses; schistosome infections in humans: Perspectives and recent findings. *Annals of Internal Medicine*, **97**, 749–50.

Nassi, H. (1978). Data on the life cycle of *Ribeiroia marini guadelupensis* n. spp., trematode sterilizing *Biomphalaria glabrata* in Guadeloupe. Maintenance of the life cycle with a view to an eventual control of the populations of molluscs. *Acta Tropica*, **35**, 41–56.

Nassi, H., Pointier, J. P. & Golvan, Y. J. (1979). Bilan d'un essai de contrôle de *Biomphalaria glabrata* en Guadeloupe á l'aide d'un Trématode stérilisant. *Annales de Parasitologie Humaine et Comparée*, **54**, 185–92.

Nelson, G. S. (1974). Zooprophylaxis with special reference to schistosomiasis and filariasis. In '*Parasitic Zoonoses*', ed. E. J. L. Soulsby, pp. 273–85. London: Academic Press.

Nelson, G. S., Teesdale, C. & Highton, R. B. (1962). The role of animals as reservoirs of bilharziasis in Africa. In *Bilharziasis: Ciba Foundation Symposium*, ed. G. E. Wolstenholme & M. O'Connor, p. 127 London: J. & A. Churchill.

Nunesmaia, H. G., Azevedo, E. S., Arandas, E. A. & Widmer, C. G. (1975). Composicao racial e anaptoglobinemia em portadores de esquistossomose mansonica forma hepatosplenica. *Revista do Instituto de Medicina Tropical de São Paulo*, **17**, 160–3.

Ongom, V. L., Ower, R., Grundy, R. & Bradley, D. J. (1972). The epidemiology and consequence of *Schistoma mansoni* infection in West Nile, Uganda. II. Hospital investigations of a sample from the Panyagoro community. *Transactions of the Royal Society of Tropical Medicine and Hygiene*, **66**, 852–63.

Ottesen, E. A. (1979). Modulation of the host response in human schistosomiasis. I. Adherent suppressor cells that inhibit lymphocyte proliferative responses to parasite antigens. *Journal of Immunology*, **123**, 1639–44.

Ottesen, E. A. (1982). Immunology: Schistosome infections in humans: Perspectives and recent findings. *Annals of Internal Medicine*, **97**, 744–9.

Ottesen, E. A. & Poindexter, R. W. (1980). Modulation of the host response in human schistosomiasis. II. Humoral factors which inhibit lymphocyte proliferative responses to parasite antigens. *American Journal of Tropical Medicine and Hygiene*, **29**, 592–7.

Palmer, J. R., Colon, A. Z., Ferguson, F. F. & Jobin, W. R. (1969). The control of schistosomiasis in Patillas, Puerto Rico. *Public Health Reports*, **84**, 1003–7.

Pannikar, M. K. (1961). Bilharziasis in St Lucia. *Journal of Tropical Medicine and Hygiene*, **64**, 151–5.

Paraense, W. L. (1975). The distribution of the molluscan vectors of schistosomiasis in the Americas. *Brasilia Médica*, **11**, 11–14.

Paulini, E. (1958). Bilharziasis control by application of molluscicides: a review of its present status. *Bulletin of the World Health Organisation*, **18**, 975–88.

Paulini, E., de Freitas, C. A. & Aguirre, G. H. (1972). Control of schistosomiasis in Brazil. In *Proceedings of a Symposium on the Future of Schistosomiasis Control*, ed. Max J. Miller, pp. 104–10. Tulane University Press.

Paulinyi H. M. & Paulini, E. (1972). Laboratory observations on the biological control of *Biomphalaria glabrata* by a species of *Pomacea* (Ampullariidae). *Bulletin of the World Health Organisation*, **46**, 243–7.

Pereira, F. E. L., Bortolini, E. R., Carneiro, J. L. A., da Silva, C. R. M. & Neves, R. C. (1979). ABO blood groups and hepatosplenic schistosomiasis mansoni (Symmers' fibrosis). *Transactions of the Royal Society of Tropical Medicine*, **73**, 238.

Pesigan, T. P. & Hairston, N. G. (1961). The effect of snail control on the prevalence of *Schistosoma japonicum* infection in the Philippines. *Bulletin of the World Health Organisation*, **25**, 479–82.

Pesigan, T. P., Harrison, N. G., Jauregui, J. J., Garcia, E. G., Santos, A. T., Santos, B. C., & Besa, A. A. (1958). Studies on *Schistosoma japonicum* infection in the Philippines. 2. The molluscan host. *Bulletin of the World Health Organisation*, **18**, 481–578.

Phillips, S. M. & Colley, D. G. (1978). Immunologic aspects of host responses to schistosomiasis: Resistance, immunopathology, and eosinophil involvement. *Progress in Allergy*, **24**, 49–182.

Pitchford, R. J. (1966). Findings in relation to schistosome transmission in the field following the introduction of various control measures. *South African Medical Journal*, **40**, Suppl.

Pitchford, R. J. (1970). Seminar on the biological aspects of bilharziasis. *Central African Journal of Medicine*, **16**, Suppl.

Pointier, J. P. (1982). Possible competitive displacement of *Biomphalaria glabrata* (intermediate host snail of schistosomiasis) by *B. straminea* in Martinique (French West Indies). *Molecular and Biochemical Parasitology, Supplement*. Abstracts of the Fifth International Congress of Parasitology, Toronto, Canada, August 1982, pp. 429–30.

Pointier, J. P., Toffart, J. L. & Nassi, H. (1981). Recolonisation of a pond in Guadeloupe (French West Indies) by a population of *Biomphalaria glabrata* following a biological control trial. *Haliotis*, **11**, 197–200.

Prata, A. (1978). Clinical experience with oxamniquine. *Advances in Pharmacology and Therapeutics*, **10**, 27–40.

Prata, A. & Schroeder, S. (1967). A comparison of whites and Negroes infected with *Schistosoma mansoni* in a hyperendemic area. *Gazette Medica de Bahia*, **67**, 93–8.

Prentice, M. A. (1970). A molluscicide formulation for the control of *Biomphalaria choanomphala* in deep water. *Organisation of African Unity Symposium on Schistosomiasis*. Addis Ababa, Ethiopia, November 1970 GS/21/1.

Prentice, M. A. (1971). A simple constant flow pesticide dispenser. *PANS Manual*, **17**, 64–6.

Prentice, M. A. (1980). Schistosomiasis and its intermediate hosts in the Lesser Antillean Islands of the Caribbean. *Bulletin of the Pan American Health Organisation*, **14**, 258–86.

Prentice, M. A. (1983*a*). Displacement of *Biomphalaria glabrata* by the snail *Thiara granifera* in field habitats in St Lucia, West Indies. *Annals of Tropical Medicine and Parasitology*, **77**, 51–9.

Prentice, M. A. (1983*b*). Field comparison of mouse immersion and cercariometry for assessing the transmission potential of water containing cercariae of *Schistosoma mansoni*. *Annals of Tropical Medicine and Parasitology*, **78**, 169–72.

Prentice, M. A. & Barnish, G. (1980). Granule formulations of molluscicide for use in developing countries. *Annals of Tropical Medicine and Parasitology*, **74**, 45–51.

Prentice, M. A. & Barnish, G. (1981). Snail infections following chemotherapy of *Schistosoma mansoni* in St Lucia, West Indies. *Transactions of the Royal Society of Tropical Medicine and Hygiene*, **75**, 713–4.

Prentice, M. A., Barnish, G. & Christie, J. D. (1977). An eco-phenotype of *Helisoma duryi* closely resembling *Biomphalaria glabrata*. *Annals of Tropical Medicine and Parasitology*, **71**, 237–8.

Prentice, M. A., Christie, J. D. & Barnish, G. (1981). A miracidial trap for use in flowing water. *Annals of Tropical Medicine and Parasitology*, **75**, 407–13.

Prentice, M. A., Jordan, P., Bartholomew, R. K. & Grist, E. (1981). Reduction in transmission of *Schistosoma mansoni* by a 4-year focal mollusciciding programme against *Biomphalaria glabrata* in Saint Lucia. *Transactions of the Royal Society of Tropical Medicine and Hygiene*, **75**, 789–98.

Pugh, R. N. H. & Gilles, H. M. (1978). Malumfashi endemic diseases research project. III. Urinary schistosomiasis: a longitudinal study. *Annals of Tropical Medicine and Parasitology*, **72**, 471–82.

Radke, M. G., Berrios-Duran, L. A. & Moran, K. (1961). A perfusion procedure suction, for recovery of schistosome works. *Journal of Parasitology*, **47**, 366–8.

Rasmussen, O. (1974). Helisoma duryi *in biological control of bilharziasis*. Danish Bilharziasis Laboratory, Charlottenlund, Denmark.

Reiner, N. E., Kamel, R., Higashi, G. I., El Naggar, A., Aquilo, M., Ellner, J. J. & Mahmoud A. A. F. (1979). Concurrent responses of peripheral blood and splenic mononuclear cells to antigenic and mitogenic stimulation in human hepatosplenic schistosomiasis. *Journal of Infectious Diseases*, **140**, 162–8.

Richards, C. S. (1963). Infectivity of *Schistosoma mansoni* for Puerto Rican molluscs including a new potential intermediate host. *American Journal of Tropical Medicine and Hygiene*, **12**, 26–33.

Richards, C. S. (1973). A potential host of *Schistosoma mansoni* in Grenada. *Journal of Parasitology*, **59**, 111.

Rijpstra, A. C. & Swellengrebel, N. H. (1962). Lateral-spined schistosome ova in a giant anteater, *Myrmecophaga tridactyla* L. (Edentata) from Surinam. *Tropical and Geographical Medicine*, **14**, 279–83.

Robart, G., Mandahl-Barth, G. & Ripert, C. (1977). Inventaire, repartition geographique et ecologie des mollusques dulcaquicoles d'Haiti (Caraibes). *Haliotis*, **8**, 159–71.

Rocklin, R. E., Brown, A. P., Warren, K. S., Pelley, R. P., Houba, V., Siongok, T. K. A., Ouma, J., Sturrock, R. F., & Butterworth, A. E. (1980). Factors that modify the cellular-immune response in patients infected by *Schistosoma mansoni*. *Journal of Immunology*, **125**, 1916–23.

Rocklin, R. E., Tracy, J. W. & El Kholy, A. E. (1981). Activation of antigen-specific suppressor cells in human schistosomiasis mansoni by reactions of soluble egg antigens nonadherent to Con A sepharose. *Journal of Immunology*, **127**, 2314–8.

Rogers, S. H. & Bueding, E. (1970). The effects of hycanthone in mice and hamsters. *Journal of Parasitology*, **56** (No. 4, Section III), 288.

Rosi, D., Peruzzotti, G., Dennis, E. W., Berberian, D. A., Freele, H. & Archer, S. (1965). A new active metabolite of 'Miracil D'. *Nature*, **208**, 1005.

Rowan, W. B. (1965). The ecology of schistosome transmission. *Bulletin of the World Health Organisation*, **33**, 63–71.

Russell, W. L. (1975). Results of tests for possible transmitted genetic effects of hycanthone in mammals. *Journal of Toxicology and Environmental Health*, **1**, 301–4.

Salam, E. A., Ishaac, S. & Mahmoud, A. A. F. (1979). Histocompatibility-linked susceptibility for hepatosplenomegaly in human schistosomiasis mansoni. *Journal of Immunology*, **123**, 1829–31.

Sandt. D. G. (1973*a*), Laboratory comparison of four cercaria recovery techniques. *Bulletin of the World Health Organisation*, **48**, 35–40.

Sandt. D. G. (1973*b*). Direct filtration for the recovery of *Schistosoma mansoni* cercariae in the field. *Bulletin of the World Health Organisation*, **48**, 27–34.

Scott, J. A. & Barlow, C. H. (1938). Limitations to the control of helminth parasites in Egypt by means of treatment and sanitation. *American Journal of Hygiene* **27**, 619–48.

Sher, A., Butterworth, A. E., Colley, D. G., Cook, J. A., Freeman, G. L. & Jordan, P. (1977). Immune responses during human schistosomiasis mansoni. II. Occurrence of eosinophil-dependent cytotoxic antibodies in relation to intensity and duration of infection. *American Journal of Tropical Medicine and Hygiene*, **26**, 909–16.

Sher, A., Heiny, S., James, S. L. & Asofsky, R. (1982). Mechanisms of protective immunity against *Schistosoma mansoni* infection in mice vaccinated with irradiated cercariae. II. Analysis of immunity in hosts deficient in T lymphocytes, B lymphocytes, or complement. *Journal of Immunology*, **128**, 1880–4.

Sherif, A. F., El Sawy, M. F., Madary, S. A. & Barahat, R. M. (1970). The chemoprophylactic aspects of antibilharzial spaced mass suppressive treatment in an endemic area. *Alexandra Medical Journal*, **16**, 169–82.

Sherman, L. R. & Carlson, T. L. (1980). A modified phenylfluorone method for determining organotin compounds in the p.p.b. and sub-p.p.b. range. *Journal of Analytical Toxicology* **4**, 31–3.

Shiff, C. J. (1973). The value of incidence for the assessment of schistosomiasis control. *Bulletin of the World Health Organisation*, **48**, 409–14.

Shiff, C. J. (1974). Focal control of schistosome bearing snails using slow-release molluscicides. In *Molluscicides in Schistosomiasis Control*, ed. T. C. Cheng, pp. 241–7. New York: Academic Press.

Shiff, C., Clarke, V. de V., Evans, A. C. & Barnish, G. (1973). Molluscicide for the control of schistosomiasis in irrigation schemes. *Bulletin of the World Heath Organization*, **48**, 299–307.

Shiff, C. J. & Evans, A. C. (1977). The role of slow-release molluscicides in snail control. *Central African Journal of Medicine*, **23** (supplement to issue 11), 6–11.

Shuval, H. I., Tilden, R. L., Perry, B. H. & Grosse, R. N. (1981). Effect of investments in water supply and sanitation on health status: a threshold-saturation theory. *Bulletin of the World Health Organisation* **59**, 243–8.

Sieber, S. M. & Adamson, R. H. (1975). Evaluation of the teratogenetic activity of hycanthone in mice and rabbits. *Journal of Toxicology and Environmental Health*, **1**,309–22.

Silva, L. C. da, Sette, H., Christo, C. H., Saez-Alquezar, A., Carneiro, C. R. W., Lacet, C. M., Ohtsuki, N. & Raia, S. (1981). Praziquantel in the treatment of the hepatosplenic form of schistosomiasis mansoni. *Arzneimittel Forschung/Drug Research*, **31**, 601–3.

Siongok, T. K. A., Mahmoud, A. A. F., Ouma, J. H., Warren, K. S., Muller, A. S., Handa, A. K. & Houser, H. B. (1976). Morbidity in schistosomiasis mansoni in relation to intensity of infection: study of a community in Machakos, Kenya. *American Journal of Tropical Medicine and Hygiene*, **25**, 273–84.

Sleigh, A., Hoff, R., Mott, K., Barreto, M., de Paiva, T. M., Pedrosa, J. de Souza, & Sherlock, I. (1982). Comparison of filtration staining (Bell) and thick smear (Kato) for the detection and quantitation of *Schistosoma mansoni* eggs in faeces. *Transactions of the Royal Society of Tropical Medicine and Hygiene*, **76**, 403–6.

Smith, D. H., Highton, R. B. & Roberts, J. M. D. (1981). Preliminary observations on the treatment of schistosomiasis mansoni with praziquantel in Kenya. *Arzneimittel Forschung/Drug Research*, **31**, 594–6.

Smith, D. H., Warren, K. S. & Mahmoud, A. A. F. (1979). Morbidity in schistosomiasis mansoni in relation to intensity of infection: study of a community in Kisumu, Kenya. *American Journal of Tropical Medicine and Hygiene*, **28**, 220–9.

Smithers, S. R. & Terry, R. J. (1976). The immunology of schistosomiasis. *Advances in Parasitology*, **14**, 399–422.

Snedecor, G. W. & Cochran, W. G. (1967). *Statistical methods*, 6th edn, p. 253. Iowa State University Press.

Sontoro, F., Carlier, Y., Borojevic, R., Bout, D., Tachon, P. & Capron, A. (1977). Parasite 'M' antigen in milk from mothers infected with *Schistosoma mansoni*. *Annals of Tropical Medicine and Parasitology*, **71**, 121–3.

Stirewalt, M. A. (1953). The influence of previous infection of mice with *Schistosoma mansoni* on a challenging infection with the homologous parasite. *American Journal of Tropical Medicine and Hygiene*, **2**, 867–82.

Stirewalt, M. A. (1956). Penetration of host skin by cercariae of *Schistosoma mansoni*. I. Observed entry into skin of mouse, hamster, rat, monkey and man. *Journal of Parasitology*, **42**, 565–80.

Strufe, R. (1963). Modified method for determining Bayluscicide in field trials. *Pflanzenschutz-Nachrichten Bayer*, **16**, 221–30.

Sturrock, B. M. & Sturrock, R. F. (1970*a*). Laboratory studies of the host–parasite relationship of *Schistosoma mansoni* and *Biomphalaria glabrata* from St Lucia, West Indies. *Annals of Tropical Medicine and Parasitology*, **64**, 357–63.

Sturrock, R. F. (1973*a*). Field studies on the transmission of *Schistosoma mansoni* and on the bionomics of its intermediate host, *Biomphalaria glabrata*, on St Lucia, West Indies. *International Journal for Parasitology*, **3**, 175–94.

Sturrock, R. F. (1973*b*). Control of *Schistosoma mansoni* transmission: strategy for using molluscicides on St Lucia. *International Journal for Parasitology*, **3**, 795–801.

Sturrock, R. F. (1974*a*). Problems associated with mollusciciding natural habitats. In *Molluscicides in Schistosomiasis control*, ed. T. C. Cheng, pp. 51–65. London: Academic Press.

Sturrock, R. F. (1974*b*). Persistence of the molluscicide Bayluscide (clonitralide) emulsifiable concentrate on mud surfaces in the tropics. *Annals of Tropical Medicine and Parasitology*, **74**, 427–34.

Sturrock, R. F. (1974*c*). Ecological notes on habitats of the freshwater snail *Biomphalaria glabrata*, intermediate host of *Schistosoma mansoni*, on St Lucia, West Indies. *Caribbean Journal of Science*, **14**, 149–61.

Sturrock, R. F. & Barnish, G. (1973). The aerial application of molluscicides with special reference to schistosomiasis control. *Bulletin of the World Health Organisation*, **49**, 283–5.

Sturrock, R. F., Barnish G. & Seeyave, J. (1974*a*). Field tests on the effect of three molluscicidal chemicals on bananas. *Pflanzenschutz-Nachrichten Bayer*, **27**, 56–61.

Sturrock, R. F., Barnish, G. & Upatham, E. S. (1974*b*). Snail findings from an experimental mollusciciding programme to control *Schistosoma mansoni* transmission on St Lucia. *International Journal for Parasitology*, **4**, 231–40.

Sturrock, R. F. & Sturrock, B. M. (1970*b*). Observations on the susceptibility of *Schistosoma* *mansoni* from St Lucia of several Caribbean strains of snails of the genus *Biomphalaria*. *West Indian Medical Journal*, **19**, 9–13.

Sturrock, R. F. & Sturrock, B. M. (1971). Shell abnormalities in *Biomphalaria glabrata* infected with *Schistosoma mansoni* and their significance in field transmission studies. *Journal of Helminthology*, **45**, 201–10.

Sturrock, R. F. & Woodstock, L. (1973). The development of fluorescent antibodies in unisexual and bisexual *Schistosoma mansoni* infections of laboratory mice. *Annals of Tropical Medicine and Parasitology*, **67**, 425–30.

Swellengrebel, N. H. & Rijpstra, A. C. (1965). Lateral-spined schistosome ova in the intestines of a squirrel monkey from Surinam. *Tropical and Geographical Medicine*, **17**, 80–4.

Tachon, P. & Borojevic, R. (1978). Mother-child relation in human schistosomiasis mansoni: skin test and cord blood reactivity to schistosomal antigens. *Transactions of the Royal Society of Tropical Medicine and Hygiene*, **72**, 605–9.

Tee-Kaw, K. & Rose, G. (1982). Population study of blood pressure and associated factors in St Lucia, West Indies. *International Journal of Epidemiology*, **11**, 372–7.

Terpstra, W. J., van Helden, H. P. T. & Eyakuze, V. M. (1975). The cellophane thick-smear technique in comparison with the filtration standing technique for the quantitative determination of *Schistosoma mansoni* ova in stools. *East African Journal of Medical Research*, **2**, 225–33.

Théron, A., Pointier, J. P. & Combes, C. (1978). An ecological approach to the problems of the responsibility of men and rats in the workings of a transmission site of *Schistosoma mansoni* in Guadeloupe (West Indies) *Annals de Parasitologie Humaine et Comparée*, **53**, 223–34.

Tikasingh, E. S. (1982). Detection of *Schistosoma mansoni* in two island populations in the Caribbean. *Molecular & Biochemical Parasitology: Supplement*. Abstracts of the Fifth International Congress of Parasitology, Toronto, Canada, August 1982, pp. 317–18.

Tikasingh, E. S., Wooding, C. D., Long, E., Lee, C. P. & Edwards, C. (1982). The presence of *Schistosoma mansoni* in Monserrat, Leeward Islands. *Journal of Tropical Medicine and Hygiene*, **85**, 41–3.

Todd, C. W., Goodgame, R. W. & Colley, D. G. (1980). Immune responses during human schistosomiasis mansoni. VII. Further analysis of the interactions between patient sera and lymphocytes during *in vitro* blastogenesis to schistosome antigen preparations. *American Journal of Tropical Medicine and Hygiene*, **29**, 875–81.

Todd, C. W., Goodgame, R. W., Colley, D. G. & Lewis, F. A. (1979). Immune responses during human schistosomiasis mansoni. V. Suppression of schistosome antigen-specific lymphocyte blastogenesis by adherent/phagocytic cells. *Journal of Immunology*, **122**, 1440–6.

Tsutsumi, H. (1972). Autopsy cases of schistosomiasis mansoni in Puerto Rico. *Kurume Medical Journal*, **19**, 227–35.

Twyford, I. T. (1975). *Geest Industries (Estates Ltd) Field Directive No. 13. Drainage of banana fields*. Mimeographed report.

Unrau, G. O. (1975). Individual household water supplies as a control measure against *Schistosoma mansoni*. *Bulletin of the World Health Organisation*, **52**, 1–8.

Unrau, G. O. (1978). Water supply and schistosomiasis in St Lucia. *Progress in Water Technology*, **11**, 181–90.

Upatham, E. S. (1972*a*). Rapidity and duration of hatching of St Lucian *Schistosoma mansoni* eggs in outdoor habitats. *Journal of Helminthology*, **3**, 271–6.

Upatham, E. S. (1972*b*). Studies on the hatching of *Schistosoma mansoni* eggs in standing-water and running-water habitats in St Lucia, West Indies. *South East Asian Journal of Tropical Medicine and Public Health*, **3**, 600–4.

Upatham, E. S. (1972*c*). Exposure of caged *Biomphalaria glabrata* (Say) to investigate dispersion of miracidia of *Schistosoma mansoni* in outdoor habitats in St Lucia. *Journal of Helminthology*, **46**, 297–306.

Upatham, E. S. (1972*d*). Effect of water depth on the infection of *Biomphalaria glabrata* by miracidia of St Lucian *Schistosoma mansoni* under laboratory and field conditions. *Journal of Helminthology*, **46**, 317–25.

Upatham, E. S. (1972*e*). Interference by unsusceptible aquatic snails with the capacity of the miracidia of *Schistosoma mansoni* Sambon to infect *Biomphalaria glabrata* (Say) under field simulated conditions in St Lucia, West Indies. *Journal of Helminthology*, **46**, 277–83.

Upatham, E. S. (1972*f*). Effects of some physico-chemical factors on the infection of *Biomphalaria glabrata* (Say) by miracidia of *Schistosoma mansoni* sambon in St Lucia, West Indies. *Journal of Helminthology*, **46**, 307–15.

Upatham, E. S. (1973*a*). Location of *Biomphalaria glabrata* (Say) by *Schistosoma mansoni* Sambon miracidia in natural standing water and running water on the West Indian island of St Lucia. *International Journal of Parasitology*, **3**, 289–97.

Upatham, E. S. (1973*b*). The effect of water temperature on the penetration and development of St Lucian *Schistosoma mansoni* miracidia in local *Biomphalaria glabrata*. *South East Asian Journal of Tropical Medicine and Public Health*, **4**, 367–70.

Upatham, E. S. (1973*c*). Effect of a waterfall on the infectivity of St Lucian *Schistosoma mansoni* cercariae. *Transactions of the Royal Society of Tropical Medicine and Hygiene*, **67**, 884–5.

Upatham, E. S. (1974*a*). Dispersion of St Lucian *Schistosoma mansoni* cercariae in natural standing and running waters determined by cercarial counts and mouse exposure. *Annals of Tropical Medicine and Parasitology*, **68**, 343–52.

Upatham, E. S. (1974*b*). Infectivity of *Schistosoma mansoni* cercariae in natural St Lucian habitats. *Annals of Tropical Medicine and Parasitology*, **68**, 235–6.

Upatham, E. S. (1975). Field studies on slow release TBTO pellets (BioMet SRM) against St Lucian *Biomphalaria glabrata*. In *Proceedings of the Controlled Release Pesticide Symposium, Wright State University, 8–10 September 1975*, ed. F. Harris, pp. 8–10. Dayton: Wright State University.

Upatham, E. S. & Sturrock, R. F. (1973). Field investigations on the effect of other aquatic animals on the infection of *Biomphalaria glabrata* by *Schistosoma mansoni*: miracidia. *Journal of Parasitology*, **59**, 448–53.

Upatham, E. S. & Sturrock, R. F. (1977). Preliminary trials against *Biomphalaria glabrata* of a new molluscicide formulation: gelatin granules containing Bayluscide wettable powder. *Annals of Tropical Medicine and Hygiene*, **71**, 85–93.

Upatham, E. S., Sturrock, R. F. & Cook, J. A. (1976). Studies on the hatchability of *Schistosoma mansoni* eggs from a naturally infected human community on St Lucia, West Indies, *Parasitology*, **73**, 253–64.

Van der Kuyp, E. (1961). Schistosomiasis in the Surinam district of Surinam. *Tropical and Geographical Medicine*, **13**, 357–73.

Van der Schalie, H. (1958). Vector snail control in Qualyub, Egypt. *Bulletin of the World Health Organisation*, **19**, 263–83.

Walsh, J. A. & Warren, K. S. (1980). Selective primary health care: an interim strategy for disease control in developing countries. *Social Science and Medicine*, **14C**, 145–61.

Warren, K. S. (1972). The immunopathogenesis of schistosomiasis: a multidisciplinary approach. *Transactions of the Royal Society of Tropical Medicine and Hygiene*, **66**, 417–34.

Warren, K. S. (1973). Regulation of the prevalence and intensity of schistosomiasis in man: Immunology or ecology? *Journal of Infectious Diseases*, **127**, 595–609.

Warren K. S., Cook, J. A., David, J. R. & Jordan, P. (1975). Passive transfer of immunity in human schistosomiasis mansoni: Effect of transfer factor on early established infections. *Transactions of the Royal Society of Tropical Medicine and Hygiene*, **69**, 488–93.

Warren, K. S., Cook, J. A. & Jordan, P. (1972). Passive transfer of immunity in human schistosomiasis mansoni: Effect of hyperimmune anti-schistosome gamma globulin on early established infections. *Transactions of the Royal Society of Tropical Medicine and Hygiene*, **66**, 65–74.

Warren, K. S., Cook, J. A., Littell, A. S., Kagan, I. G. & Jordan, P. (1973a). Immunologic diagnosis of schistosomiasis. II. Further studies on the sensitivity and specificity of delayed intradermal reactions. *American Journal of Tropical Medicine and Hygiene*, **22**, 199–204.

Warren, K. S., Kellermeyer, R. W., Jordan, P., Littell, A. S., Cook, J. A. & Kagan, I. G. (1973b). Immunologic diagnosis of schistosomiasis. I. A controlled study of intradermal (immediate and delayed) and serologic tests in St Lucians infected with *Schistosoma mansoni* and in uninfected St Vincentians. *American Journal of Tropical Medicine and Hygiene*, **22**, 189–98.

Warren, K. S. & Mahmoud, A. A. F. (1976). Targeted mass treatment: a new approach to the control of schistosomiasis. *Transactions of the Association of American Physicians*, **89**, 195–204.

Warren, K. S., Mahmoud, A. A. F., Cummings, P., Murphy, D. J. & Houser, H. B. (1974). Schistosomiasis mansoni in Yemeni in California: Duration of infection, presence of disease, and therapeutic management. *American Journal of Tropical Medicine and Hygiene*, **23**, 902–9.

Warren, K. S. & Peters, P. A. (1967). Quantitative aspects of exposure time and cercarial dispersion on penetration and maturation of *Schistosoma mansoni* in mice. *Annals of Tropical Medicine and Parasitology*, **61**, 294–300.

Webbe, G. (1962a). The transmission of *Schistosoma haematobium* in an area of Lake Province, Tanganyika. *Bulletin of the World Health Organisation*, **27**, 59–85.

Webbe, G. (1962b). Population studies on intermediate hosts in relation to transmission of bilharziasis in East Africa. In *Bilharziasis: Ciba Foundation Symposium*, ed. G. E. Wolstenholme & M. O'Connor, pp. 7–22. London: J. & A. Churchill.

Webbe, G. & Jordan, P. (1966). Recent advances in knowledge of schistosomiasis in East Africa. *Transactions of the Royal Society of Tropical Medicine and Hygiene*, **60**, 279–312.

Webbe, G. & Sturrock, R. F. (1964). Laboratory tests of some new molluscicides in Tanganika. *Annals of Tropical Medicine and Parasitology*, **58**, 234–9.

Weir, J. M., Wasif, I. M., Hassan, F. R., Attia, S. D. M. & Kader, M. A. (1952). An elevation of health and sanitation in Egyptian villages. *Journal of the Egyptian Public Health Association*, **27**, 55–122.

Wells, A. V. (1959). Antibodies to poliomyelitis viruses in St Lucia. *West Indian Medical Journal*, **8**, 161–70.

Wells, A. V. (1961). Malaria eradication in St Lucia, WI. *West Indian Medical Journal*, **10**, 103–11.

White, G. F., Bradley, D. J. & White, A. V. (1972). *Drawers of water. Domestic water use in Africa*. Chicago, Illinois, USA: University of Chicago Press.

Wikler, M., Demeur, C., Dewasme, G. & Urbaine, J. (1980). Immunoregulatory role of maternal idiotypes, ontogeny of immune networks, *Journal of Experimental Medicine*, **152**, 1024–35.

Woodstock, L., Cook, J. A., Peters, P. A. & Warren, K. S. (1971). Random distribution of schistosome eggs in the faeces of patients with schistosomiasis mansoni. *Journal of Infectious Diseases*, **124**, 613–18.

Wright, W. H., Dobrovlny, C. G. & Berry, E. G. (1958). Field trials of various molluscicides (chiefly sodium pentachlorphenate) for the control of aquatic intermediate hosts of human bilharziasis. *Bulletin of the World Health Organisation*, **18**, 963–74.

Wyler, D. J. (1983). Regulation of fibroblast function by products of schistosomal egg granulomas: Potential role in the pathogenesis of hepatic fibrosis. In *Cytopathology of Parasitic Disease: Ciba Foundation Symposium*, ed. D. Evered & G. M. Collins, pp. 99, 109–206. London: J. & A. Churchill.

Yokagawa, M. (1972). Control of schistosomiasis in Japan. In *Proceedings of a Symposium on the Future of Schistosomiasis Control*, ed. Max J. Miller, pp. 129–32. Tulane University Press.

INDEX